The Pilates Guidebook

Pilates Mat exercises & theory for teachers & enthusiasts

Richard A. Brown

Integrated Movement & Manual Therapist (IMMT)
Osteopathy (MSc)
Certified Structural Integration (ATSI)
Professional Certificate Orthopaedic Manipulative Therapy
Clinical Diploma Acupuncture
Founder :   Bodyworks Studios (China)
              Sino-British Academy
              SOMAT-X® System
              Tower of Power®
              CoreFormer®

First Published in 2024
by Zhonghao Publishing

11 Carroll Place
Llandudno
Conwy LL30 2AL
Wales, United Kingdom

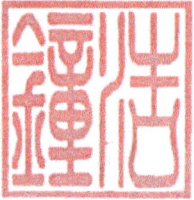

Email: zhonghaobrown123@me.com

ISBN 978-0-9955087-2-9

Disclaimer

Every effort has been made to include the most up to date and accurate information in this publication. However the author would be grateful for any errors to be brought to his attention. The author can not take any responsibility for any loss or injury and/or damage to persons or property relating to any use of material in this publication. It is the responsibility of the the individual to obtain permission from his or her healthcare professional before undertaking any forms of physical activity and undertake of of the exercises presented in this publication in a responsible manner.

To the fullest extent of the law neither the Publisher nor the authors, contributors or editors assume any liability for any injury and/or damage to persons or property as a matter of negligence or otherwise from any use of any methods, instructions or ideas contained in the material herein.

The individual is always recommended to seek medical clearance from the appropriate medical professional before beginning any exercise program of any form.

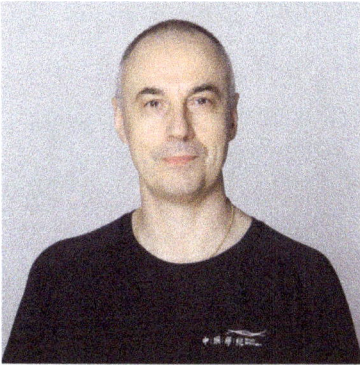

About the Author

Before teaching Pilates Richard was deeply engaged in Martial Arts and Manual Therapy having opened with his partner the first full time Martial Arts based fitness studio in Hong Kong in 1997. After gaining interest in Pilates based programs through one of his students Richard relocated to Shanghai in 2003 where he opened one of the first Pilates studios in China in 2005.

Richard is the founder of the Bodyworks® (BaoWo) Studio in China and the Co Founder of the Sino-British Academy, a certification and training organisation providing courses and workshops nationally around China in Anatomy, Pilates, Feldenkrais and Osteopathic based programs as well as other sports and movement related workshops.

Richard is also the founder of the SOMAT-X® system and inventor of specialized equipment such as the CoreFormer ®, Core Suspension® and Tower of Power®.

"Dedicated with love & affection to my long suffering wife,

son & 3 beautiful daughters"

Introduction from Pat Guyton - 2nd Generation Master Pilates Instructor

Richard and I first met at a conference in Guangzhou, China. We were both guest teachers at a Pilates conference. As Pilates studio owners and directors of teacher training programs, we were aware of the growing interest in Pilates education. The enthusiasm of a younger generation was inspirational. We could project the need for qualified teachers would be immediate. Both of us understood this could lead to a Pandora's box. The conundrum would be how to open studios to meet demand with quality. The purchase of the equipment would be the easy part. The struggle would be staffing a Pilates studio while maintaining the integrity of the method. Pilate is a practice first and foremost. Joe Pilates wrote about health and fitness as a prerequisite for leading a healthy and productive life. Ideally personal study should precede entrance into a teaching program. Richard and I were aware that the world of technology has altered how the younger generations relate to education and to business. While apprenticeship is the most effective and satisfying way to study, we were concerned that this may not be realistic at this juncture. We commiserated over many conversations and concluded that maybe we should change our attitudes. How could we honor the method and create an open door for educational opportunity for all aspiring teachers?

Richard is determined to provide the younger Pilates generation a guide for study. The anatomy section is robust. We both share the belief that functional movement within the Pilates exercises is not a detraction from Joe Pilates' vision. All Pilates educators have an imperative responsibility for our generation to bequeath a lineage that is both archival and informed by science. The book format for learning the exercises is adroitly presented. There are in color coded boxes for easy content reference, corresponding text, clear photos, and directions for cuing. There are QR codes that present the visual demonstration for each exercise. My generation did not have these resources. The information is detailed but it is also incremental. The student can select sections for study as the teacher experience develops. Hopefully Pandora's box has treasures that will inspire further study and promote Joe Pilates's vision that the whole world would be doing his work. I will be adding this book to my recommended study for my training program.

Pat Guyton
Master Pilates Instructor

Director:
Pat Guyton Pilates Conservatory®

Dedication:

This book is dedicated with love to my son and three beautiful daughters, as well as my ever-supportive wife. Without them, I have no idea where or what I would be doing in life!

Acknowledgements:

Reflecting on the past 30 years of teaching, I have been fortunate to meet and share stories and experiences with people from all walks of life. Each of these individuals has had some form of influence, big or small, in shaping the person I have become today and indirectly or directly guiding me to write this book.

While the names and number of these people are too many to mention, some deserve particular recognition:

You never forget your first teacher! Thank you, Ron Claessen (Australia), for introducing me to the martial arts. Master teacher Chen Chang from Hong Kong, who showed me the ways of Chen Tai Chi and QiGong. Hiroaki Isumi (Rocky), followed by Ray Panter, who oversaw my development in Aikido.

My late partner in Hong Kong, Pierre Ingrassia, who helped generate the confidence for me to open one of the first Pilates studios in China.

Duncan Wong and Tiffany Hua, who gave me the opportunity to open the first Bodyworks studio in the Namaste Yoga Shala in Shanghai.

Roger Hsieh, whose generosity allowed my wife and me to open our first studio together in Shanghai.

Dan Shen, who was not only my wingman to protect me from excessive amounts of Baijiu (Chinese rice wine) on my wedding night but also instrumental in helping us open the first Bodyworks Studio in Shanghai.

Master Instructor Pat Guyton deserves special mention as a mentor, brilliant instructor, and awesome human being! Pat has immense knowledge of many things Pilates and Beyond, which she manages to teach in a simplified version that makes it easy for students to understand.

She personifies the saying, "Any old idiot can make something sound complicated, but it takes a true genius to make it simple." She is indeed a true genius at getting information across in such an engaging and wonderful manner.

Madeline Black is another wonderful mentor whom I consider it a pleasure to have learned from. Madeline has the unique ability to combine the knowledge and practical aspects of Movement with Manual Therapy techniques that I have not seen or known in any other teacher.

A huge thank you goes out to Kerry D'Ambrogio and Kerry Fung ("Kerry West & Kerry East"), who have taught me so much in regards to manual therapy and whom I consider to be master practitioners that inspire others.

A big thank you goes to my amazing Osteopathic teachers Jaime Camarasa, Ignacio Diaz Cerrado, and Pablo Llanes, who possess incredible knowledge of the body and how it moves, enough to fill an entire library.

In 2001, I embarked on a journey at the Rolfing Institute, Boulder, into the treatment and movement concepts of a little-known body tissue called 'fascia'! Many years later, I finally completed a full certification in the USA, thanks to Thomas Myers, one of Ida Rolf's original students.

Subsequently, through Thomas Myers, I was lucky to be introduced to James Earls, who remains a significant mentor and teacher for me in understanding how the body 'actually moves'.

I would also like to thank Vicky and Lee for agreeing to be the models in the book. Vicky is not only a friend of many years but also a valuable member of the Sino-British Academy teaching team.

Many of you may wonder who the amazing lady in the book's images is, the one who beautifully performs the exercises for you to see after scanning the QR codes. Her name is Rebecca Zhu, and she has been an amazing long-term friend since my arrival in China. She is also known as the 'Mother of Pilates in China,' having helped us establish the Bodyworks brand and teaching Pilates to both students and teachers for many years.

There is, of course, one person in particular who has had a significant influence on the Pilates market in China, without whom many individuals pursuing a career in Pilates and reading this book would not have a job! That person is the delightful and gorgeous actress Sun Li. I don't believe there is anyone else who has achieved or promoted the benefits of Pilates in China to such an extent as Sun Li. Without her perseverance and dedication to health and wellbeing, the name Pilates would still be almost unheard of in China. I am honored that she agreed to write a foreword for the Chinese version of the book.

And of course, no acknowledgement would be complete without two further mentions:

Firstly, my beautiful family consisting of my long-suffering wife Julianne, my three beautiful daughters Zhade, Zhenna, Zhai, and my son Nathan, who continually inspire me to pursue new things in life. Seeing my daughters first thing in the morning uplifts my soul and fuels my drive to accomplish new things.

Lastly, the biggest thanks of all must go to all the brave and unsuspecting souls who have walked through my door in Hong Kong and Shanghai over the last 30 years. Without the faith and trust of all the people I've had the immense good fortune to meet, I would not have achieved everything I have, and certainly, this book would not exist!

As one of my mentors, Mr. Brian Scura, remarks, "It's good to pay it forward" (a wonderful movie by that name). It would give me immense pleasure and humble satisfaction if this book can help the reader, in whatever small way, personally or as a coach or instructor, to 'pay it forward' for the benefit of those seeking health and wellbeing.

I sincerely hope you enjoy reading the following pages and, above all, I hope it may help you in some way to maintain or restore vitality to your life.

With Gratitude

Richard Brown

2024

contents

CHAPTER

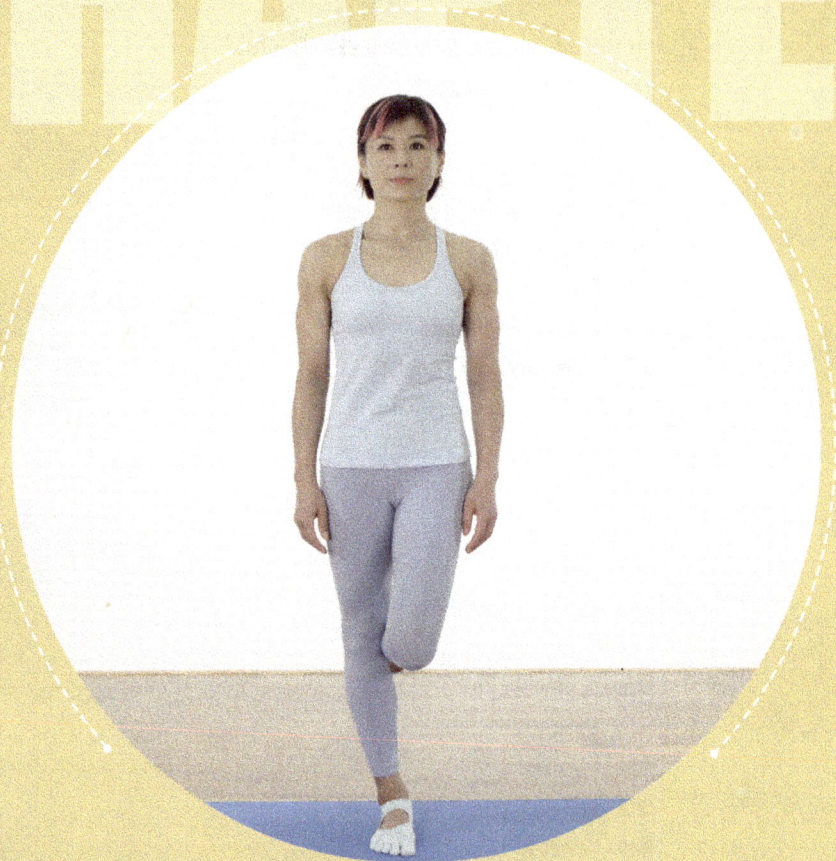

ONE

Introduction

1.1 ▸ Who is this book for ?

The purpose of this book is to introduce the reader to a repertoire of Pilates Mat and related exercises as taught by the Sino-British Academy based in Shanghai, China.

This handbook is suitable for :

Anyone wishing to start Pilates as a means of exercise or become a Pilates teacher. It should also be useful for existing Pilates Instructors or people already practicing Pilates mat exercises as part of his / her exercise routine.

1.2 ▸ Why you should read this book :

For the 'Instructor'

It is hoped that the book will introduce you to many of the fundamental skills to learn and teach Pilates Mat and Pilates derived exercises to your clients in an effective and safe manner.

For the 'Enthusiast'

It is hoped, that the reader will be encouraged to take more responsibility for his or her own physical wellbeing thus promoting the concept of healthy exercise that is both interesting, challenging and more importantly both viable and productive in today's environment of stress and expectations of immediate results.

This book does not intend to re-invent the wheel through 'special' or 'secret' exercises. It is a simple honest introduction to some of the concepts of Pilates exercise whilst merging other principles of body mechanics and functional movement and corrective exercises that we teach in the Sino-British Academy and Bodyworks Studios across China.

Pilates is probably best known as a bunch of exercises that a person performs on a mat to increase abdominal strength and flexibility. However the mat exercises comprise only a part of the Pilates repertoire as there are a whole bunch of machines and equipment that no self respecting Pilates studio would be without.

These include :

Trapeze Table (or Cadillac)
Reformer
  Split Chair or Wunda Chair
Spine Corrector
Ladder Barrel
Guillotine
Armchair
Ped-O-Pull

The total number of exercises on the Pilates apparatus is too many to count and each exercise has its' own combinations or variations in terms of progression or regression (ie make the exercise easier or harder).

1.3 ▸ Exercises in this Book

The purpose of this book is to focus on 'Preparatory Mat' and Pilates Mat exercises I consider are the most practical and important movements to teach as a Pilates Mat teacher or learn as a person new to exercising. This is by no means a comprehensive list of exercises. For instance the experienced practitioner will notice there are 10 omissions from the original sequence of 37 exercises as follows :

The Hundred

Rollover

Corkscrew

Neck Pull

Jack Knife

Boomerang

Seal

Crab

Rocking on Stomach

Control balance

However for the sake of a sense of completion for the exercises the reader can refer to Appendix I where you will find both a list of the original Pilates Mat Sequence as well as associated QR codes to watch the related video of the movement.

There are some important considerations for the omissions of some of the exercises as follows :

Pareto's Law

Otherwise know as the 80/20 principle it basically means that 80% of an outcome comes from 20% of its causes.

For instance a business or studio owner may realise that 80% of all income is coming from only 20% of clients.

Another example may be in relation to pain where 80% of back pain may be coming from emotional stress which accounts for only 20% of the physical condition of a person.

For instructors what this means is that if you were to learn 100 exercises then 80% of the time you will only be teaching 20 of those exercises. The other 80 exercises will make an appearance from time to time however your 'core curriculum' of exercises will be reduced to only 20. It makes sense therefore that you should become proficient in these 20 exercises and know them extremely well as you will be teaching

these most of the time.

Principles

As stated previously my opinion is that a teacher should become competent and experienced in teaching a sufficient 'base number ' of exercises before considering to go on with more advanced movements.

What I mean by competent is really in fact the ability to understand and identify basic 'movement principles' within a certain exercise. Once the teacher has identified and understands these principles it is relatively easy to transfer these principles into other exercises or movement patterns.

An example would be the Boomerang exercise which can be seen as a combination of the Spine Stretch, Teaser and Rollover exercises so therefore it makes sense that a person should only be attempting this exercise after he or she is competent in the afore mentioned three exercises.

Another example is the 'Hundred' exercise. Literally thousands of teachers around the world are probably opening a Pilates mat class with the traditional Hundred exercise which is considered by many as a 'warm up' exercise. However when one looks at the pre requisite skills needed for this movement one may observe that the performer needs :

1 *A good connection through the latissimus dorsi muscles to the core,*

2 *Strong and effective deep flexors of the neck to hold the head in position*

3 *Effective articulation through the cervical and thoracic vertebrae*

4 *Good strength and organisation of the lumbo-pelvic-hip complex and core to hold the legs in position.*

Unfortunately the vast majority of individuals do not have these requirements and consequently perform this exercise with the result of getting lower back or neck pain.

Many teachers will 'regress' this exercise by shortening the leg lever (bend the legs) or maybe even allow the head to stay on the floor however this does not 'teach' the student the necessary skills needed to perform the exercise adequately. Perhaps another exercise which incorporates the appropriate skills may be an alternative.

Another factor in the choice of exercises is that of safety. In the traditional Pilates sequence the Rollover is the third exercise in the sequence. Given the fact that 80% of the time we are teaching or working with clients whom do not regularly exercise it would be simply impractical and irresponsible to expect them to perform a Rollover with very little preparation. Another limiting factor here is a very common pattern that is seen time and time again in fitness centers across the world. This is the impact of 'sitting for prolonged periods' creating tension and tightness in what Dr Vladimir Janda termed the tonic or postural muscles of the body contributing to tension and muscular imbalances throughout the body.

Simply focusing on the so called 'Core Strength' for the client is most likely going to be met with failure. One rational in the above exercise would be the dominance of the lower erector spinae muscles over the abdominal muscles leading to the inability to perform an appropriate flexion (articulation) movement through the spine. This would inherently place possible damaging forces through the spine and into the neck area if the client tries to perform some of the above listed exercises.

There is another realization that many persons do not seem to understand and that is the fact that simply performing the same exercise over and over again is most likely NOT going to improve it ! A faulty or dysfunctional movement pattern is not going to disappear simply because we 'try harder' or repeat the movement 100 times.

And herein lies one of the major aspects of Pilates that many people seem oblivious towards. Whilst the exercises in the Pilates repertoire may indeed be great for giving a person a 'work out' it is important to remember to ask what level the individual is starting out on his or her exercise program. It is important to acknowledge what Master Teacher Pat Guyton terms as 'the person in front of us' and treat him or her as an individual that has specific needs and requirements (even though of course there are many common reoccurring patterns that present themselves) starting with building a base level of skill that all other movements and exercises can be built on. Thus we set ourselves and our clients up to succeed in the long term even if we have to go slow at the beginning.

My optimistic and very sincere wishful outcome of this book therefore is twofold :

1 *I hope that by writing this book it will be useful in helping develop a meaningful, safe and effective approach to Pilates Mat training.*

2 *It would be fantastic if somebody were able to pick up this book as a beginner or instructor from another movement system and work his or her way through it and become familiar enough to use the information for his or her own practice as well as being able to pass on the information to others.*

1.4 So Why Did I Write This Book ?

Over the years of teaching I have quite often been asked the question, "Can you tell me the name of a good book for me to learn Pilates ?" Teaching Pilates should be very much a 'hands on' methodology. Books are great for imparting knowledge but no matter how much you read about learning to drive it's not going to help much without literally sitting behind a wheel and feeling how the clutch works with the gear shift. That being said it should make it easier to work the clutch with the gear selector once there is an understanding of the relationship between the two.

So similarly it makes sense that anyone wishing to learn subjects such as Pilates that he or she would also gain benefit from being able to read and study about the exercises and underline anatomy alongside or before working with a teacher or student.

So as much as the above question comes up I always struggle for an answer to advise on any particular book that contains the necessary criteria I think should be in such a publication.

So please allow me to explain by listing out some of the criteria that I personally think should be included in any handbook for instructors.

"The longest journey begins with a single step."

1.5 Anatomy

The above quote may be rather a cliche one but it's also one I consider extremely pertinent to the study of the human body and movement.

As responsible and professional instructors it should be our duty to be as informed and educated as possible in 'things that make the body work'. This includes a sound basis in the anatomy and physiology of the musculoskeletal and other systems of the body.

I once heard a teacher tell me " I judge the ability of an instructor by whether or not he can give an appropriate session to my 16 year son as well as my 70 year old mother"

I have in fact 'stolen' his quote over the years to give the exact statement to many students in that a good teacher should recognise the needs and differences between different populations and prescribe an effective and safe exercise protocol appropriately.

To do this one must have a good knowledge in anatomy and basic physiological concepts such as heart rate, precautions and contraindications as well as the ability to assess " The Body in Front of You"

At the very least therefore it should be our responsibility as professional movement coaches to have an understanding of the basic 'structural' knowledge of the musculoskeletal system and for this reason I consider any 'Instructors handbook ' should include these references.

Most of the muscle illustrations in the book are printed with permission from the anatomy app from Vesal.

1.6 'Beginner or Advanced' ?

You may have been a little confused in the introduction stating that this book is both for the beginner and advanced practitioner or teacher. However, in my experience it is the 'basic' things that can 'make or break' a movement in being safe and / or effective. The basic things include such things as :

Verbal cues

Tactile cues

Appropriate set up (note the term appropriate as opposed to 'correct')

Knowing 'What' the movement is supposed to accomplish

Knowing 'How' this should be performed

Understanding how an exercise or movement may be modified to suit the requirements of the practitioner.

I find all the above requirements sadly lacking in many classes and quite often if I ask a teacher "Why are you doing this exercise " ? Or "What is the intended outcome for this movement" ? The instructor is more often than not unable to give a clear logical explanation. Surely however this should be the basic requirement for a teacher ? Please note however that I'm not trying to be condescending with an inability to answer, however the truth is that in real life more often than not we learn something by copying and in turn use this to teach what we think we have 'learned'.

Consequently we usually end up in a situation of relying on what we think we have learned and remembered and slowly over time this information itself becomes diluted and usually ends up in a distorted retelling or teaching of the original version.

If we had perfect memory for all the things we think we have learned this would not be enough either as it would only be a 'copy' version of the information and not an embodiment of the knowledge through putting into practice what we have learned visually, audibly and spatially.

Therefore the ability to present or teach an exercise or movement as simply as possible, in my opinion, becomes one of the hallmarks of a master teacher.

However this begs the question " Does the teacher teach this in a simple manner because of all the things he or she does not know or does the teacher teach in a simple manner because of the years of mastery behind the technique !"

Perhaps another way to say it is to ask "Do you teach what you don't know or are you teaching an abbreviated version of the large amount of things you do know ?"

So if we now come back to the first remarks above regarding the basics it will be seen that the basics are the first things we learn but also the first things we forget. It is the experienced instructor that is able to both understand and apply the basics to set a student up to succeed. Therefore the most basic things become the most advanced.

In regards to the above points this book endeavours to somewhat address these issues through the use of colour coded boxes which refer to various aspects of the exercise or movement.

The boxes are arranged as follows :

Rose Box	Contraindications and precautions
Pink Box	Benefits of the exercise
Green Box	The general principles behind the movement
Blue Box	Cues to help the instructor or student perform the movement
Yellow Box	Questions

Precautions & Contraindications

A 'precaution' is generally described as something to watch out for in terms of safety and may refer to a medical condition or an aspect of the exercise that needs special attention.

A contraindication is generally referred to as a medical condition which would make this exercise not suitable for the individual to perform.

Benefits

Muscles targeted, specific or general movement dysfunctions that the exercise may help. A specific dysfunction would be 'bulging disc' whereas a general dysfunction may simply be termed as 'back pain'.

Therapeutic & Functional **Benefits** from the exercise :

Therapeutic : Strengthens the hamstring muscles
Functional : Helps improve squatting and standing

Principles

Pilates based exercises are very good for targeting aspects of movement through a terminology not commonly used by teachers of other movement styles. As an example the 'Swan' exercise may be seen as targeting a 'spinal articulation in extension' whereas in the gym we may refer to it as 'toning our back muscles'. An understanding of the terminology of the principles is crucial to effective and safe instruction.

Cues

Tactile Cues

A tactile cue uses 'touch'. The instructor will touch the student appropriately to help promote the desired outcome for the movement. Tactile cues tend to be of 3 kinds :

Instructive - for example the teacher touches a particular vertebra on the students spine to indicate where the movement may be blocked or wants to be initiated from.

Assistive - for example the teacher supports the students feet when going into a Teaser position

Resistive - for example the teacher presses into the students feet to give proprioceptive feedback for the student to press back against to help the movement.

Verbal Cues

The use of imagery and clear instructions may have significant benefit for the student or practitioner and more often than not create a movement pattern much more applicable to the desired one than a protocol of instructions broken down move by move that does more to hinder a required movement than actually encourage it.

A verbal cue should always come before a tactile cue.

Questions

Some comments or questions for the reader to help experiment and explore the movement in order to understand it's value and meaning better

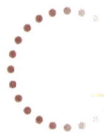

A common critique of the Pilates Mat repertoire is that it is 'two dimensional' and that the movements are emphasized in a 'sagittal plane' (forwards and backwards) and there is not enough sideways and rotational movement patterns in the system.

I personally agree with this view and indeed in the Bodyworks Studios around China we teach many exercises that are not to be found in any classical or self help Pilates books but instead use exercises based in 'therapeutic' or 'functional' movement patterns of how the body moves safely and efficiently. For instance, the Side Kick series of exercises on the mat have a wonderful therapeutic effect but are functionally lacking as the body predominantly does not use the targeted muscles in this way.

I therefore consider it to be the obligation of the instructor to understand these limitations and consequently integrate more 'functional' exercises into their respective sessions with the clients.

In an effort to keep this book accessible to as many persons as possible I have refrained from simply introducing the 'complete exercise' as it is commonly taught in many studios across the world but rather focus on the elements that I consider to be of importance when teaching or introducing certain exercises to an individual who is new to exercising.

1.7 ▶ A note on the exercises

This book contains elements of both traditional and modern interpretations of recognised 'Pilates Mat' exercises as well as 'non Pilates' corrective exercises. The concept behind this selection is to combine what I call 'Therapeutic exercises' with what I term 'Functional exercises' which is how we move in our everyday lives in real life movement.

An example of this is the Pilates standing roll down exercise which can hardly be described as a 'Functional movement'. However the ability to move through each vertebra in the spine on a roll down ensures minimal 'splinting' of the vertebrae (grouped or block movements) which would in turn allow maximal mobility for each joint which can only be described as a good thing !

This mobile and healthy spine can then be used more efficiently and effectively in an appropriate functional movement such as a tennis serve, golf swing or simply putting your luggage into the rack on an airplane !

I sincerely hope you enjoy reading and practicing the movements in this book. I would personally love to hear any feedback with constructive comments on things the reader likes or dislikes in the book. I especially would love to hear of any suggestions for improvements or corrections the reader feels should be made.

Most of all I sincerely hope you find the information useful and helpful and the contents help you in your daily life in terms of the reason why you bought the book in the first place. Whether you suffer from some form of physical impairment or ailment or simply wish to improve your posture and or improve your sporting performance I hope there is something of use for you in these pages.

With Gratitude

Richard Brown

CHAPTER

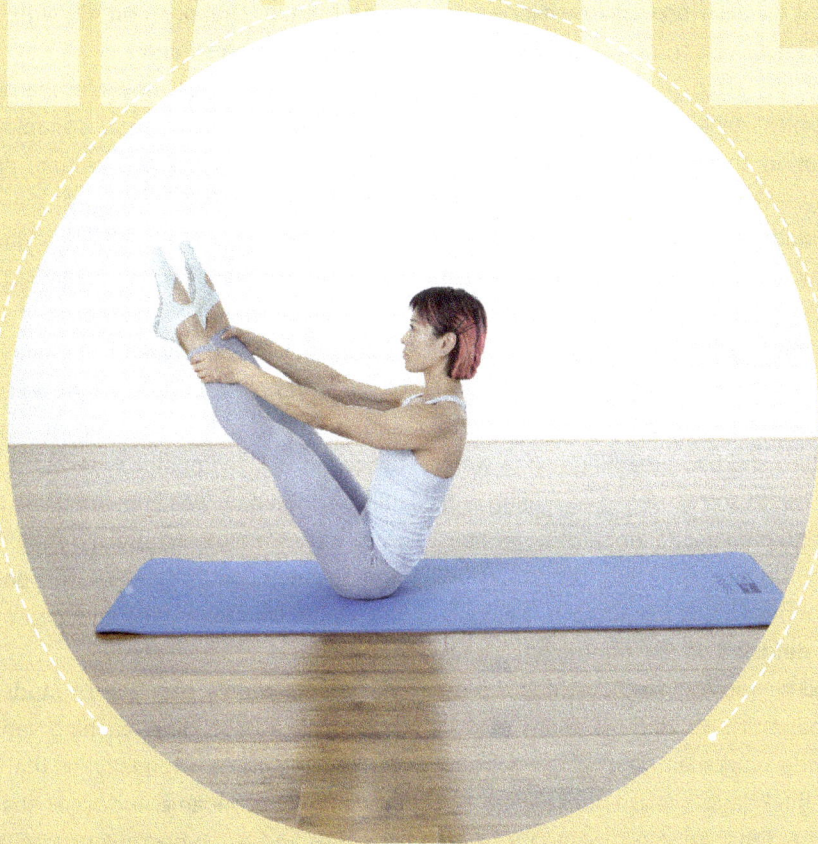

Two

History of Pilates

Pilates is a form of exercise originally developed by Joseph Hubert Pilates which he originally called 'Contrology'. After his death in 1967 some of his students and 'disciples' decided to carry on his work and called it Pilates in honour of the founder of the system.

Born in Monchengladbach in1883 it is said that Joseph Pilates was often sick as a child and so dedicated his life to improving his health and physical strength. His father was a gymnast and interested in body building and so introduced Joseph to these systems.

Pilates came to believe that modern lifestyle traits such as poor posture and bad breathing habits were at the root of poor heath and so began designing and using pieces of equipment and apparatus to help with his training methods.

In 1912 Pilates moved to England but being a German he was detained in an internment camp during the first world war. It is said that it is during this time Pilates began to develop his series of mat exercises and spring equipment that would later be synonymous with the Pilates system of exercise.

After the war Joseph returned to Germany but being uncomfortable with the political and social conditions of the country he emigrated to USA in about 1925 via a cruise ship. It was on this ship that he met his future partner Clara and upon their arrival in New York they opened a studio and began teaching to anyone who would come and learn. The original focus of his system Contrology was on key concepts of Breathing, Concentration, Control, Centering, Flow and Precision. These same concepts are well known today with various differing vocabulary such as 'spinal articulation', 'core control' etc...

Joseph and Clara soon gained a following from the local dance community and would receive students from Martha Graham and George Balanchine for training and rehabilitation.

Joseph Pilates is well known for the publication of the book 'Return to Life through Contrology' published in 1945 which contains the written principles of his methodology as well as many of the exercises which today make up much of the 'Pilates Mat' repertoire. The exercises are presented as controlled movements for an exercise workout and not a therapy. Practiced consistently it is advocated that these Pilates exercises improve flexibility, build strength and develop control and endurance in the whole human body.

Joseph was also constantly inventing apparatus and invented the now well known pieces of equipment of Reformer, Cadillac (Trapeze table), Ladder Barrel, Wunda Chair and Ped-O-Pull. It is said however that the 'Spine Corrector' was invented by his wife Clara !

Many of Joseph's and Clara's students went on to open their own studios teaching variations or trying to preserve the authenticity of the method. These students later became known as the 1st generation disciples and (in no particular order) are principally :

Eve Gentry
Ron Fletcher
Carola Trier
Mary Bowen
Kathy Grant
Lolita San Miguel
Jay Grimes
Audrey May
Romana Kryzanowska

Joseph Pilates died in 1967 at the age of 83 in New York.

Defining Classical vs Modern Pilates

These days there are many schools of Pilates derived from Josephs original teachings and each school or style may have a different emphasis on a particular methodology of teaching. School 'A' for instance may be heavily influenced by the physical therapy school of thought whilst school 'B' may be characterized by the 'Fitness/Gym' approach. Classical schools tend to have an emphasis on the 'Dance' aspect of Pilates.

It is not possible to say which style is 'more correct' than the other as they offer different approaches which will appeal across a variety of people. Also exercises within these 'systems' will have very subtle or major changes in the way they are taught such as the Mermaid exercise which can be found to have a variety of differences depending on the school teaching it.

As a rule of thumb I'm going to go out on a limb here and state that 'Modern Pilates is an amalgamation of the evolution of Pilates whilst Classical Pilates aims to preserve the original work as Joseph Pilates taught it.

The original teachings of Joseph held on to a number of principles. For instance it is said that Joseph thought that the lumbar spine should be straight like a newborn baby and this view was upheld by a vast majority of his followers even through to today. However nowadays many practitioners consider this to be detrimental to the health of the spine due to the unwanted pressure placed into the discs and a possible consequence of loss of natural curvature of the spine.

Other principles are much less problematic and still actively encouraged. Indeed the favoured methodology for breathing recommended by Joseph is now commonly known as a 'Pilates breath'.

After the death of Joseph Pilates Romana Kryzanowska was tasked with the job of organising the teachings of Joe into a system among which required detailing the principles of Pilates. Romana can probably be credited with writing the now established 6 principles as originally taught in Pilates as follows :

1. *Concentration*
2. *Control*
3. *Center*
4. *Flow*
5. *Precision*
6. *Breathing*

Concentration

Pilates demands intense focus: In Pilates the way that exercises are performed is more important than the exercises themselves.

Control

"Contrology" was Joseph Pilates' preferred name for his method, and it was based on the idea of muscle control. "Nothing about the Pilates Method is haphazard. The reason you need to concentrate so thoroughly is so you can be in control of every aspect of every moment."

Centering

The center is the focal point of the pilates method. These days we commonly refer to the 'core' and many of the older teachers will call it the 'Powerhouse'. All movement in Pilates should begin from the powerhouse and flow outward to the limbs. This is the main focus of Pilates and the process to help strengthen the rest of the body.

Flow

Referring to the 'efficiency of movement' Pilates aims for elegant sufficiency of movement, using just enough effort to get the job done in a smooth and efficient manner. Once precision has been achieved, the exercises are intended to flow within and into each other in order to build strength and stamina.

Precision

Precision is essential to correct pilates: as Joseph said : "concentrate on the correct movements each time you exercise, lest you do them improperly and thus lose all the vital benefits of their value". The focus is on doing one precise and perfect movement, rather than many halfhearted ones. This is more akin in philosophy to the martial arts as opposed to the fitness culture of the West. The goal is for this precision to eventually become second nature and carry over into everyday life as grace and economy of movement.

Breathing

Breathing is fundamental to a myriad of spiritual and physical disciplines and Pilates is no exception. In Return to Life, Pilates devotes a section of his introduction specifically to breathing as "bodily house-cleaning with blood circulation". He saw considerable value in increasing the intake of oxygen and the circulation of this oxygenated blood to every part of the body. Proper full inhalation and complete exhalation were key to this. Joseph saw forced exhalation as the key to full inhalation and he advised people to squeeze out the lungs as they would wring a wet towel dry. These days we may refer to the action of the Transversus Abdominus muscle and associated 'local core muscles' in helping this function in order to keep the lower abdominals close to the spine with the breathing directed laterally, into the lower rib cage. A Pilates breath is described as posterior lateral breathing , meaning that the practitioner is instructed to breathe deep into the back and sides of his or her rib cage. When practitioners exhale, they are instructed to note the engagement of their deep abdominal and pelvic floor muscles and maintain this engagement as they inhale. Pilates attempts to properly coordinate this breathing practice with movement, including breathing instructions with every exercise.

"Above all learn to breathe correctly ."

CHAPTER

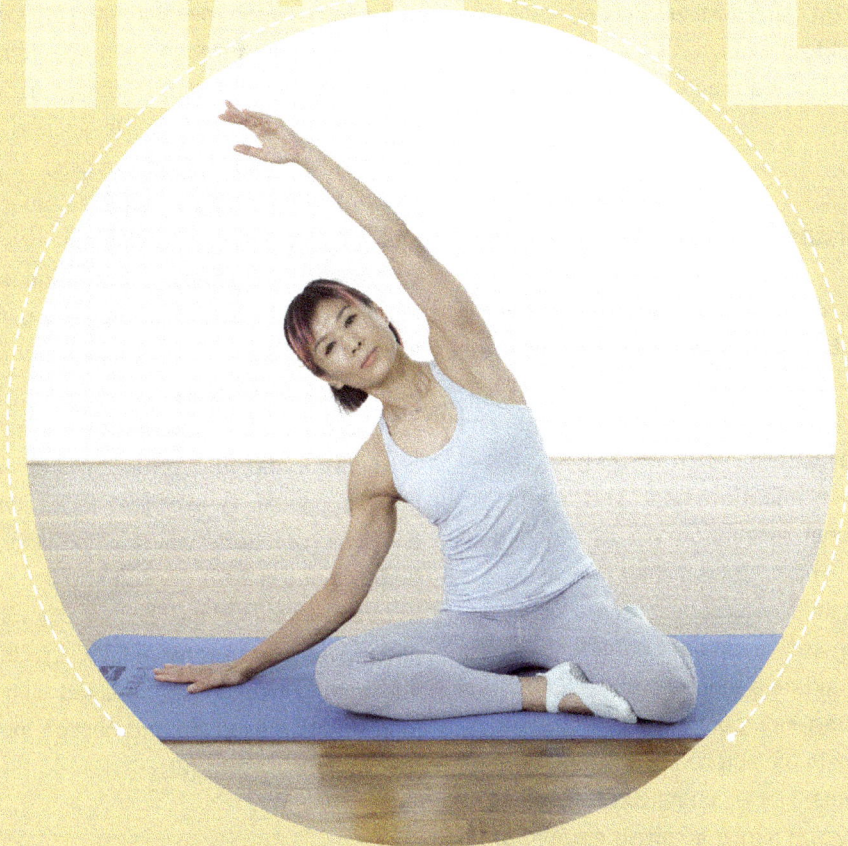

Three

Important Questions about this book

So before we go any further delving into the exercises let's get to the nitty gritty of what you may achieve from reading and practicing the exercises in this book.

3.1 ▶ Does Pilates Make You Lose Weight ?

Umm good question. The short quick fire answer is 'no'. But wait ! Before you put the book down in disappointment - please read on.......

The exercises in this book are designed and explained in a way to help improve ones posture, self awareness, mobility and movement. This is a far cry from the traditional gym approach of working at maximum effort. The emphasis therefore is on the wellness and not the fitness aspect for the individual. Certainly if you can become competent in the exercises presented here then it would be a natural progression to start incorporating more challenging exercises leading to an increase of work in terms of duration and or intensity which may in turn lead to a more toned body and hence a certain amount of fat loss.

What I have found from personal experience and working with clients over the years is that the Pilates method will in fact help change the body shape due to the changes in breathing patterns and posture which will in fact give the appearance of having lost some excess baggage around the waist or elsewhere in the body.

However one should remember the facts. A person of say 65 kg kilos and average athletic ability running on a treadmill everyday for 1 hour at approximately 9 km per hour will burn approximately 500 calories in that hour. So if one pound of fat equals 3,500 calories it can be seen that the individual would need to run for 1 hour every day for 7 days in order to burn 1 lb

of fat. A common mistake made by many beginners to exercise is to then increase food intake and especially carbohydrate intake in an effort to maintain his or her energy levels and thus negating any benefits made by the exercise.

In terms of pure fat loss exercise programs involving high intensity interval training may give considerable cardiovascular benefits. That being said though a common mistake is to jump in too fast too soon leading to a higher risk of injury and energy fatigue due to lack of recovery.

A consistent Pilates program whether it be by itself or incorporated into other training regimes in my humble opinion is excellent for reducing tiredness and risk of injury whilst improving posture and performance in ones chosen sport.

In terms of fat loss the number one most consistent and proven way to achieve fat weight loss is to adjust your eating habits accompanied with low intensity long duration exercise and/or high intensity interval training.

3.2 How Often Should a Person do the exercises ?

How often should you move ? All day everyday is the answer.

Here's another answer. A good friend of mine was working in our studio in Hong Kong after just arriving from the Ivory Coast. He was a body building champion and later became a world Muay Thai champion so he was used to working out very regularly. He had been at the studio for about a week when one day he came up to me with a look of total surprise. He said to me " Richard". "Did you know that there are some people - they go the whole day without exercise " !

He was totally shocked to come to this realisation after so many years of dedicated hard work himself ! So the answer is quite simply as often as you possibly can.

3.3 ▶ Are These Exercises For Rehabilitation?

The word rehabilitation is seen as having a medical context and as Pilates instructors we should never claim to have any form of medical benefits. Interestingly enough Joseph Pilates used to work with a great deal of injured dancers and supposedly became very frustrated with the lack of acceptance and recognition of his system in the medical industry. Back in those days there was no such thing as sport science or protocols for rehabilitation after surgery so it was not surprising he never received the recognition many people think he deserved.

However there are a huge number of clinical examples and personal stories from people you meet in the 'Pilates world' that swear by its' efficiacy helping people with all manner of physical disabilities and dysfunctions. Probably the most commonly heard examples are those people that have found Pilates of great benefit for knee, hip, back and shoulder problems.

To avoid misconceptions with the medical fraternity a popular phrase used these days is 'Prehabilitation' or 'prehab'. That is the act of practicing or receiving an exercise or treatment in order to help prevent the need for rehabilitation. Added to this many doctors are now even recommending prospective patients to go on a course of prehab in order to help the recovery period after an operation.

This being said though if you are thinking of starting a Pilates program to help any form of physical or medical condition it is absolutely essential that you should have an appropriate medical check beforehand. This book does not promote or encourage the idea of following the exercises here as a replacement for medical treatment !

Posture

One of the most common themes that tend to crop up in our trainings is that of posture. It seems that indeed Pilates has a very good reputation when it comes to describing some of the benefits of practicing Pilates as ' improved posture' is a term that is used with Pilates training a lot. The term posture can be seen in relation to the body held in a static position as well as a dynamic movement. Most clients and students consider posture to be that of the former whereas a person may stand in front of her instructor and have a static postural assessment made. And whilst this may be of benefit for many persons there is still a debate as to how much static posture contributes to dysfunction.

However I think it is safe to assume for the most part people have a sense of what an aesthetically good posture should look like and how it relates too many factors such emotional state, self-confidence etc regardless of how much you may consider the posture to contribute towards dysfunction and/or pain.

Experienced teachers will most probably tell you that the majority of their clients come from a sedentary background and exhibit patterns commonly found as a direct or partial result from habitual patterns with a lack of movement.

Some of the more common patterns you will find amongst your clients that may be helped through Pilates exercises include person is with :

1️⃣ *Short tight lower back and hip flexors - arched lower back*

2️⃣ *Short tight chest and neck muscles - forward head posture*

3️⃣ *Forwards shifted ribcage - arched lower back & forward head posture*

4️⃣ *Forward pelvis - sway back posture*

5️⃣ *Side shift of ribcage - Possible leg length discrepancy*

6️⃣ *Rotation of upper body - possible leg length discrepancy and/or scoliosis*

7️⃣ *Flat back - tucked pelvis*

It would be rather simplistic to think that we can alter a lifetime of habitable movements to completely change somebody's posture using just the mat exercises. However the exercises you will find in this book should go someways at least to building a foundation from which a person can embark on a more specialised program with greater success.

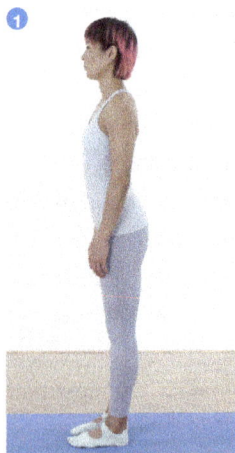

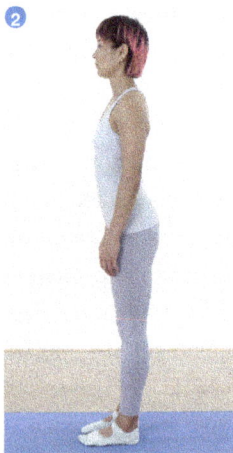

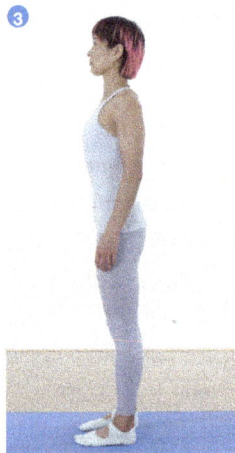

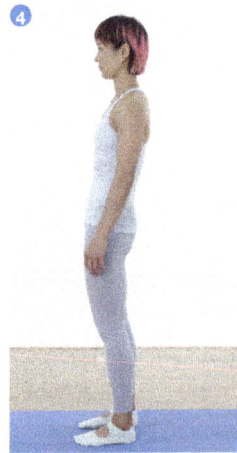

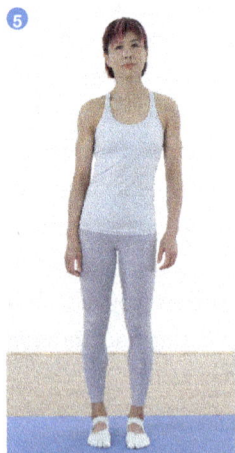

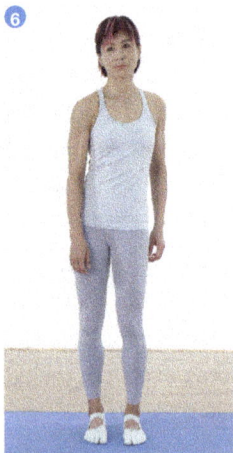

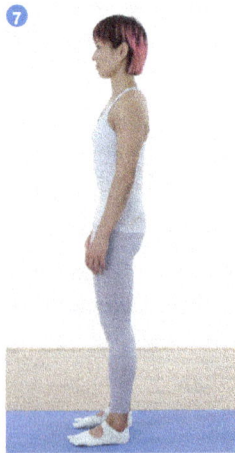

CHAPTER

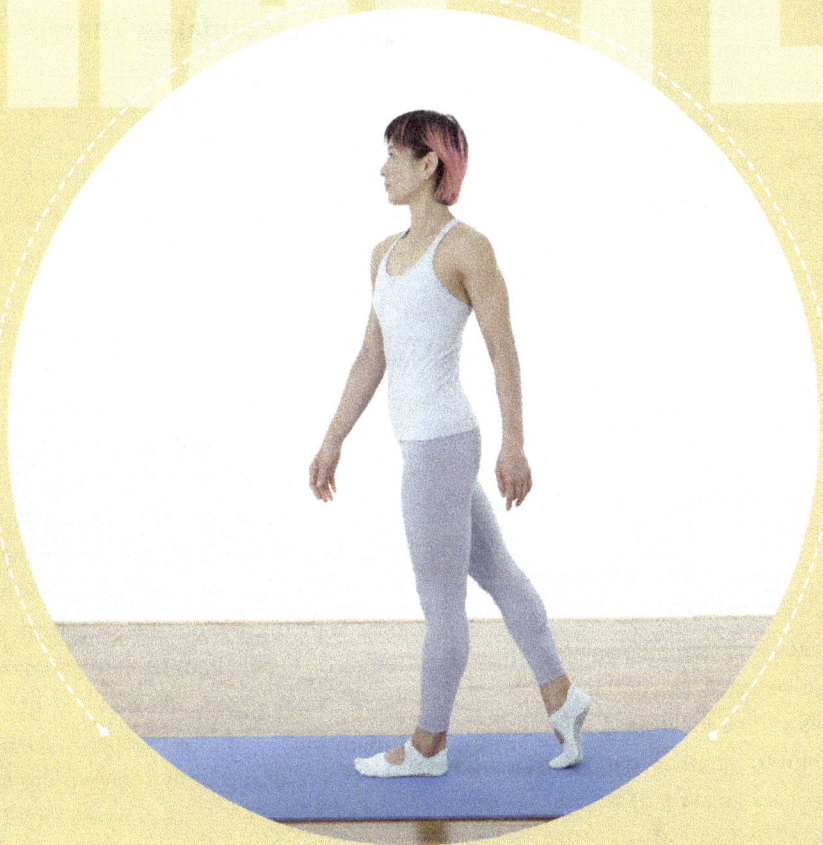

Four

Pilates & 'Functional Training'

A term that is often bandied around these days is 'Functional Training'. However a quick search on the internet of the term 'Functional Training' will most likely yield disappointing results for a clear definition. However I consider it important that professional movement instructors and educators should have a clear and basic knowledge of what comprises a database of 'Functional Anatomy' in order to facilitate 'Functional Movement' training. This in turn usually comes about as a result of further education and courses in various movement disciplines as well as Manual Therapy or 'structural modalities. For instance James Earls (author of various books such as Born to Walk, and Understanding The Human Foot) illustrates a simple example of how inversion and eversion of the right foot will contribute to thoracic rotation.

The study of 'fascia' is an increasingly popular subject and can give great illustrations as to how movements or pain at one location in the body may have a relationship to another part of the body nowhere near the first location. Through his book Anatomy Trains, Thomas Myers has almost singlehandedly introduced the concepts and practical applications of fascia to the world of physical therapists, personal trainers and movement specialists. This has spawned a whole new genre of 'fascial fitness' within the fitness industry and can be used limitlessly to illustrate and explain many so called 'functional movement' patterns.

I encourage the reader of this book to further his or her own knowledge and depth of understanding through the pursuit of study in associated disciplines in order to better understand some of the exercises and principles behind the movements in this book.

A list of recommended reading is in the appendix at the back of this book.

4.1 Functional vs Therapeutic

So let's get this straight off the bat - I don't consider Pilates Mat exercises as being 'Functional Exercises'. This is a consideration that I believe many practitioners are unable to make a distinction about and thus transfer this information appropriately to the student.

As human beings we are bipedal in nature - that is we move and operate on two legs. So without going into the whole evolutionary thing I would hope it is suffice to say we are primarily designed to operate in an upright position that requires an organization within gravity. To be able to distribute and direct the resultant forces though posture and movement we need to be able to organize an optimal structure of the body to deal not only with gravity but the resulting ground reaction forces that result from posture and movement.

More simply put, if we do not have optimal organization of the bones, tissues and other structures of the body then we are setting ourselves up for a lack of efficiency of movement. The result of this lack of efficiency is a need to compensate which over time puts stress on the tissues and may lead to dysfunction and or injury.

A functional movement therefore may be considered as one that is similar to an everyday movement which includes the parameters of gravity and ground reaction force. Running would be an obvious example of a 'functional movement'. However this begs the question "does more running improve running "? As a general rule of thumb the answer would be no. Human beings are habitual animals that look for the easiest and most efficient way to do things even if they are clearly not the most efficient ! Watch a young child turn off a light switch and you will see the whole body move to bring the hand towards the switch. Observe an adult performing the same task and you will see minimal amount of body movement with usually a lift of the arm and a press with the finger with little connection through the body. Repeat this movement hundreds or thousands of times as during a lifetime and you will achieve an energy saving but very inefficient method of moving the upper limb.

In terms of the spine a good example would be the role down exercise against the wall. I was once on a corrective exercise course in Hong Kong where the instructor ridiculed the exercise as non-functional Pilates s***. There is much research to suggest that flexion movements of the lumbar spine are not healthy movements due to the compression exerted onto the disc between the vertebra and thus over time may lead to the soft gel like substance inside the disc being pushed outwards the back of the vertebra where it may impinge or make contact with a nerve - hence a bulging disc. The logical conclusion to this is hard to refute as it is physically not possible for one vertebra to move on the one below it without using bone below as a pivot point (actually the true pivot point is on the disc). I think that is is now pretty well much accepted that the traditional 'crunch' or 'sit up' in the gym is considered a contraindicated form of exercise due to the pressure and shearing force exerted onto the discs.

However most people are unaware of how much pressure is being exerted onto his or her discs when they are performing such movements. One of the benefits of Pilates is for the individual to discover and explore new movement patterns that bring an awareness to the spine and other areas of the body and in doing so help to improve the movement pattern. An important consideration here is that many of the movements and exercises are taught on a piece of equipment or on a mat which reduces the impact of gravity and a ground reaction force and thus enables the practitioner to achieve greater self awareness in his or her movements which may then be transferred to a specific sport or more functional setting.

In Pilates we call the ability of one vertebra to move on the one below it articulation. If there is reduced articulation between two or more parts of the spine then another part of the spine will have to compensate by not only increasing its own specific range of movement but in fact will have to do so with an increase in shearing and other forces directed at the joint/s. The Roll Down from the wall exercise becomes a great therapeutic movement that enables the individual to focus and become aware of areas of the spine that do not move so well.

Another example which I very often give my students is that of a mixed martial arts expert that came to my studio many years ago thinking he would learn 'core training techniques'. This guy was around one hundred kilos in weight and had legs the size of tree trunks. One of the exercises he practiced was the Supine Leg in Springs on the Trapeze table. He was using the yellow springs (weak springs) and suffering big time making humongous efforts to produce the movements I asked him to perform. After a few minutes he thought he had achieved a great work out ! As luck would have it my next client that day was a young, rather skinny girl of around 12 years of age whom came for help with her scoliosis. She had already been a regular for over a year and was very familiar with the exercise. I asked her to demonstrate for the martial artist and she duly obliged performing the movements with little apparent effort. The martial artist was totally blown away and couldn't understand how this little girl could perform something so easily that he had struggled so much to deal with. What he failed to realize was that for all the effort he was making with the muscles of his inner thighs his outer thighs muscles were equally matching the resistance and hence he was in a constant battle with himself leading to huge effort and very little efficiency. Whilst the young girl was able to focus on the muscles needed to produce the movement and in effect 'turn off' the muscles opposing the movement.

Traditional gym exercises have also received criticism as being 'non functional' however many strength building exercises are in fact very good at targeting specific muscle groups whilst minimizing the stress on other muscle groups in the kinetic chain. Whilst this may not sound very functional there would indeed be a positive benefit of 'strengthening the link in the chain'. However it should be noted that once this individual link may be improved it is important to 're connect' the link into the myo-fascial arthrokinetic chain to improve functional performance.

So whilst many of the Pilates Mat exercises are not considered 'Functional' in their own right they are most certainly very 'Therapeutic' and it's this therapeutic nature that has enabled the Pilates

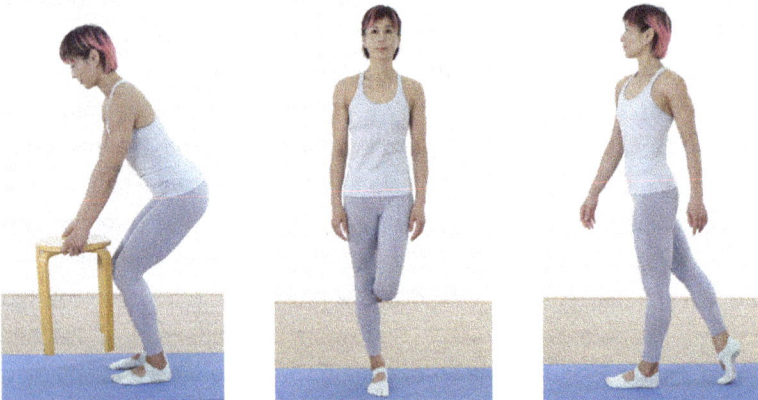

Good kinesthetic awareness and connection through the myo-fascial kinetic chain is essential for safe efficient functional movement.

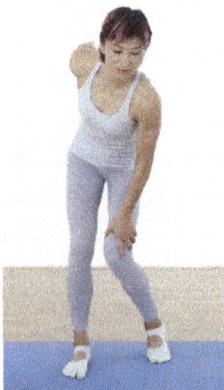

A lack of kinesthetic awareness and / or poor connection through the myo-fascial kinetic chain may lead to dysfunction, inefficiency of movement, pain and injury.

system to gain a reputation for any or all of the following :

- *Core strength*
- *Strength without the 'bulk'.*
- *Flexibility with strength*
- *Rehabilitation for the spine*
- *Balanced muscle tone and strength*

Finally in regards to the above list I should make a note about the first benefit of 'Core Strength'. In fact I actually believe the term core strength to be a very misleading term and one that is most commonly used for marketing and promotional purposes. I personally become quite agitated when someone comes to my studio and says that he or she has been told by the doctor or physiotherapist that they have to improve their core strength. To me this has actually no real meaning as this would be akin to saying that the young girl in the previous example was 'stronger' than the martial artist. Common sense tells us that a hundred kilogram man is going to be stronger than a 40 kilogram young girl.

One such description for 'efficient core control' in this regards may be as follows :

"The ability to use the myofascial chain of muscle and tissue in an efficient manner that maximizes the individuals use of muscle pattern firing and sequencing to pre contract at the appropriate moment, stabilize at the appropriate moment and produce a resulting required appropriate movement"

The definition of strength however is the ability to move a mass with a singular maximum amount of effort through contraction of the muscle fibers.

So if an individual is actually suffering from back pain because of his or her 'core muscles' it is going to be because of dysfunctional movement patterns and not because of the lack of strength . As previously mentioned in the introduction Dr Vladimir Janda puts forward a very good theory on how the 'tonic' (postural) muscles of the body can easily inhibit the 'phasic' moving muscles which is a good explanation of how the erector spinae muscles in the back can inhibit the abdominal muscles from working. So no matter how much you work on your so called 'core strength' you will be set up to fail without finding some release through the tonic muscles first. The habitual overuse of the right iliocostallis lumborum muscles is a great example of this !

Studies have showed that it only takes less than ten per cent of effort to use the core musculature for stabilization of daily exercises".

There is no one universal exercise for trunk control that would account for the specific needs of all activities. What is needed is re-education of the musculature to work in an efficient and cohesive manner to minimize effort and produce optimal performance.

Welcome to Pilates (& Beyond).

CHAPTER

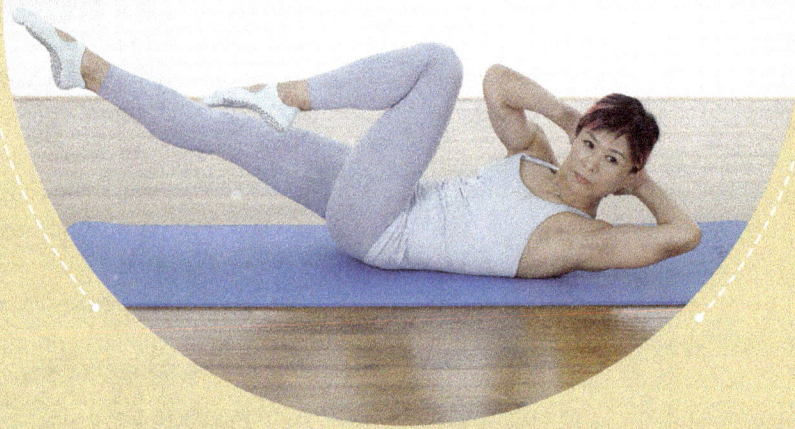

Five

Foundations of Anatomy for Movement

5.1 Introduction - physiology of cells, tissue & organs

Cells

To live they must be bathed in fluid:

Intracellular fluid:

Also called cytosol and is found within the cell.

Extracellular fluid:

a. Found outside the cells. Includes lymph (74%), blood plasma (25%), transcellular fluid (1%), such as eye, digestive etc.
b. The extracellular matrix also contains collagen and elastin fibres.
c. The extracellular matrix has the ability to turn from a gel-state to a more solid like state.

Tissues (Groups of Cells !)

1) Epithelial tissue – cover and line surfaces
2) Nerve tissue – communicate areas of body
3) Muscle tissue – moves things
4) Connective tissue – connect structures

Epithelial tissue

Covers various body surfaces and forms the lining of body cavities as well as parts of various glands of the body. The cells that make up the epithelial tissue are simple and can reproduce quickly in areas that are subject to damage such as the skin and mouth.

Nerve Tissue

Comprised of the brain, spinal cord and nerves. Conducts nerve impulses throughout the body. Nerve cells are also called neurons.

Muscle Tissue

3 types of muscle tissue:
1) Skeletal – striated and used for voluntary movement
2) Smooth – non-striated and involuntary movement in internal organs
3) Cardiac – Striated, involuntary and found in the heart.

Connective Tissue

Classification of Connective Tissue
1) Loose Connective Tissue
   a) Areolar
   b) Adipose
   c) Reticular
2) Elastic connective tissue
   Forms walls of arteries, lung tissue, trachea and bronchiole tubes.
3) Cartilage
   a) Hyaline – articular cartilage, septum of nose, costal cartilages of ribcage, throat.
   b) Fibrocartilage – very tough. Forms the intervertebral discs, menisci of knee joint and pubis symphysis.
   c) Elastic cartilage – Found in ears
4) Bone (osseous tissue)
   Mostly collagen fibers and very rigid. Embedded within the fiber matrix is fluid matrix where the minerals to from the bone are located.
5) Liquid connective tissue
   This is the blood where the cells are suspended in a liquid called the blood plasma.
6) Dense connective tissue (Fascia)
   a) Dense regular – makes up tendons, ligaments, aponeuroses.
   b) Dense irregular – organised lake a basket weave found in fascia of muscle, deep/investing fascia,

periosteum of bones and perichondrium of cartilage.
Fascia is a major limiting factor of flexibility !
Connective tissue develops in response to the
demands imposed on it !

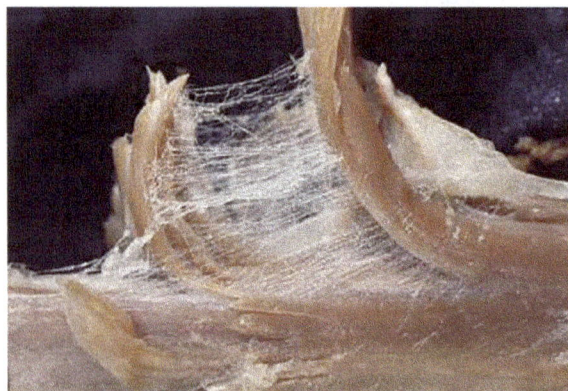

Reproduced with kind permission from the Author Ron Thompson

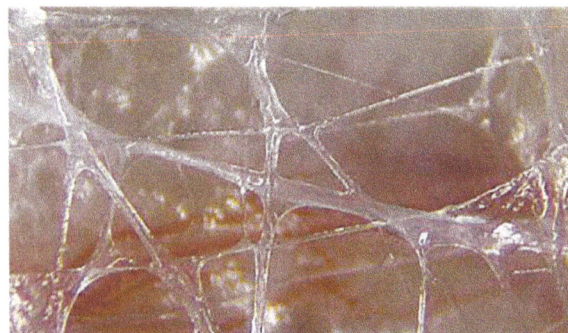

Reproduced with kind permission from the Author J.C
Guimberteau MD, Endovivo VideoProductions, France

Where is Fascia ?

Superficial Fascia

Lies directly below the skin and covers the body

storing fat and has various nerves, vessels and
lymphatics passing through at this level.

Deep Fascia

Lines the body and surrounds every anatomical
structure down to the cellular level including muscle,
bones, nerves, organs, blood vessels and lymph
vessels.

Myo-Fascia (part of the deep fascia)

Myo relates to muscles and facial relates to fascia
which is the strong connective tissue within which
muscles, nerves and organs of the body are encased.

Deepest Fascia

Lies within the dural membrane of the cranial sacral
system and encases the central nervous system of
the brain and spinal cord.

Arrangement of Fascia

Fascia runs in a '3 dimensional cobweb type matrix'
from head to foot and wraps and envelopes organs,
muscles, bones, joints and even down to a cellular
level.
Fascia creates space for nerves, lymph and arteries
to pass through.
The majority of fascia is arranged longitudinally
through the body from head to toe. Horizontally
arranged fibers can be seen to separate the body
into sections at the cranial base, hyoid, thoracic inlet,
respiratory diaphragm and pelvic diaphragms. If
these 'horizontal structures' or diaphragms are
restricted the longitudinal energy of the body (blood,
lymph, 'chi') will be affected.

Molecular Structure of Fascia

Collagen

Gives fascia its strength and resistant to tearing
Collagen fibers are considered in manual therapy to be able change their orientation thus changing the 'directional resistance' and shape of the fascia.
Collagen fibers may be stretched 5% of their length.

Elastin

Helps to absorb tensile forces.
Has cross linkage fibers in the same way as collagen to give strength.
Has the ability to return to its original state after stretching
Can stretch up to 150% of their length.

Ground Substance

Ground substance fills the spaces between the fibers.
Fascia experiences different levels of blood supply, nerve innervation and tensible ability throughout the day. In the fascia of a muscle (myofascia) there is a material called ground substance which has various ranges of consistency. When changing from a liquid form, to a gel, and then into its more solid state, the myofascia tightens, thus tensing the muscle.
In a healthy state, your ground substance has a fluid or springy consistency, so that it can absorb the forces that are created through trauma or when you move. When the ground substance hardens, its' absorbency vastly diminishes causing stress by transmitting force further along the 'line' to associated muscles and joints.
By returning the ground substance to a healthier state, the tensile (strength giving) collagen fibers within the fluid are released and able to move to where they are needed for support ie: arranging the body within gravity.
If however the tissue remains in a shortened or even lengthened position, it will maintain it's 'hyper-innervated' state severely affecting the ability of the muscle (group) to contract or relax leading to both physical and mental fatigue.
Fascia is also the material that forms adhesions and scar tissue. Consequently relaxing the fascia may not only make a muscle more functional but also help restore stability and health to associated joints.

Fascial Tensions for Movement

Bow String Theory

Think of the spine as a bow
The string of the bow can be represented by the anterior fascia of the body and relates to the anterior, longitudinal interconnected fascia which helps maintain a anterior/posterior balance and in turn relates to the 3 major functions of standing upright : eyes, vestibular system and soles of the feet.
If the string is too tight the body can not straighten – Extension movements now become almost impossible without unwanted stress or dysfunction at various levels of the spine (typical hyperlordotic and excessive kyphotic posture).

Bio Tensegrity

Bio relates to the body and tensegrity relates to a construction principle which can be traced to Buckminster Fuller. In a tensegrity construction there is no direct contact between solid components. Instead there is a dynamic balance of tension made through cables and rods.
However the body also consists of sliding surfaces and sectioned cavities/chambers which can be sealed off.

In a bio-tensegrity model the body can be seen to be interconnected throughout so that when force is applied at one specific area the whole system reacts or is affected by the force and distributive tension.

For example a person may complain of shoulder pain but in actual fact the pain may be caused by fascial tension coming from the hip (or any other number of areas of the body).

Causes of Fascial Tension

- *Physical Trauma*
- *Inflammation*
- *Infection*
- *Structural imbalance*
- *Muscle imbalance*
- *Burns*
- *Osseous restrictions*

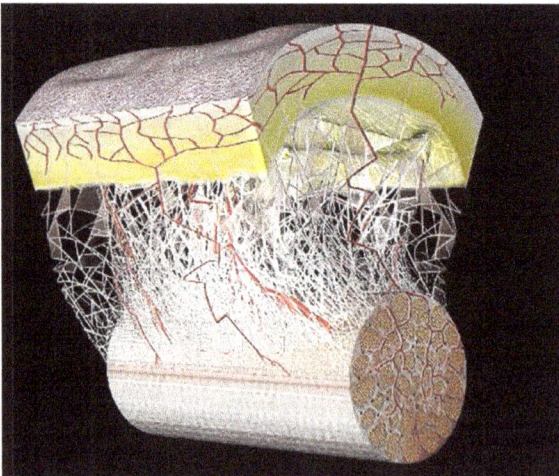

Reproduced with kind permission from the Author J.C Guimberteau MD, Endovivo VideoProductions, France

- *Muscle guarding*
- *Poor posture*
- *Body positioning*
- *Surgery – scar tissue*
- *Mental stress – emotions.*

It is important to note that numerous layers of dysfunction accumulate over a lifetime and hence may take years to address.

Organs

An organ is defined as two or more tissues working together to perform a specific function in the body.

Organ Systems

1) Integumentary – hair, nails, sweat glands, skin
2) Nervous – brain, spinal cord and nerves
3) Endochrine – ductless glands that secrete hormones
4) Digestive – organs of alimentary canal
5) Respiratory – organs of the air passageways and lungs.
6) Circulatory – heart, blood vessels and blood
7) Lymphatic – lymph vessels, nodes, lymph, thymus gland and spleen.
8) Urinary – kidneys, ureters, bladder and urethra
9) Reproductive – male and female reproductive organs
10) Skeletal – bones, ligaments and cartilages
11) Muscular – muscles and tendons

Skeletal System

Bone is a type of connective tissue infused with calcium salts and have their own system of blood and lymph vessels and nerves.

Functions

1) Structural support
2) Protection of softer tissues
3) Act as levers for muscular system
4) Manufacture blood cells
5) Store inorganic salts

Contains

1) Osteoblasts – bone producing cells
2) Osteoclasts – bone dissolving cells
3) Osteocytes – maintain bone but don't produce new bone matter

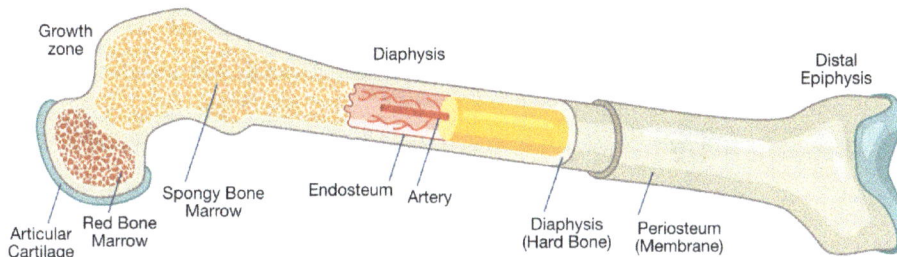

Bone structure

Diaphysis – shaft of the bone, compact
Epiphyses – Expanded 'spongy' ends and separated from shaft by epiphyseal growth line.
Medullary cavity – hollow section of shaft containing yellow marrow and reduces weight
Cancellous bone – spongy bone with honey combed structure containing red marrow
Compact bone – hard dense bone making the diaphysis and outer layer of short, flat or irregular bones.
Articular cartilage – covers the end of the epiphyses
Periosteum – outer sheave covering diaphysis and bound strongly to the bone. The place where tendons and ligaments attach.
Endosteum – thin layer of connective tissue lining the medullary cavity.

Bone growth

Bone develops at the epiphyseal disc until late teens or twenties when it ossifies.
The growth in girth occurs under the periosteum.
Osteoblasts and osteoclasts continually produce and dissolve bone matter throughout life called 'remodeling'.
Two factors affecting this are hormonal control and mechanical stresses and loads including gravity.

Muscular System

Structure

1) Myofibril – bundles of myofilaments
2) Fiber –a bundle of myofibrils
3) Fascicle – a bundle of muscle fibers.
4) Muscle belly - A bundle of fascicles.
5) Connective tissue / fascia
a) endomysium surrounds individual fibers
b) perimysium – surrounds the fascicle
c) epimysium – surrounds muscle belly
The tendon is the convergence of all these 3 layers.

They give the muscle its directionality.

The fascia is a major determinate of flexibility

Internal structure of muscle fiber

1) myofibrils – containing the myofilaments of actin and myosin.

2) Sarcomere – functional section of muscle cell with Z-lines marking the end of each section.

3) Sarcoplasmic reticulum – surrounds the myofibrils and stores calcium ions

4) T-tubules – tubes connecting sarcoplasmic reticulum to outside of sarcolemma

Muscles Fiber Arrangement

The arrangement of fibers within a muscle can be broadly categorized as being 2 distinct types of architecture; Parallel and Pennate:

a. Parallel

Fibers are arranged on a longitudinal axis of the muscle in line with the tendon. These fibers can shorten considerably and move the body segment through a longer range of motion than the pennate fibered muscles. eg; sartorius, rectus abdominis and biceps brachii

b. Pennate

In this arrangement the fibers sit at an angle to the longitudinal axis of the muscle and at an angle to the tendon. The shape can be seen to be similar to a feather. When the fibers contract the angle of attachment increases and exerts less force through the tendon and into the bone it moves. Pennate arrangements however allow for more muscle fibers per unit of muscle and can thus transmit more force than parallel arrangements. eg; tibialis posterior, rectus femoris and deltoid muscles.

Types of muscle fiber

There are 2 main types of muscle fiber:

I) Slow twitch (ST) or Slow Oxidative (SO)

IIa) Fast Twitch (FTa) or Fast Oxidative / Glycolytic (FOG)

IIb) Fast Twitch (FTb) or Fast Glycolytic (FG)

Slow Twitch – Slower to contract adapted to low intensity, long duration.

Fast Twitch / or Type II -Fast contraction time and generate greater force of contraction.

Fast Oxidative Glycolytic Type IIa - Mixture of oxidative and glycolytic properties.

Type II c fibers - Usually accounts for less than 5% of muscle fibers and possible result of Type IIb being converted to Type IIa.

Contraction of muscles

1) At rest the proteins tropomyosin and troponin stop the cross bridges of myosin binding with actin.

2) Acetylcholine is released at neuromuscular junction.

3) Action potential travels along sarcolemma and enters cell via T-tubules

4) Calcium ions are released into muscle fiber sarcoplasm

5) Calcium ions remove inhibitory effect of tropomyosin and troponin.

6) Heads of myosin move the actin filaments like a ratchet

7) Z-line are pulled closer together at each end of the sarcomere

8) Muscle fibers are thus shortened

9) Upon relaxation the calcium is removed back to the sarcoplasmic reticulum.

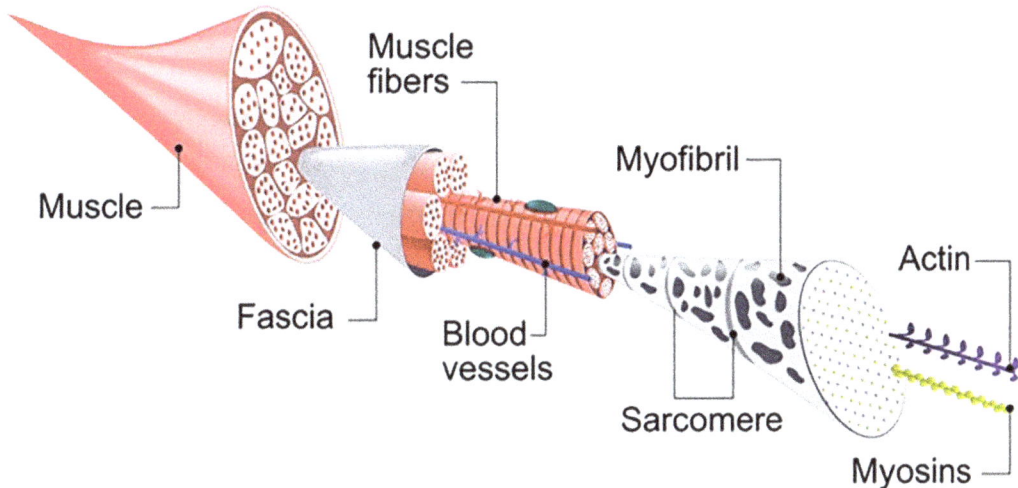

Muscle fibers

Muscle

Fascia

Blood vessels

Myofibril

Sarcomere

Actin

Myosins

5.2 ▸ Motor Units

A muscle fiber is stimulated by motor nerves containing motor neurones.

The neurone and it's fibers supplied are called a motor unit.

There may be as little as 5 fibers per unit (eye muscles) or as many as 2000 (quadriceps).

Type I or Type II muscle fibers are determined by the type of neurone supplying the muscle

Motor neurones end with a plate called the neuromuscular junction.

When an impulse arrives acetylcholine is released between the sarcolemma of the fiber and the plate of the neurone.

A wave of electricity is conducted which if strong enough will cause the fibers in the unit to contract. If it is not strong enough but comes at a high enough frequency the summation of the discharges at the presynaptic membrane (sarcolemma) will be strong enough to initiate contraction.

Muscle Fatigue

Interruption of neuromuscular events
a. Depletion of acetylcholine
b. Imbalance of sodium and potassium ions
c. A reduced amount of calcium ions

Depletion of energy source

a. If ATP can not be replaced fatigue will result.
b. Reduction in glycogen results in levels not being maintained.
c. Depletion of Carnitine

Body fluids

a. Lack of water will disturb ion balance
b. Insufficient blood supply will contribute to all factors leading to fatigue.

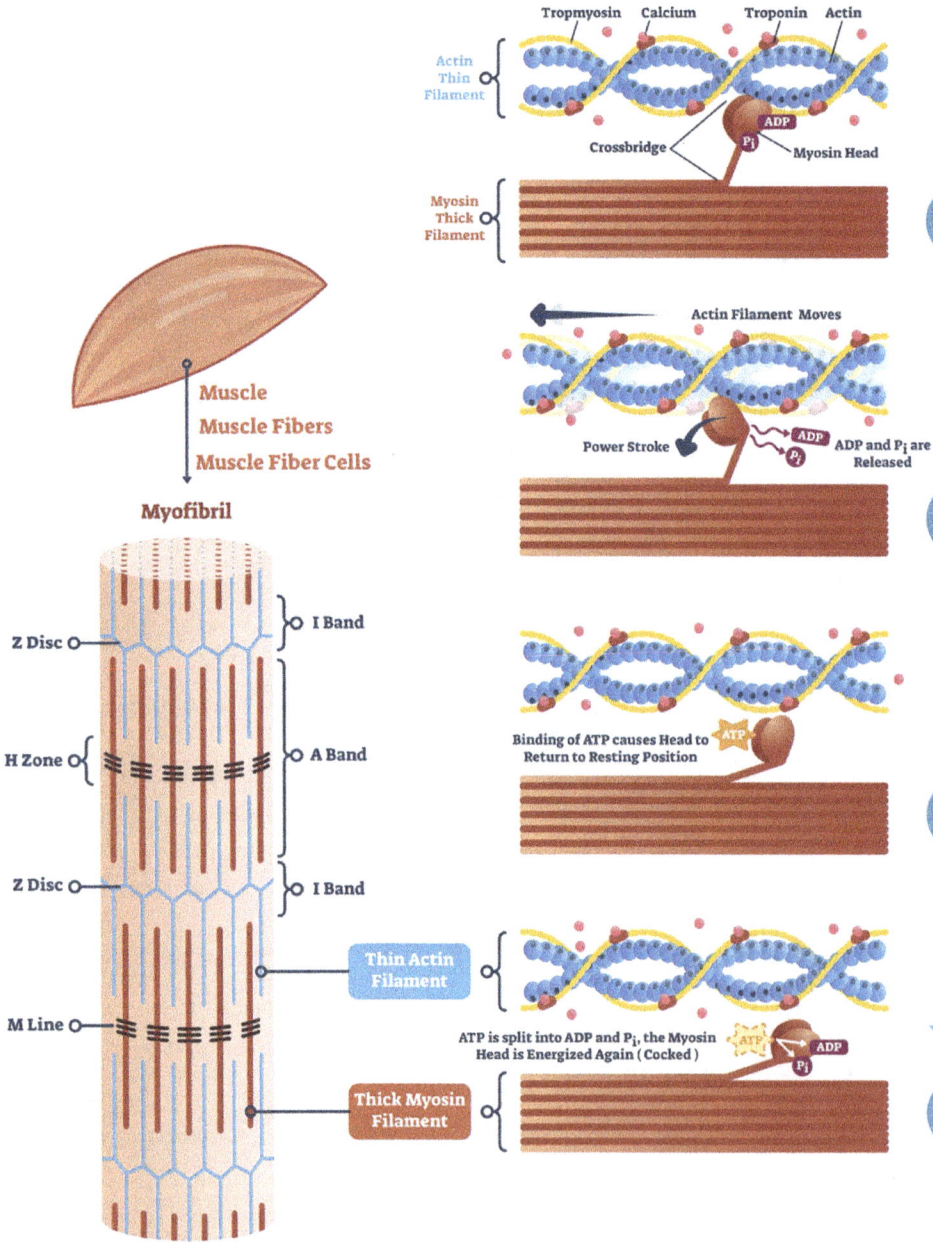

Muscle
Muscle Fibers
Muscle Fiber Cells

Myofibril

Z Disc
I Band
H Zone
A Band
Z Disc
I Band
M Line

Thin Actin Filament

Thick Myosin Filament

Tropmyosin   Calcium   Troponin   Actin

Actin Thin Filament

Crossbridge   Myosin Head

ADP
Pi

Myosin Thick Filament

1

Actin Filament Moves

Power Stroke   ADP and Pi are Released

ADP
Pi

2

Binding of ATP causes Head to Return to Resting Position

ATP

3

ATP is split into ADP and Pi, the Myosin Head is Energized Again (Cocked)

ATP   ADP
Pi

4

Mechanoreceptors

There are 3 categories of sensory perception :
  • Baroreceptors
  • Tactile
  • Proprioceptors

Baroreceptors

Baroreceptors are located in the carotid sinus and the aortic arch. They sense the blood pressure and relay the information to the brain, so that a proper blood pressure can be maintained.

Tactile Receptors

In the skin there are 4 types of tactile mechan-oreceptors :

Merkels disks

Respond to light touch and are found in the upper layers of the skin. They are especially prevalent in the finger tips and lips. Together with Meissener's corpuscles they allow for fine touch and detail.

Meissener's corpuscles

These are found in the upper layers of the skin and respond quickly to pressure and low frequency vibration being also found in the eyelids. Together with Merkels Disks they allow for fine touch and detail.

Ruffini endings

Occur deeper in the skin layer. They detect skin stretch and deformation in the skin allowing for feedback for gripping objects and contribute to kinesthetic awareness. They also detect warmth and because they are situated deeper in the skin layer than the cold receptors humans detect cold faster than they do heat.

Pacinian corpuscle

Located in the deep layer of the skin, periosteum of the bone, joint capsules, viscera and genitals. They detect deep, changing pressure and high frequency vibration through compression.
Note: There is a 5th type of mechanoreceptor, Krause end bulbs, in specialized regions which detect cold.

Mechanoreceptors in Fascia

Golgi Tendon Organs (GTO's)

Situated at the junction of the a muscle and tendon they detect the amount of stretch in a tendon and stimulate the activation of the antagonist muscle whilst inhibiting the contracting muscle.

Pacinian corpuscle

Located at myotendinous junctions, spinal ligaments, investing muscular tissues they respond to rapid pressure changes and vibrations. They give a sense of kinesthesia for movement control.

Ruffini endings

Occuring in the peripheral joint ligaments, dura mater, and other tissues associated with stretching the respond to sustained as opposed to changing pressure. Stimulation may result in inhibition of sympathetic activity.

Interstitial

Found almost everywhere including inside bones and especially the periosteum. They respond to both rapid and sustained pressure changes resulting in changes to vasodilation.

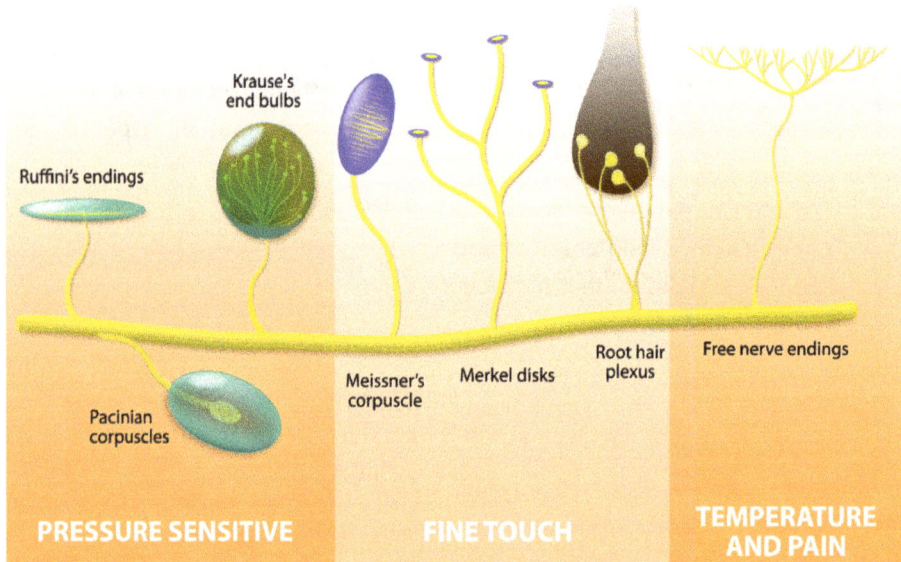

Krause's
end bulbs

Ruffini's endings

Pacinian
corpuscles

Meissner's
corpuscle

Merkel disks

Root hair
plexus

Free nerve endings

PRESSURE SENSITIVE   **FINE TOUCH**   **TEMPERATURE
AND PAIN**

Proprioceptors

Muscle Spindle

Consists of 3 modified fibers with sensory and motor neurones.

Contracton or extension of the spindle is detected by the sensory nerve endings and relayed to the central nervous system.

Contraction of a muscle can be made via the alpha neurons directly or through the muscle spindles via the gamma neurons.

Activation via the alpha neurons is faster than the gamma loop but if both pathways are utilised at the same time the muscle contraction will produce greater force.

A Stretch Reflex may be activated when the muscle spindle perceives a stretch to be unsafe.

Reciprocal Inhibition – stimulation to a muscle to contract leads to the inhibition of the opposing muscle

Proprioceptive Neuromuscular Facilitation (PNF) Stretch

A technique used to relax and /or stretch a muscle that utilises the muscle spindles and golgi tendon organs to facilitate a relaxation of the muscle and tendon in order for the muscle to release tension and thus be able to be 'stretched' further.

Stretched Muscle

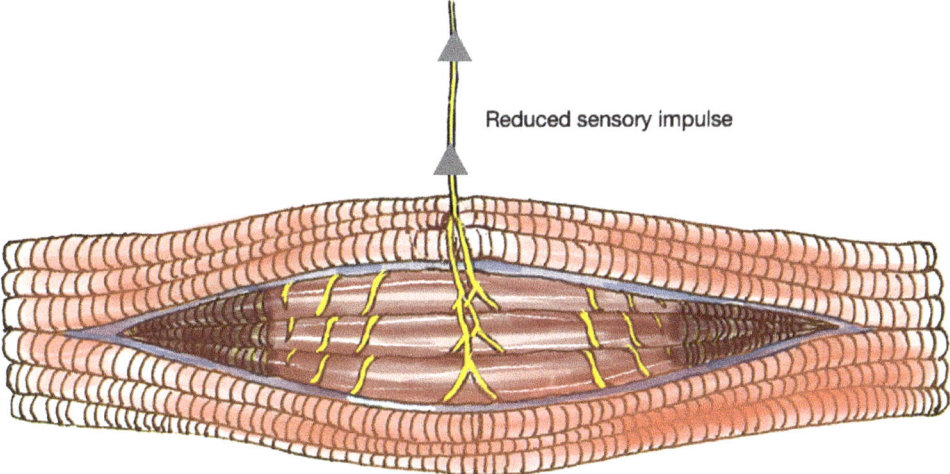

Reduced sensory impulse

Contracted Muscle

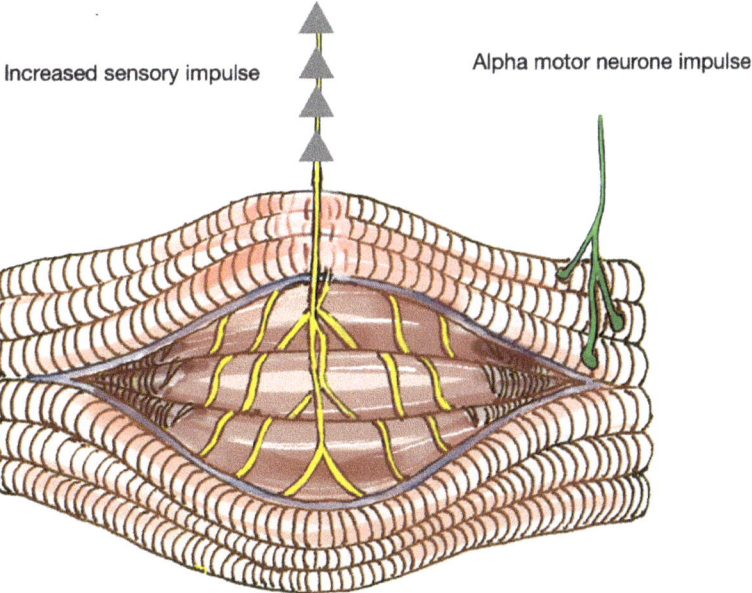

Increased sensory impulse

Alpha motor neurone impulse

Muscle Spindle Apparatus

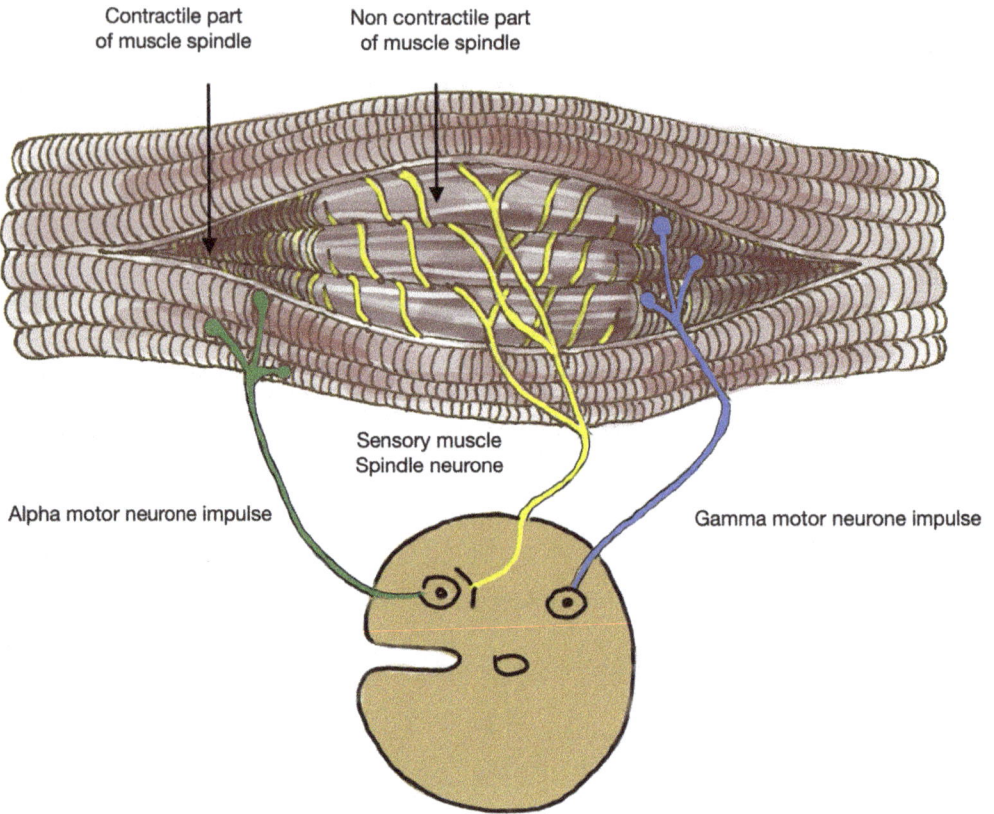

Contractile part
of muscle spindle

Non contractile part
of muscle spindle

Sensory muscle
Spindle neurone

Alpha motor neurone impulse

Gamma motor neurone impulse

Energy Supply Systems

All energy for the muscular system comes from the breakdown of glucose. The glucose molecule is broken down into usable energy in the mitochondria which are the organelles in the cell where cellular respiration takes place. Mitochondria are often referred to as "the powerhouse of the cell".

The mitochondria breaks the glucose down to form (amongst things- depending on the energy system used), a nucleotide called Adenosine Triphosphate, which is the actual 'fuel' used to power the muscle.

A nucleotide is the basic building block of nucleic acids and consist of a sugar molecule attached to a phosphate group and a nitrogen-containing base.

There are essentially 3 systems that supply the ATP or energy to the muscles :

1) Phosphocreatine system
2) Anaerobic system
3) Aerobic system

Phosphocreatine system (PC)

Stores of ATP are limited but ALL energy must be channeled through ATP and replenished as soon as it is used up.

ADP + Phosphocreatine = ATP + Creatine

No lactic acid is produced but the PC can only be regenerated using ATP which is unavailable at maximal exercise intensity.

ATP is also regenerated via other sources as well as the PC system:

a) Energy from lactic anaerobic respiration.

b) Aerobic oxidation of glycogen, FFAs and blood glucose although carbohydrates are also needed to help completely break down fats.

Anaerobic Glycolysis

Anaerobic respiration generates 2 ATP molecules from each glucose molecule.

Pyruvic acid is used to oxidize (remove 2 hydrogen atoms) NAD2H, which in turn becomes lactic acid.

Lactic acid is removed by:

a) Sweat
b) Urine
c) Reconversion to glycogen
d) Aerobic oxidation to carbon dioxide and water. (About 3 hrs after exercise)

Delayed Onset Muscle Soreness (DOMS)

Pain and tenderness that occurs in the muscles of a novice or untrained athlete usually 1 -2 days after exercise. Thought of as being due to an increase of pressure within the muscle tissue due to the microtrauma of muscle fibers caused by the eccentric phase of exercise.

Aerobic system

If there is sufficient oxygen available to the pyruvic acid it will carry on into the cell to the mitochondria to be broken down into carbon dioxide and water via the Krebs Cycle.

One molecule of glucose may yield 38 molecules of ATP

5.3 ► The Human Skeleton

There are 206 bones in the body although it is possible to slightly vary. The skeleton can be divided into 2 sections : axial and appendicular skeleton

Axial Skeleton

Skull : the cranium and facial bones
Hyoid bone
Vertebral column : divided into : 7 cervical vertebrae, 12 thoracic vertebrae, 5 lumbar vertebrae
Ribcage : consisting of 12 pairs of ribs and the sternum (manubrium, body and xiphoid process)
Sacrum: 5 fused bones
Coccyx: 3-5 fused bones

Appendicular Skeleton

Pectoral girdle : clavicle and scapula (shoulder blade)
Upper limb : humerus, ulna, radius, carpal bones (8 each hand), metacarpal bones (5 each hand) and phalanges (14 per hand)
Pelvic girdle : 2 coxal bones which are 3 bones fused together (ilium, ischium and pubis)
Lower limb : femur, patella (knee cap), tibia, fibula, tarsal bones (7 each foot), metatarsal bones (5 per foot) and phalanges (14 per foot).
It should be noted that the 'Pelvis' is different to the 'Pelvic girdle'. The pelvis consists of the pelvic girdle plus the sacrum and coccyx.

Structural Anatomical Terms

Head : enlargement at end of bone
Crest : ridge
Condyle : rounded process usually articulates with another bone
Epicondyle: process above a condyle.

Ramus : branch like structure coming off another bone
Spine : 'pointy' type projection
Styloid process : sharp, spiky projection
Trochanter : large process
Tuberosity : 'rough' area of bone usually for muscle attachment
Facet : small almost flat surface
Foramen : a hole in the bone
Fossa : depression
Sinus : cavity or hollow space

Joints

A joint is a junction between 2 or more bones and are classified in 3 groups as to the type of movement available.

Synarthroses

Immovable joints are separated by fibrous tissue with no space between the joints or 'active' movement. eg: cranial bones

Amphiarthrosis

Slightly moveable joints are separated by a fibro-cartilage disc. eg: pubic symphysis, intervertebral joint and sacral illiac.

Diarthrosis

More commonly known as synovial joints or freely moveable joints. The end of each bone is covered with hyaline cartilage which is incased within a joint capsule. Ligaments surround the joint capsule to give it support and inner layer has a synovial membrane to secrete synovial fluid which acts to lubricate the joint.
There are 6 types of diathroses
1) Hinge - allows for flexion and extension
2) Ball & socket - allows movement in all planes and

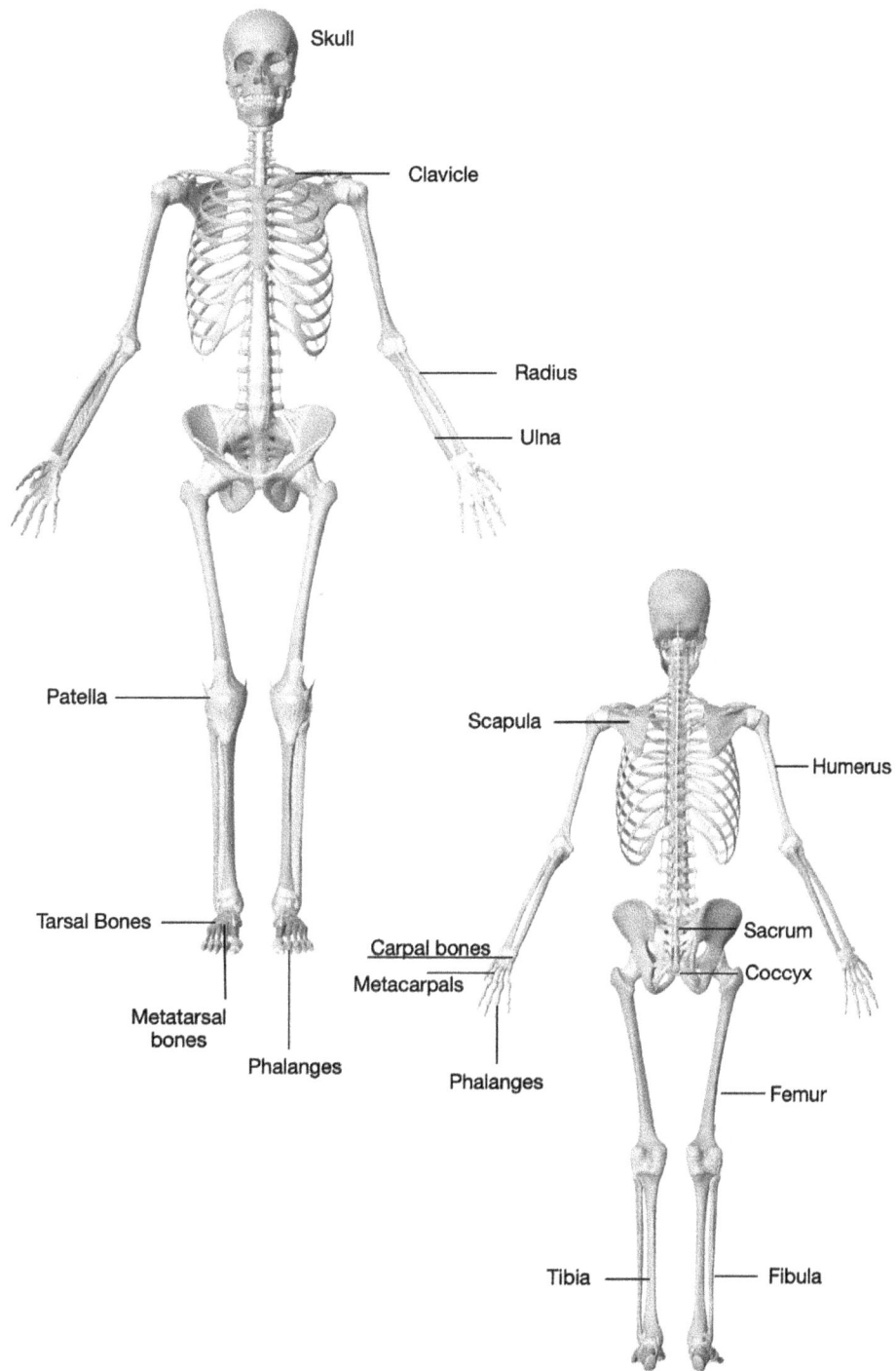

Skull

Clavicle

Radius

Ulna

Patella

Scapula

Humerus

Tarsal Bones

Carpal bones

Sacrum

Metacarpals

Coccyx

Metatarsal
bones

Phalanges

Phalanges

Femur

Tibia

Fibula

is the most moveable.

3) Pivot - bone sits within a ring formed by another bone allowing rotation

4) Ellipsoid - rounded end fits inside a hollow or cavity of another joint allowing flexion/extension and abduction/adduction in 2 planes

5) Saddle - 2 saddle shaped ends fit together for movement in 2 planes

6) Gliding - flat surface allowing for non-axial or limited movement

Ligaments

Fibrous tough connective tissue connecting articulating bones and blending in with the periosteum of the bone. Ligaments stabilize the joint and have very poor blood supply resulting in a very long recovery time if injured.

Tendons & Aponeurosis

Dense regular connective tissue which connects a muscle with its bony attachment blending in with the periosteum of the bone. An aponeuroses is a flattened or expanded sheet of tendon. A tendon and aponeuroses have better blood supply than a ligament but it is still very poor resulting in prolonged recovery time.

Diagram of a Synovial Joint

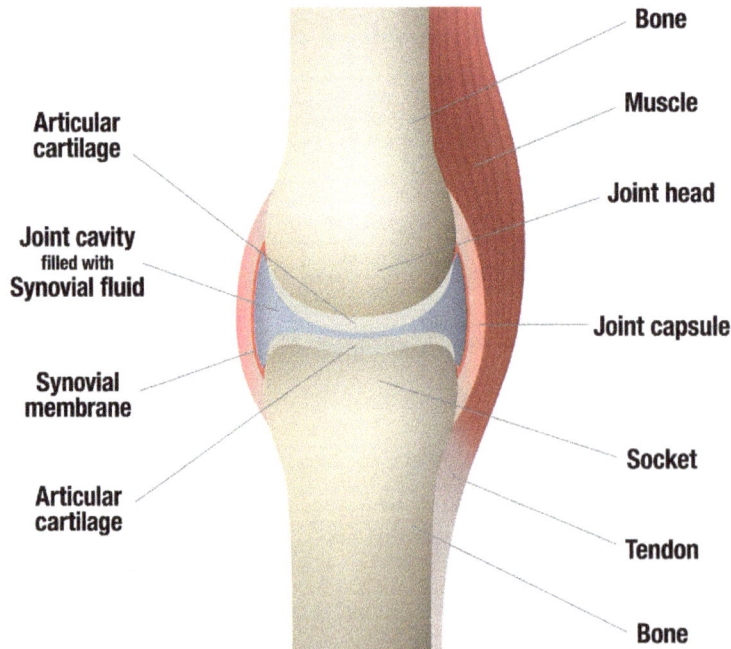

Articular cartilage

Joint cavity filled with Synovial fluid

Synovial membrane

Articular cartilage

Bone

Muscle

Joint head

Joint capsule

Socket

Tendon

Bone

Bursa

A sac filled with synovial fluid and situated between a tendon and bone acting as a sort of pulley for the tendon and excretes synovial fluid to lubricate the joint.

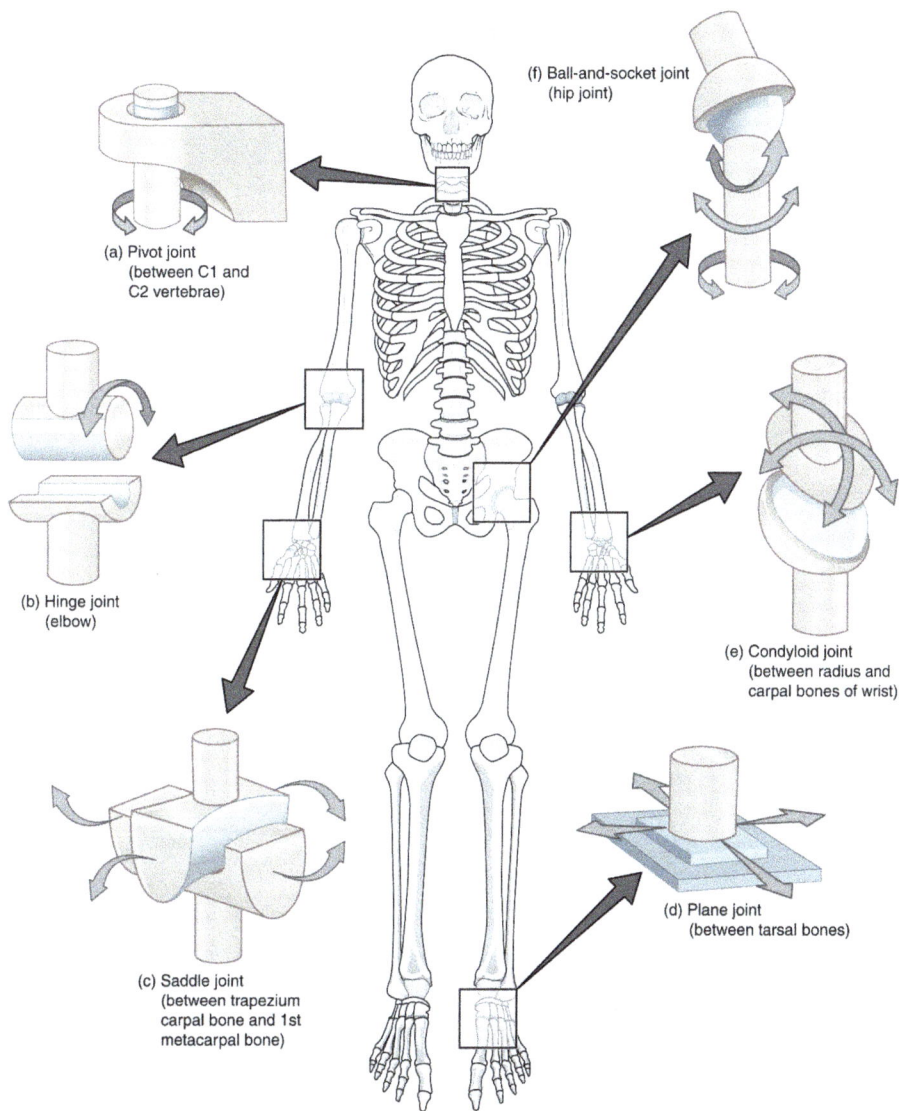

(f) Ball-and-socket joint (hip joint)

(a) Pivot joint (between C1 and C2 vertebrae)

(b) Hinge joint (elbow)

(c) Saddle joint (between trapezium carpal bone and 1st metacarpal bone)

(d) Plane joint (between tarsal bones)

(e) Condyloid joint (between radius and carpal bones of wrist)

Types of Synovial Joints esp.jpg" by OpenStax College/licensed under CC

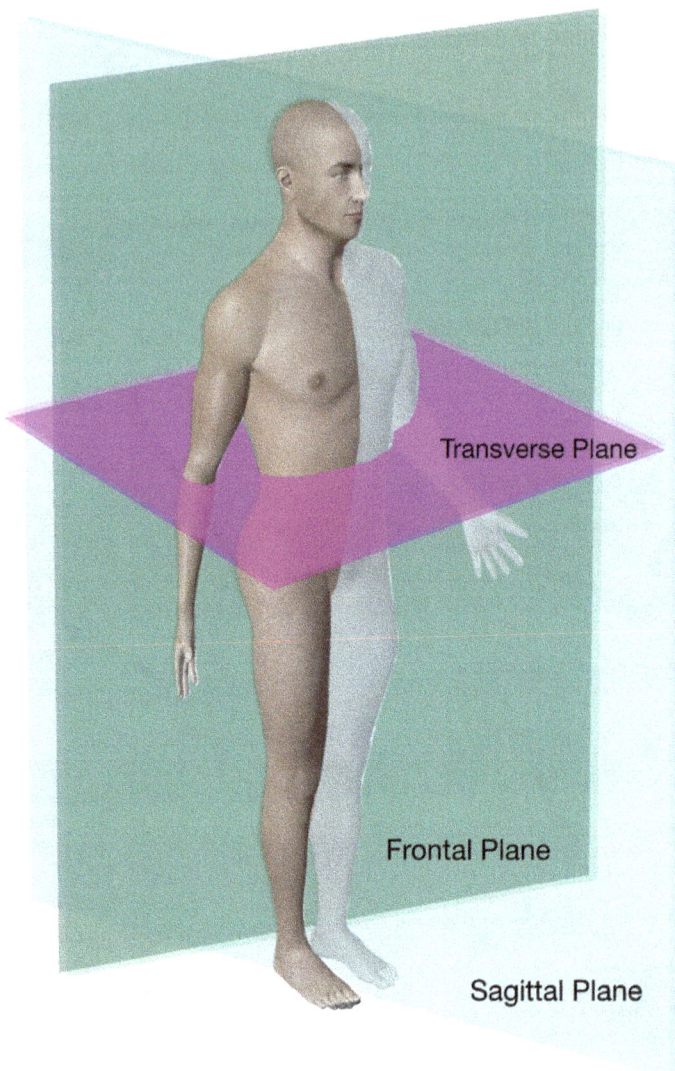

Transverse Plane

Frontal Plane

Sagittal Plane

5.4 ► Classifications of Movement

An axis is an imaginary line about which motion occurs and is helpful to denote the plane of movement for a joint.

Planes of movement

• Frontal / Coronal plane – as in lifting arms out to the side
• Sagittal plane – as in bending forwards or back
• Transverse plane – rotation - as in twisting around

Movements in Sagittal plane

Flexion – angle of joint decreases as body parts moved together
Extension – return from flexion move
Hyper extension – continuation of extension beyond start position or straight line
Dorsiflexion – bending foot at ankle towards the shin
Plantar flexion – pointing foot away from shin (extension)
Protraction – forward movement of body part or return from retraction
Retraction – backward movement of body part or return from protraction.

Movements in Frontal plane

Abduction – sideways movement away from body
Adduction – return from abduction
Elevation – raising a body part
Depression – lowering a body part
Inversion – turning the foot so the sole faces medially
Eversion – turning the foot so the sole faces laterally
Lateral flexion – sidebending trunk or neck
Upward rotation of scapula – bottom of scapula rotates outwards and up
Inward rotation of scapula – return from upward

Movements in Transverse plane

Rotation – turning around to the side
Lateral rotation – arm or leg rotates outwards
Medial rotation – arm or leg rotates inwards
Lateral rotation of knee – occurs only when knee flexed
Medial rotation of knee – occurs only when knee is flexed
Supination – turning palms upwards
Pronation – turning the palm downwards
Horizontal abduction – when arm is flexed to 900 the arm moves away from midline
Horizontal adduction – when arm is flexed to 900 the arm moves towards midline.

All 3 planes (oblique plane)

Circumduction – swinging arms or legs in a circle

Muscle Terminology

Myo – anything to do with muscle
Origin – immovable attachment of the muscle
Insertion – the attachment that moves
One joint / two joint – A muscle will cross either one or two joints between attachments
Agonist – prime mover produces most of the force in a movement.
Antagonist – opposes the agonist and must lengthen to allow movement. Important for protection or 'braking / deceleration' to prevent injury
Synergist – help agonists overcome resistance
Stabilizer – fixes body segment to allow 'correct' movement to occur
Neutralizer - helps prevent unwanted action of agonist.

Note:

Throughout this manual muscle attachments are labelled simply as 'Attachments'. The terminology of 'Origin' & 'Insertion' is considered to now be outdated and replaced with the following terms :

- *Axial attachment /*
- *Appendicular attachment /*
- *Proximal attachment /*
- *Distal attachment /*

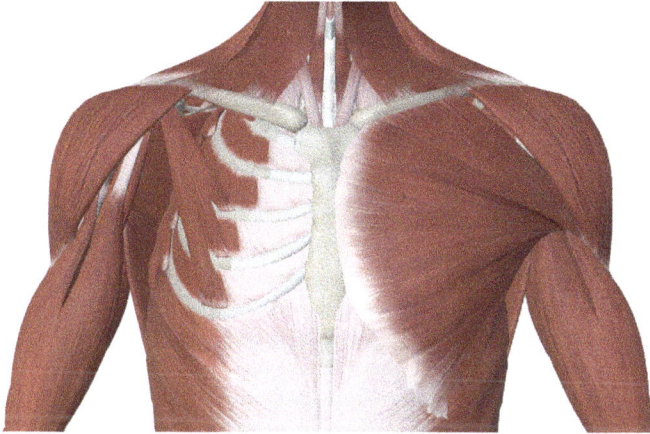

Bones:

1. Clavicle
   a. Sternal end
   b. Acrominal end

2. Scapula
   a. Axillary border
   b. Glenoid fossa
   c. Medial border
   d. Coracoid process
   e. Inferior & Superior angles
   f. Spine
   g. Infraspinous fossa
   h. Supraspinous fossa
   i. Subscapula fossa
   j. Acromium

3. Humerus
   a. Head
   b. Greater & Lesser tubercles
   c. Bicipital groove
   d. Deltoid tuberosity
   e. Lateral epicondyle
   f. Medial epicondyle
   g. Capitulum
   h. Trochlea
   i. Olecranon fossa

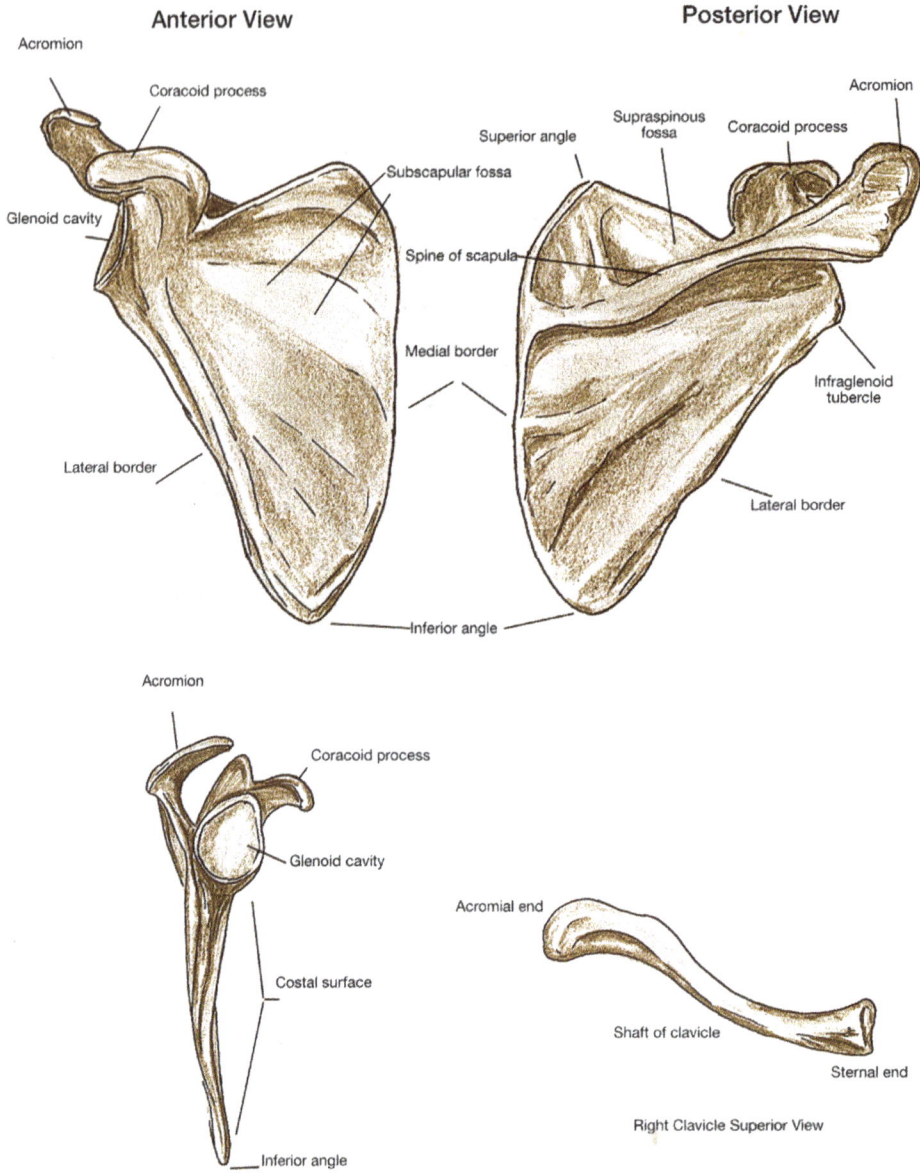

Anterior View

Acromion

Coracoid process

Glenoid cavity

Subscapular fossa

Spine of scapula

Medial border

Lateral border

Inferior angle

Posterior View

Superior angle

Supraspinous fossa

Coracoid process

Acromion

Infraglenoid tubercle

Lateral border

Inferior angle

Acromion

Coracoid process

Glenoid cavity

Costal surface

Inferior angle

Acromial end

Shaft of clavicle

Sternal end

Right Clavicle Superior View

Humerus

Greater Tuberosity

Head of humerus

Lesser Tuberosity

Inter tubercular Groove

DeltoidTuberosity

Anterior View

Posterior view

Radial Fossa

Coronoid fossa

Medial Epicondyle

Lateral Epicondyle

Groove for ulna nerve

Trochlea

Trochlea

Capitellum

Olecranon

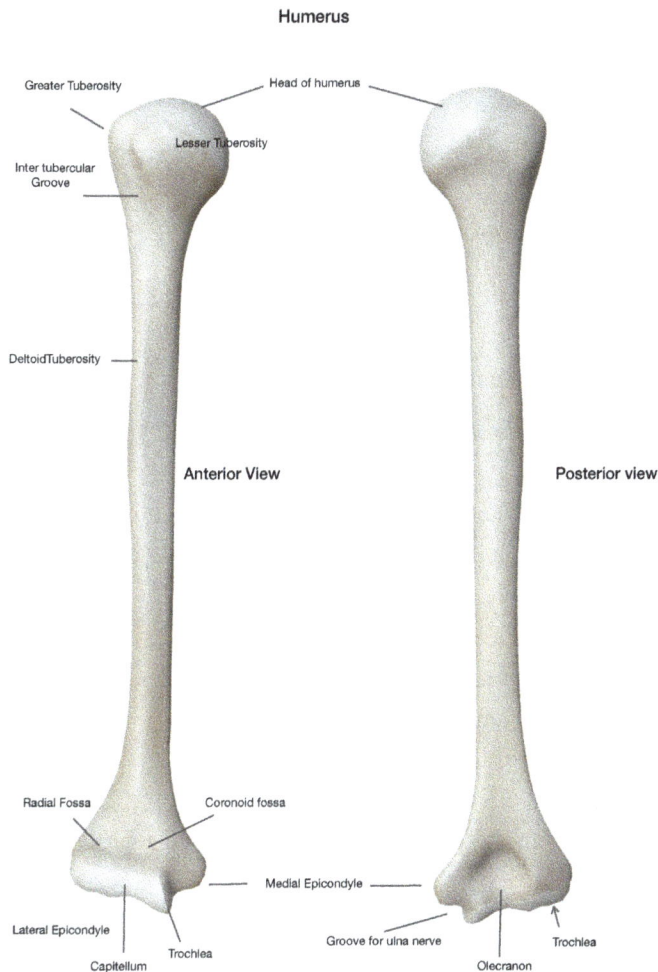

Joints and Ligaments

Sternoclavicular joint - is the only bone to bone connection between the whole shoulder girdle and the axial skeleton. Allows for a gliding movement.

Acromioclavicular joint - gliding joint often stressed through improper 'pushing'
movements or falling on an outstretched arm/hand.

Glenohumeral joint - the 'shoulder joint'. Similar to the hip joint but less stable due to a more shallow fossa. Stability is greatly enhanceed through the 'rotator cuff muscles'. Repetitive movements and incorrect shoulder girdle movement patterns can cause various pathologies for this joint.

Nuchal Ligament - Connective tissue from base of skull to the C7 vertebra dividing the posterior neck muscles.

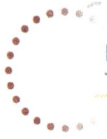

Muscles

Axial to Appendicular

1) Latissimus dorsi

Attachments

Thoracolumbar aponeurosis from T7 to iliac crest

Anterior proximal shaft of humerus

(in between teres major and pec major)

Action

Extends, adducts and medially rotates humerus

Note

Forms the posterior wall of the axillary cavity

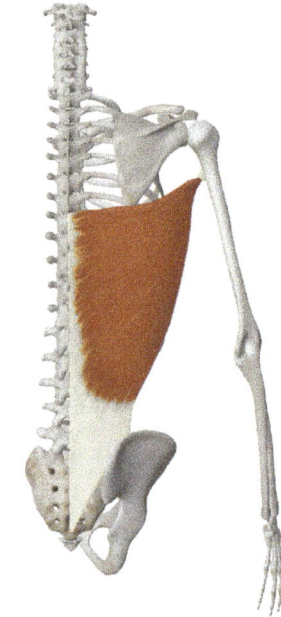

2) Trapezius

Attachments

Occiput, nuchal ligament and SP's of C7 to T12.

Upper Traps: lateral clavicle and acromium

Middle Traps: Spine of scapula

Lower Traps: root of spine of scapula

Action

Upper Traps: Elevation and upward rotation of
scapula

Middle Traps: Retraction of scapula

Lower Traps: depression and upwards rotation of
scapula

Note

Also works to stabilize scapulae and act as
neutralizer .

Cause of many tension headaches and severely
affected by improper posture such as sitting for
prolonged periods.

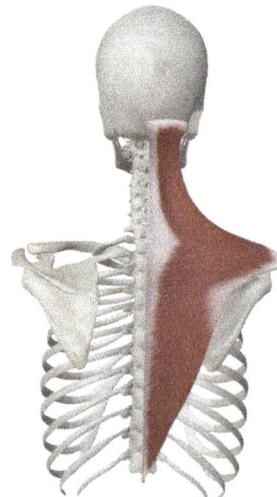

3) Rhomboid Major

Attachments

SP's of T2 to T5

medial border of scapula between the spine and inferior angle of scapula.

Action

retraction and downward rotation of scapula

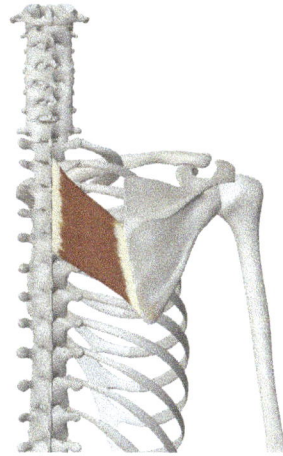

4) Rhomboid Minor

Attachments

SP's C7 to T1

upper portion of medial border of scapula at level of spine of scapula.

Action

retraction and downward rotation of scapula

Note

lies under the trapezius and can become weak and tight due to overuse of the traps due to improper posture such as 'pulling back the shoulders'

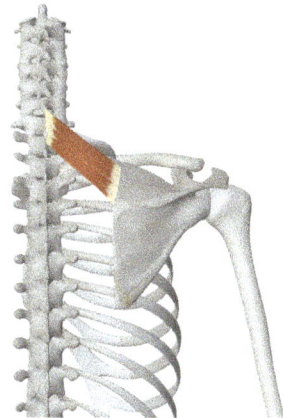

5) Levator Scapula

Attachments

TP's of C1 to C4

superior angle of scapula

Action

elevation and downward rotation of scapula

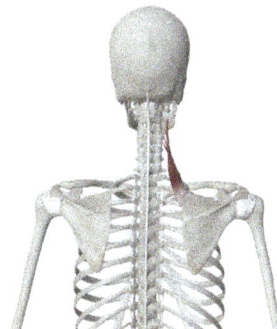

6) Serratus Anterior

Attachments

anterolateral surface of first 8 ribs

anterior surface of medial border of scapula

Action

protraction and upward rotation of scapula upper
fibres produce downward rotation of scapula lower
fibres depress scapula

Note

Major muscle used for stabilization for pushing
movements

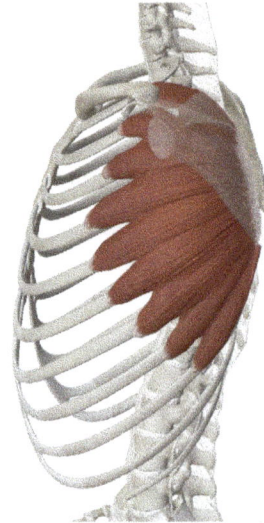

7) Pectoralis Major

Attachments

medial half of clavicle sternum and cartilages of
superior 6 ribs both heads attach to proximal shaft
of humerus

Action

flexes, adducts and medially rotates humerus
(clavicular head) extends, adducts and medially
rotates humerus (sternal head)

Note

major agonist muscle used for pushing movements
common tendon flips over on itself before insertion
on humerus

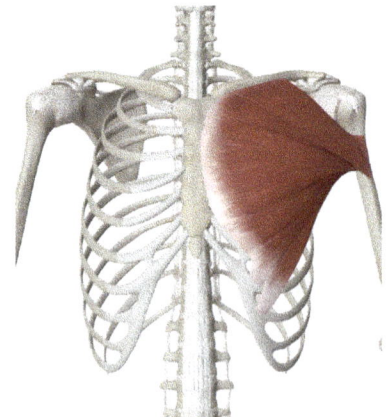

8) Pectoralis Minor

Attachments

anterior surface of 3rd , 4th and 5th ribs

coracoid process of scapula

Action

protraction, depression and downward rotation of
scapula

Note

can also aid forced inspiration by raising ribcage

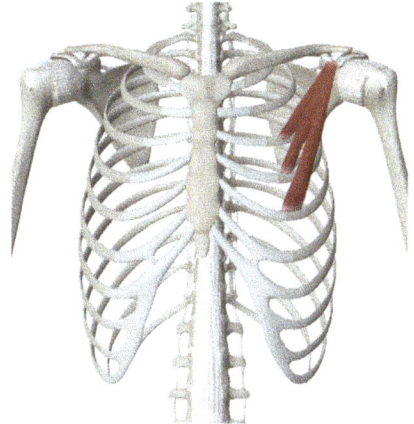

9) Subclavius

Attachments

medial end of first rib inferior shaft of lateral 2/3 of
clavicle

Action

depression and stabilization of clavicle

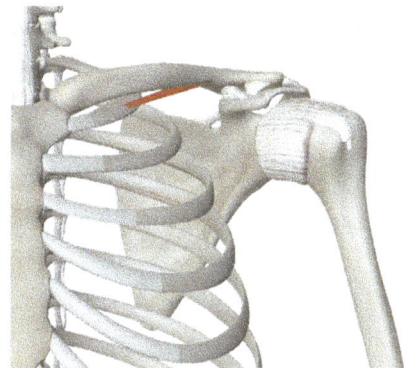

Appendicular to Appendicular

1) Supraspinatus (rotator cuff muscle)

Attachments

supraspinous fossa

top of greater tubercle

Action

initiates abduction

Note

common pathology for rotator cuff problems
(tendonitis)

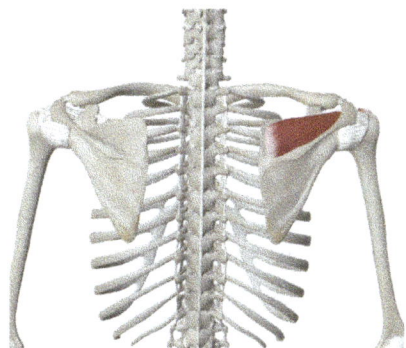

2) Infraspinatus (rotator cuff muscle)

Attachments

infraspinous fossa

posterior surface of greater tubercle

Action

lateral rotation and adduction of humerus

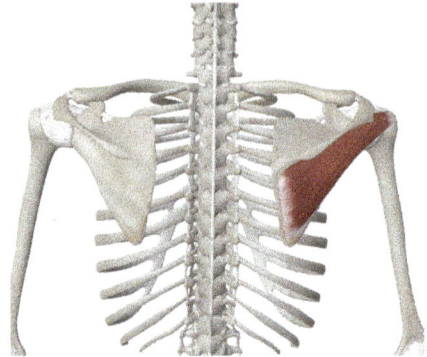

3) Teres Minor (rotator cuff muscle)

Attachments

posterior inferior lateral surface of scapula

posterior head of greater tubercle below

infraspinatus

Action

lateral rotation and adduction of humerus

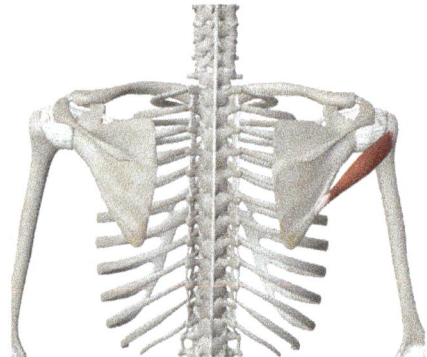

4) Subscapularis (rotator cuff muscle)

Attachments

subscapula fossa

anterior surface of lesser tubercle

Action

medial rotation and adduction of humerus

Note

All the above 'rotator cuff' muscles act to stabilize

the head of the humerus in the glenoid fossa

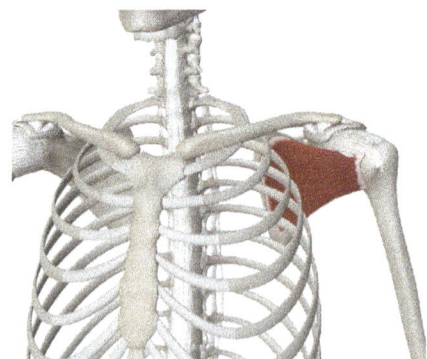

5) Teres Major

Attachments

inferior angle of scapula

medial lip of bicipital groove of humerus

Action

extends, adducts, and medially rotates
humerus

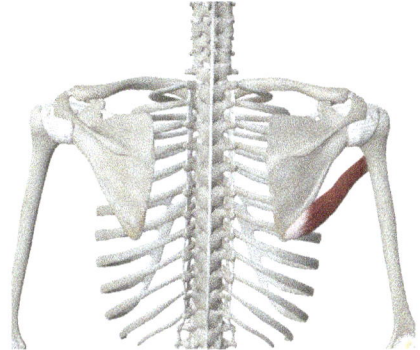

6) Deltoid (3 heads)

Attachments

lateral third of clavicle (anterior head)

lateral edge of acromium (middle head)

spine of scapula (posterior head)

deltoid tuberosity of humerus (all 3 heads)

Action

flexion, medial rotation and horizontal
adduction of humerus (anterior)

abduction to 90° (middle)

extension, lateral rotation and horizontal
abduction of humerus (posterior)

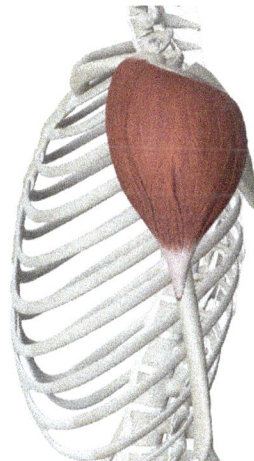

7) Biceps Brachii (2 heads)

Attachments

supraglenoid tubercle of scapula above
glenoid fossa (long head)

coracoid process of scapula (short head)

radial tuberosity of radius

Action

flexion of elbow and supination of forearm (long
head)

Helps flex humerus at shoulder joint

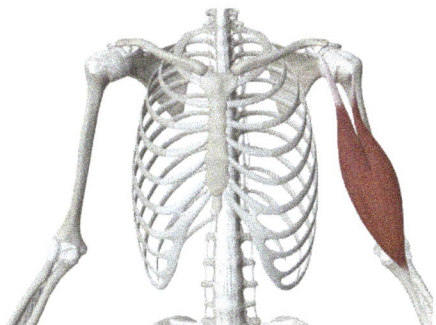

8) Triceps Brachii (3 heads)

Attachments

infraglenoid tubercle of posterior scapula (long head)

middle shaft of posterior humerus (lateral head)

lower 2/3 of posterior shaft of humerus (medial head)

olecranon process of ulna

Action

extends elbow, extends humerus, assists adduction (long head)

extends elbow (lateral head)

extends elbow (medial head)

Note

the long head crosses 2 joints

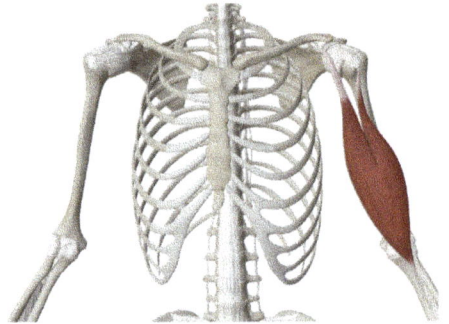

9) Coracobrachialis

Attachments

coracoid process of scapula

middle medial border of humeral head

Action

flexion and adduction of humerus

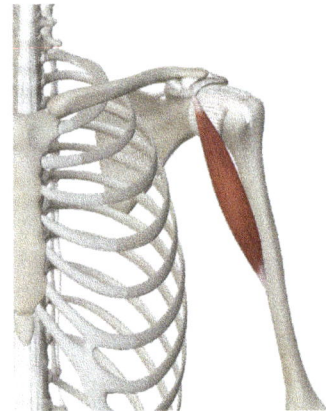

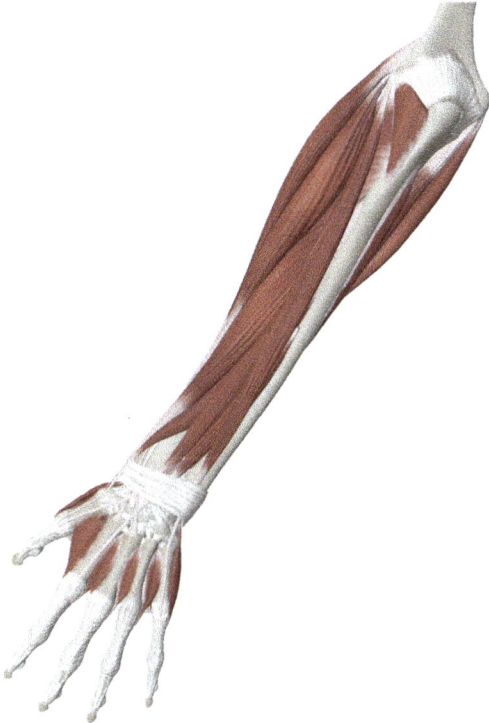

2. Radius
   a. shaft
   b. head
   c. tuberosity
   d. styloid process
   e. ulnar notch
3. Carpal bones
   a. scaphoid
   b. lunate
   c. triquetrum
   d. pisiform
   e. trapezium
   f. trapezoid
   g. capitate
   h. hamate
4. Metacarpals I-V
   a. base
   b. shaft
   c. head
5. Phalanges (proximal, middle, distal)
   a. base
   b. shaft
   c. head

Bones:

1. Ulna
   a. shaft
   b. olecranon process
   c. coronoid process
   d. trochlear notch
   e. radial notch
   f. tuberosity
   g. head
   h. styloid process

Joints and ligaments

1. Humeroulna : hinge between the trochlea of the humerus and semilunar (trochlear) notch of the ulna. Flexion and extension

2. Radiohumeral: disc-like head of radius and capitulum of humerus. Allows gliding movement in flexion and extension as well as rotation for supination and pronation.

3. Proximal radioulna: head of radius articulates with radial notch of the ulna allowing supination and pronation

4. Distal radioulna: head of ulna articulates with ulna notch of radius allowing for movement during supination and pronation

5. Radiocarpal: the wrist joint.

6. Intercarpal (IC): gliding joint of the carpals

7. Carpometacarpal (CM): saddle joint at thumb but other 4 joints gliding.

8. Intermetacarpal (IM): gliding joints

9. Metacarpalphalangeal (MP): the knuckles hinge joints allowing flexion, extension, adduction and abduction

10. Interphalangeal (IP) : the finger hinge joints

Carpal Tunnel

The carpal bones form a 'tunnel' which is bottomed by a retinaculum (ligament) running from the hook of hamate to the trapezium. Through this space runs the flexor tendons and median nerve which can all become impinged if the tunnel space becomes narrower.

Anterior View of right radius & ulna

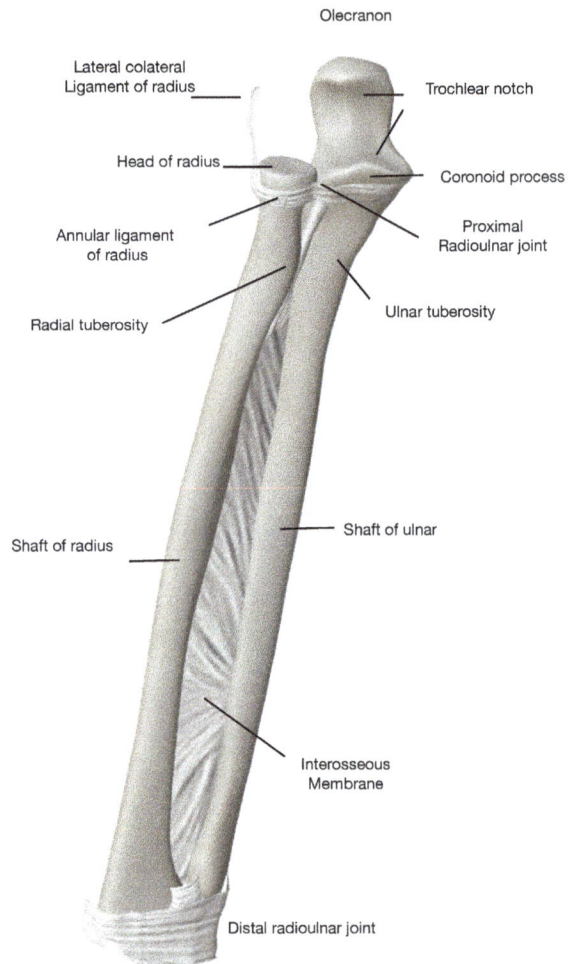

Olecranon

Lateral colateral
Ligament of radius

Trochlear notch

Head of radius

Coronoid process

Annular ligament
of radius

Proximal
Radioulnar joint

Radial tuberosity

Ulnar tuberosity

Shaft of ulnar

Shaft of radius

Interosseous
Membrane

Distal radioulnar joint

Right Hand Anterior View

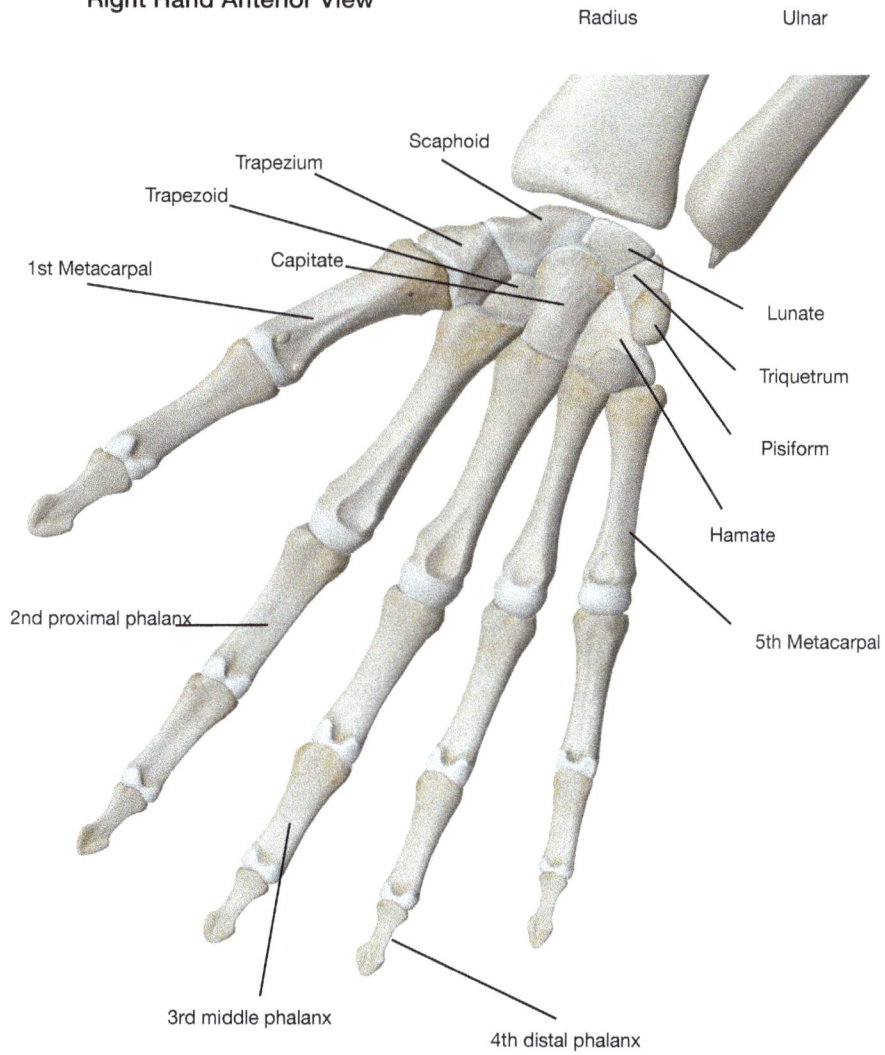

Radius

Ulnar

Scaphoid

Trapezium

Trapezoid

1st Metacarpal

Capitate

Lunate

Triquetrum

Pisiform

Hamate

2nd proximal phalanx

5th Metacarpal

3rd middle phalanx

4th distal phalanx

Muscles

1) Biceps Brachii (2 heads)

Attachments

supraglenoid tubercle of scapula above glenoid
fossa (long head)

coracoid process of scapula (short head)

radial tuberosity of radius

Action

flexion of elbow and supination of forearm (long
head)

Helps flex humerus at shoulder joint

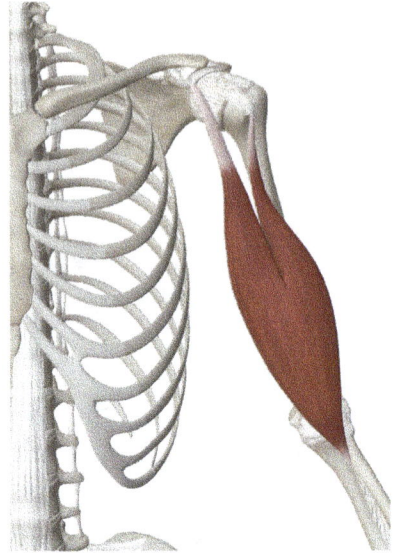

2) Triceps Brachii (3 heads)

Attachments

infraglenoid tubercle of posterior scapula (long
head)

middle shaft of posterior humerus (lateral head)

lower 2/3 of posterior shaft of humerus
(medial head)

olecranon process of ulna

Action

extends elbow, extends humerus,
assists adduction (long head)

extends elbow (lateral head)

extends elbow (medial head)

Note

the long head crosses 2 joints

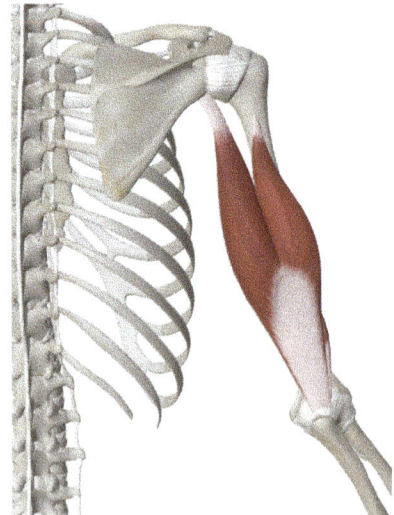

3) Brachialis
Attachments
distal half of anterior shaft of humerus
coronoid process and tuberosity of ulna
Action
main flexor of elbow

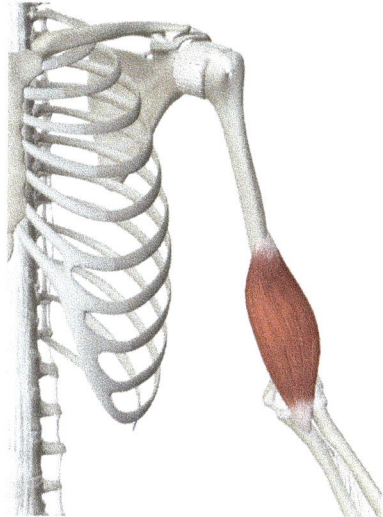

4) Anconeus
Attachments
posterior lateral epicondyle of humerus
olecranon process of ulna
Action
extension of ulna at elbow

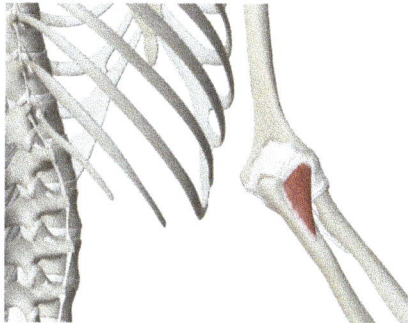

5) Brachioradialis
Attachments
lateral supracondylar ridge of humerus
styloid process of radius
Action
flexion of forearm
Extensors of Wrist & Hand

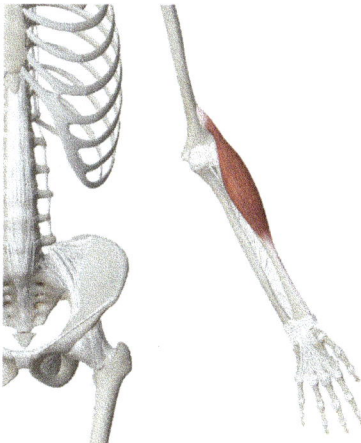

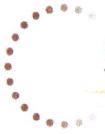

6) Extensor Carpi Radialis Longus and Brevis

Attachments

Lateral supracondylar ridge of humerus

Longus

Base of 2nd metacarpal

Brevis

Base of 3rd metacarpal

Action

Extend & abduct the wrist

Assist elbow flexion

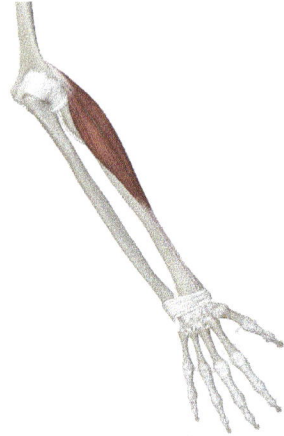

7) Extensor Carpi Ulnaris

Attachments

Lateral epicondyle of humerus

Base of 5th metacarpal

Action

Extend the wrist

Adduct the wrist

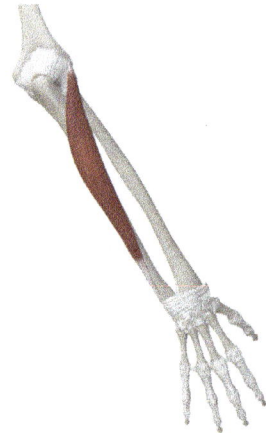

8) Extensor Digitorum

Attachments

Lateral epicondyle of humerus

Middle and distal phalanges of 2nd to 5th fingers.

Action

Extend 2nd - 5th fingers

Assist wrist extension.

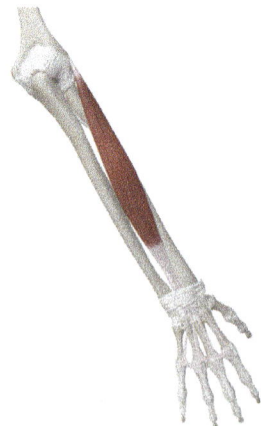

9) Extensor Indicis

Attachments

Posterior surface of distal shaft of ulna and interosseous membrane.

Tendon of extensor digitorum at level of 2nd metacarpal.

Action

Extend the 2nd finger

Assist adduction of 2nd finger

Note

Tension in these extensor muscles is a main cause of 'tennis elbow' and contributes to 'carpal tunnel' syndrome.

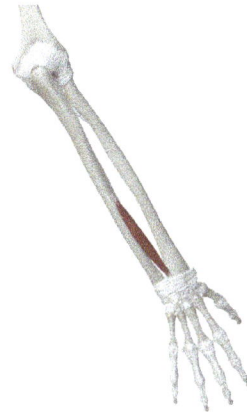

Forearm Flexors

10) Flexor Carpi Radialis

Attachments

Medial epicondyle of humerus

Base of 2nd and 3rd metacarpals

Action

Flex the wrist

Abduct the wrist

Flex the elbow

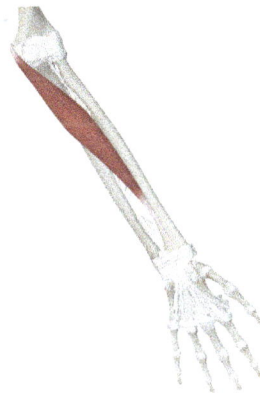

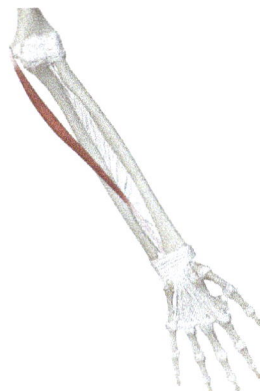

11) Palmaris Longus

Attachments

Medial epicondyle of humerus

Flexor retinaculum & palmar aponeurosis

Action

Tense the palmar fascia

Abduct the wrist

Flex the elbow

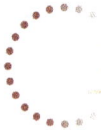

12) Flexor Carpi Ulnaris

Attachments

Humeral Head

Medial epicondyle of humerus

Ulnar Head

Posterior surface of proximal half of ulnar shaft.

Pisiform

Action

Flex the wrist

Adduct the wrist

Assist elbow flexion

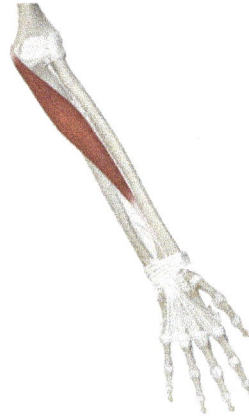

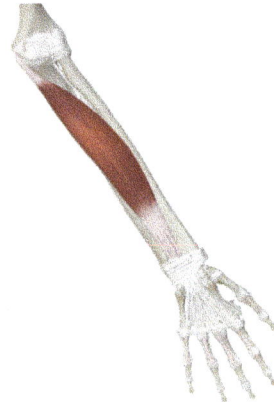

13) Flexor Digitorum Superficialis

Attachments

Medial epicondyle of humerus, ulna

collateral ligament, coronoid process of ulna

and shaft of radius.

Sides of middle phalanges of 2nd to 5th fingers.

Action

Flex the wrist

Adduct the wrist

Assist elbow flexion

14) Flexor Digitorum Profundus

Attachments

Anterior medial surface of proximal 3/4 ofulna

Base of distal phalanges on palmar surface of 2nd

to 5th fingers

Action

Flex 2nd to 5th fingers

Assists wrist flexion

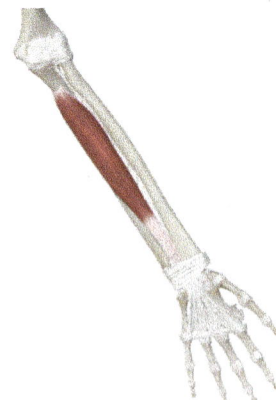

15) Supinator

Attachments

Posterior medial surface of proximal ulna

Wraps laterally around to anterior medial surface of proximal 1/3 of radius

Action

Supinates forearm

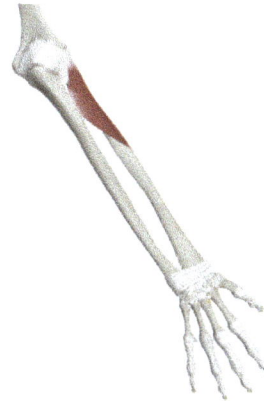

16) Pronator Teres

Attachments

Posterior medial epicondyle of humerus

Middle of lateral shaft of radius

Action

Pronation of forearm

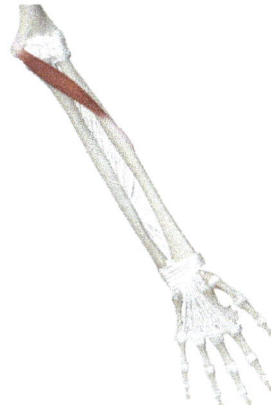

17) Pronator Quadratus

Attachments

Distal ¼ of anterior shaft of ulna

Distal ¼ of anterior shaft of radius

Action

Pronation of forearm

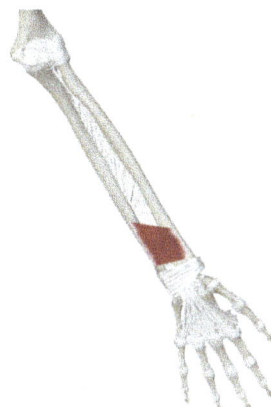

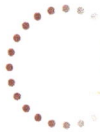

5.7 The Pelvis

Functions of the Pelvis

The strong and rigid pelvis is adapted to serve a number of roles in the human body. The main functions being:

Transfer of weight from the upper axial skeleton to the lower appendicular components of the skeleton, especially during movement.

Provides attachment for a number of muscles and ligaments used in locomotion.

Contains and protects the abdominopelvic and pelvic visera.

The Greater and Lesser Pelvis

The osteology of the pelvic girdle allows the pelvic region to be divided into :

- *The true pelvis*
- *The false pelvis*

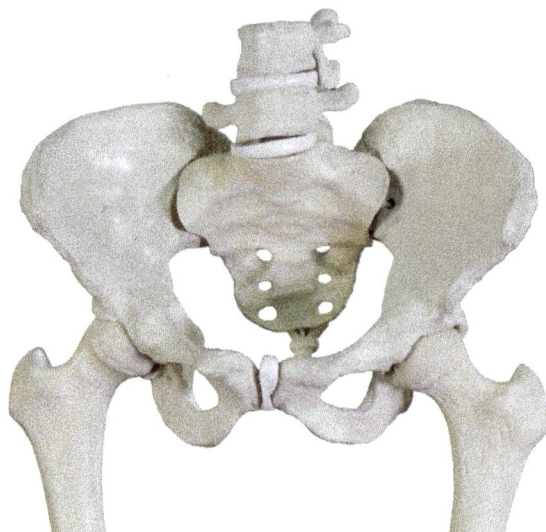

Pelvic Girdle

The pelvic girdle is a ring-like structure, located in the lower part of the trunk. It connects the axial skeleton to the lower limbs and consists of 2 innominate bones but does NOT include the sacrum. The bony pelvis however consists of the two hip bones (innominate or pelvic bones), sacrum and coccyx.

There are four articulations within the pelvis:

Sacroiliac Joints (x2) – Between the ilium of the hip bones, and the sacrum

Sacrococcygeal symphysis – Between the sacrum and the coccyx.

Pubic symphysis – Between the pubis bodies of the two hip bones.

Ligaments attach the lateral border of the sacrum to various bony landmarks on the bony pelvis to aid stability.

The superior portion of the pelvis is known as the greater pelvis (or false pelvis). It provides support for the lower abdominal viscera (ileum and sigmoid colon).

The inferior portion of the pelvis is known as the lesser pelvis (or "true" pelvis) within which resides the pelvic cavity and pelvic viscera.

The junction between the greater and lesser pelvis is known as the pelvic inlet. The outer bony edges of the pelvic inlet are called the pelvic brim.

Pelvic Inlet

The pelvic inlet marks the boundary between the greater pelvis and lesser pelvis. Its size is defined by its edge, the pelvic brim.

The borders of the pelvic inlet:

- *Posterior: The sacral promontory (the superior portion of the sacrum).*
- *Lateral: The arcuate line on the inner surface of the ilium, and the pectineal line on the superior ramus.*
- *Anterior: The pubic symphysis.*

The pelvic inlet determines the size and shape of the birth canal, with the prominent ridges key areas of muscle and ligament attachment.

Some alternative descriptive terminology can be used in describing the pelvic inlet:

- *Linea Terminalis – Refers to the combined pectineal line, arcuate line and sacral promontory.*
- *Iliopectineal line – Refers to the combined arcuate and pectineal lines.*

Pelvic Outlet

The pelvic outlet is located at the end of the lesser pelvis, and the beginning of the pelvic wall. Its borders are:

- *Posterior: The tip of the coccyx*
- *Lateral: The ischial tuberosities and the inferior margin of the sacrotuberous ligament*
- *Anterior: The pubic arch (the inferior border of the ischiopubic rami).*

The angle beneath the pubic arch is known as the sub-pubic angle and is of a greater size in women.

The Pelvis

Bones:

1. Coxal bone
Made from the fusion of 3 bones; ilium, ischium and pubis
  a. Ilium
    i. iliac crest
    ii. anterior superior iliac spine (ASIS)
    iii. anterior inferior iliac spine (AIIS)
    iv. posterior superior iliac spine (PSIS)
    v. posterior inferior iliac spine (PIIS)
    vi. greater sciatic notch
  b. Ischium
    i. ischial tuberosity (sitz bone)
    ii. ischial spine
    iii.lesser sciatic notch
    iv. ramus of ischium
  c. Pubis.
    i. pubic symphysis
    ii. pubic tubercle
    iii. superior ramus
    iv. inferior ramus
  d. Acetabulum
  e. Obturator foramen
2. Sacrum : five fused bones
  a. Base - the 'top'. Acts as a base for the spinal vertebrae
  b. Apex - articulates with the coccyx
  c. Auricular surface - the sides which articulate with the os coxa (sacroiliac joint)
3. Coccyx : 3 to 5 bones act as the insertion for major pelvic floor muscles
4. Femur
  a. head
  b. neck

c. greater trochanter

d. lesser trochanter

e. gluteal tuberosity

f. linea aspera

g. medial condyle

h. lateral condyle

i. medial epicondyle

j. lateral epicondyle

Pelvis Anterior View

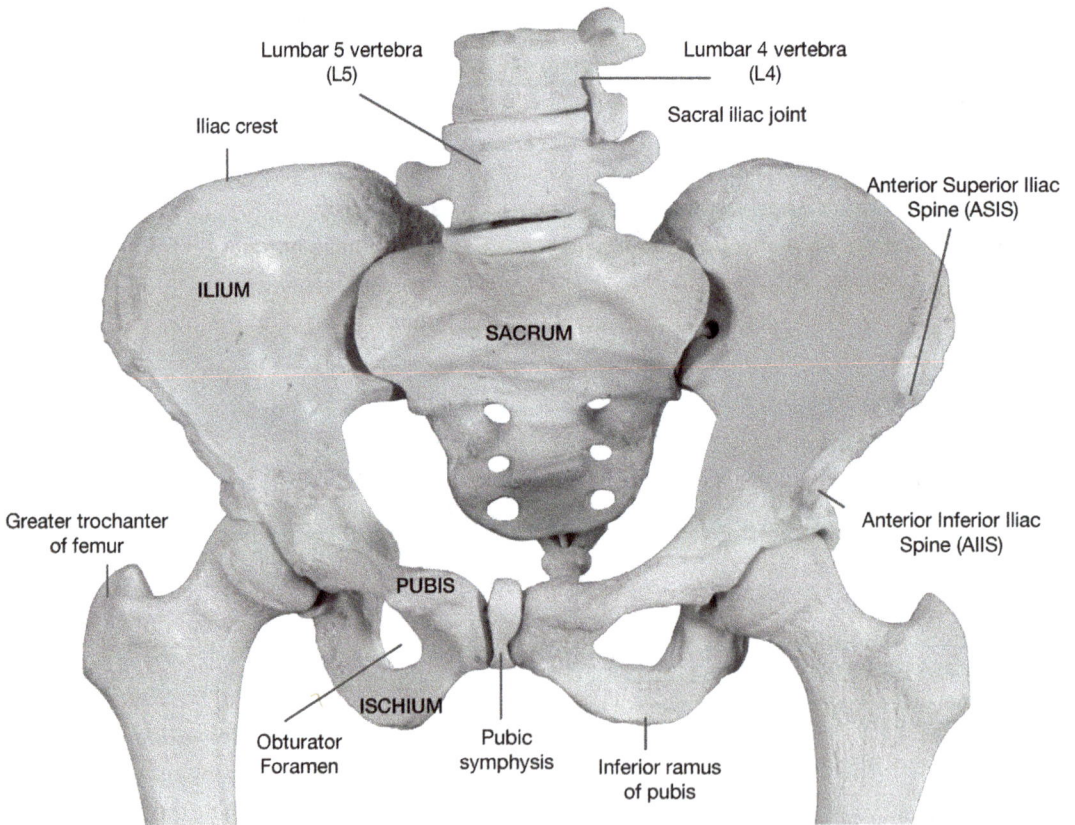

Lumbar 5 vertebra (L5)

Lumbar 4 vertebra (L4)

Iliac crest

Sacral iliac joint

Anterior Superior Iliac Spine (ASIS)

ILIUM

SACRUM

Greater trochanter of femur

Anterior Inferior Iliac Spine (AIIS)

PUBIS

ISCHIUM

Obturator Foramen

Pubic symphysis

Inferior ramus of pubis

Pelvis Posterior View

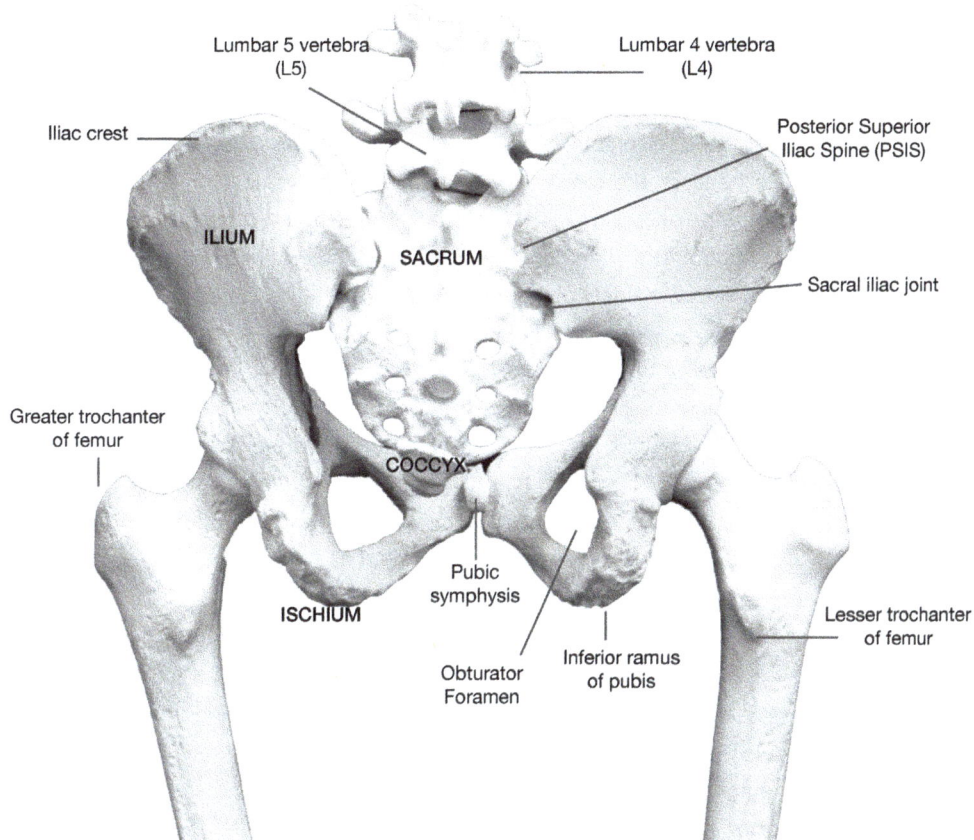

Lumbar 5 vertebra (L5)

Lumbar 4 vertebra (L4)

Iliac crest

Posterior Superior Iliac Spine (PSIS)

ILIUM

SACRUM

Sacral iliac joint

Greater trochanter of femur

COCCYX

Pubic symphysis

ISCHIUM

Lesser trochanter of femur

Obturator Foramen

Inferior ramus of pubis

Note. The pelvis is divided into two sections of :
a. Greater or 'false' pelvis - the superior 'bowl'
b. Lesser or 'true' pelvis - the inferior 'bowl'
The Pelvic Brim or Linea Terminalis is the dividing line between the 2 sections.

The superior aperture of the pelvic brim is oval in females but heart shaped in males

Joints and Ligaments

1. Pubic Symphysis : slightly moveable joint with a fibrocartilaginous disc between the two articulating pubic bones.

2. Sacroilliac Joint (SI joint) : 2 joints joining the ilium and sacrum and important for being able to transfer loads between the axial and appendicular skeleton. Lack of good 'form' and/or 'force' closure of these joints greatly contributes to low back pain.

3. Hip joint : ball and socket with head of femur held in acetabular socket from 3 main ligaments of pubofemoral, ischiofemural and iliofemural.

4. Sacrotuberous ligament : from ischial tuberosity to lateral border of sacrum blending in with the fibres of other sacral ligaments.

5. Sacrospinous Ligament : runs from iscial spine to sacrum and resists posterosuperior movements of sacrum

6. Iliofemoral, pubofemoral and ischiofemoral Ligaments : twist around the head of the femur to resists extension of femur but relax on flexion.

7. Sacroiliac Ligaments : numerous ligaments running on the anterior and posterior sides of the ilium and sacrum.

8. Iliolumbar Ligaments : from TP's of L5 to crest of ilium and extremely strong causing L5 to function more like an extension of sacrum. Possibly consisting of more muscle fibres when young.

9. Inguinal Ligament : from ASIS to pubis and forms a tube through which the spermatic cord runs in men.

Muscles & Fascia

The muscles and fascia of the pelvis form the pelvic floor in the pelvic outlet and the pelvic wall. The region directly below the pelvic floor within the pelvic outlet is known as the perineum with it's base being skin and fascia and the roof being the pelvic floor. Looking up at the perineum superiorly it can be seen to be diamond shaped with the four corners being the pubic bone (top), coccyx (bottom) and the 2 ischial tuberosities (left and right).

The pelvic floor (pelvic diaphragm) muscles are made up of

1. Levator Ani : (consists of)
• Pubococcygeus - runs from pubis to the coccyx
• Illiococcygeus - runs from the ilium to the coccyx
• puborectalis, Illiosacralis, puboanalis, pubovaginalis (female), levator prostate (male)
Coccygeus - (wag the tail muscle) from ischial spine

to coccyx (NOT part of levator ani)

2. The pelvic wall consists of :
Sacrotuberous ligament
Sacrospinous ligament
Tendonous arch (obturator Internus muscle) – tendonous thick fascia on the medial surface of the wall where pubococcygeus and iliococcygeus muscles attach.
Piriformis muscle - forms part of the posterior portion of the muscular bowl of the internal pelvis
Iliacus muscle - fills the sides of the pelvic bowl

3. Perineum
The diamond shaped boundaries of the perineum are the pubic symphysis, ishiopubic ramus, ischial tuberosity (sitz bone) and sacrotuberous ligament.
The perineum is divided into two triangles bisected by a 'line' between the 2 ischial tuberosities. These are known as the urogenital and anal triangles.

4. Urogenital Triangle
This contains the urethra, penis and scrotum in males and the urethra, clitoris and vagina in females. It also includes the urogenital diaphragm composed of the deep transverse perineal muscle and superficial perineal space containing the ischiocavernosus and bulbospongiosus muscles. These muscles aid in the erection of the penis and clitoris.
The Superficial Transverse Perineal muscles stabilize the perineal body and act as a form of divisional line between the Urogenital and Anal Triangle.

5. Anal Triangle
This consists of the levator ani muscle, anus, ischiorectal fossa and the external sphincter ani muscle which is secured posteriorly by the anococcygeal ligament.

6. Fascia lata : fascia of the thigh which lies under the superficial fascia and wraps all around the outside of the thigh.

7. Iliotibial tract (ITT) or band (ITB) : a thickening of fascia lata and runs along lateral aspect of thigh from crest of ilium to tibia. A major culprit in knee pathologies.

8. Femoral Triangle : bordered by Sartorius, Adductor Longus and Inguinal Ligament. Pectineus and Iliopsoas lie deep in the triangle

Functional Movements of the Pelvic Bones & Pelvic Floor

The Pubic Symphysis and Sacral Iliac joints of both innominate bones make 4 joints of the pelvis and operate in a closed chain – that is; if a movement occurs at one joint then movement must occur or is effected at all other 3 joints.

The sacrum is attached to the coccyx which is also a joint which causes a change in tension of the pelvic floor muscles when the coccyx moves.

When the ischial tuberosities come together the ASIS's move apart

The Pelvic Floor Muscles - Viewed from Below

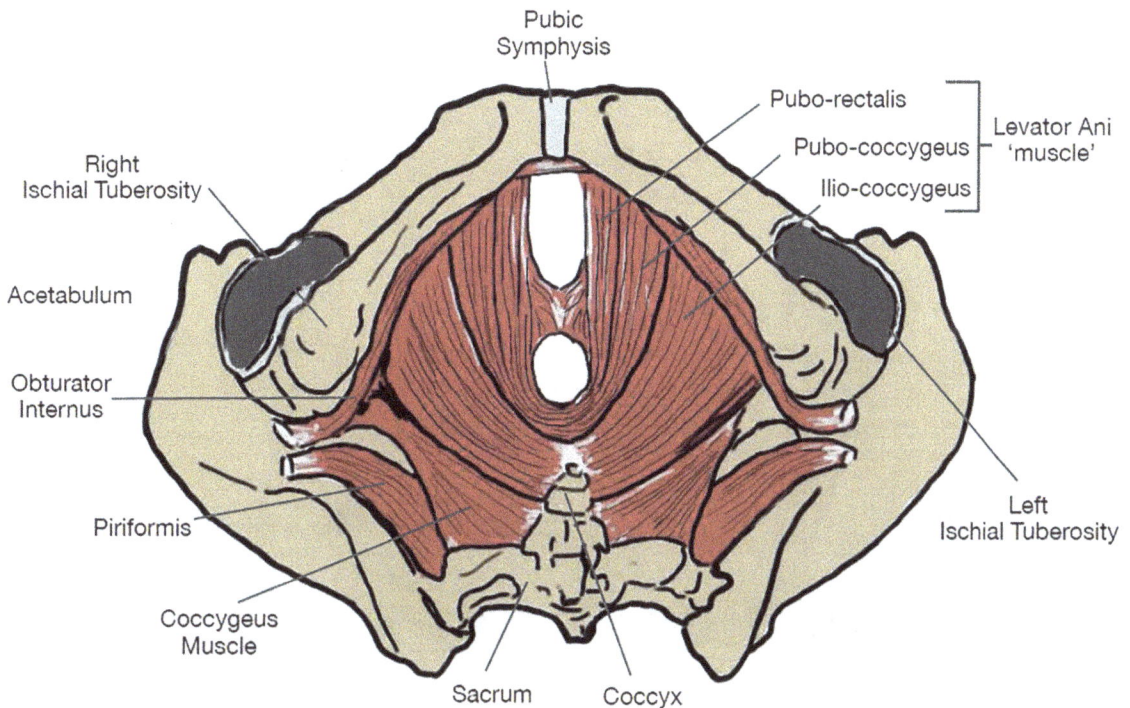

When the ischial tuberosities move apart the ASIS's come together

Straightening the legs promotes the ischial tuberosities to come together

Bending the legs helps promote the ischial tuberosities to move apart

Whilst bending the knees:

The sacrum nutates

Ischial tuberosities move apart

ASIS's move towards each other

When straightening the legs:

The sacrum counter nutates

Ischial tuberosities move towards each other

ASIS's move apart

• Anterior rotation of the right innominate bone produces spinal rotation left

• Anterior rotation of left innominate bone promotes spinal rotation right

Cross Section of Right Thigh - Viewed from Above

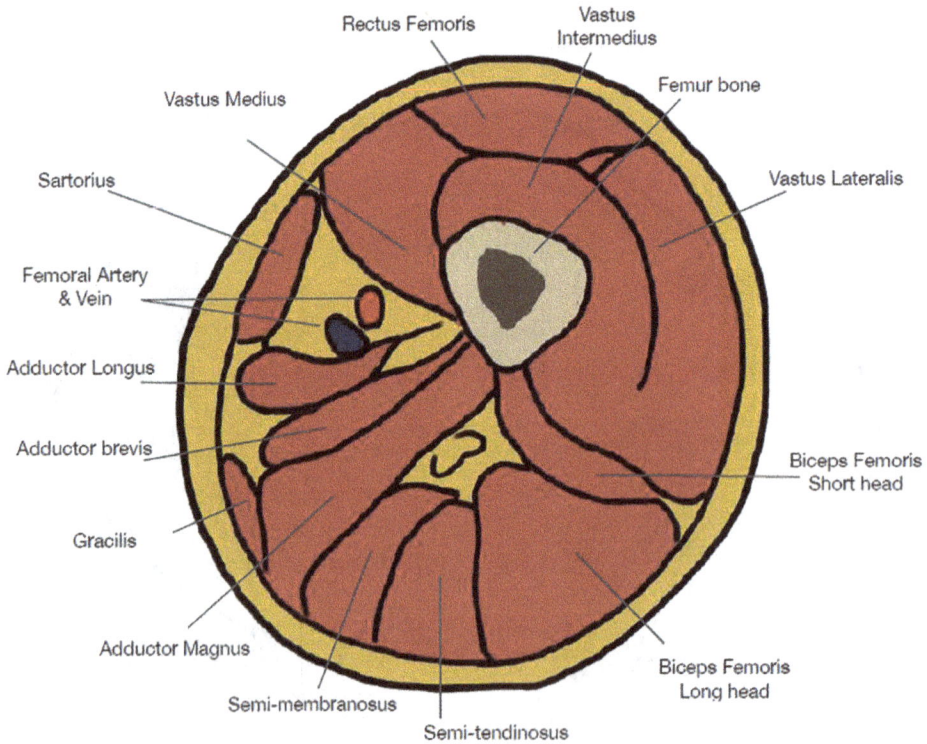

Rectus Femoris

Vastus Intermedius

Vastus Medius

Femur bone

Sartorius

Vastus Lateralis

Femoral Artery & Vein

Adductor Longus

Adductor brevis

Biceps Femoris Short head

Gracilis

Adductor Magnus

Biceps Femoris Long head

Semi-membranosus

Semi-tendinosus

1) Tensor Fascia Lata

Attachments

iliac crest just posterior to ASIS

into the ITB which continues to lateral condyle of tibia

Action

flexion, medial rotation and abduction of femur.
Stabilizes extended knee when walking.

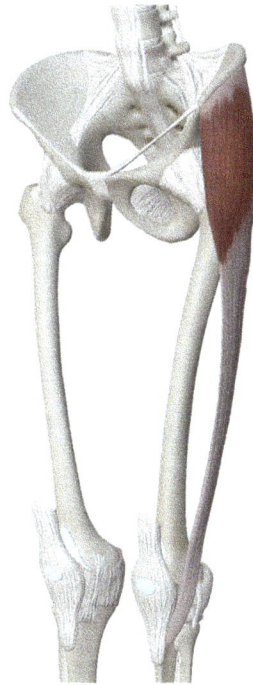

2) Gluteus Maximus

Attachments

PSIS and down lateral aspect of sacrum onto sacrotuberous ligament

ITB and gluteal tuberosity of femur

Action

extends femur at hip Lateral rotation of extended hip joint, assists in abduction of hip whilst deep fibers (gluteal tuberosity) assist in adduction.

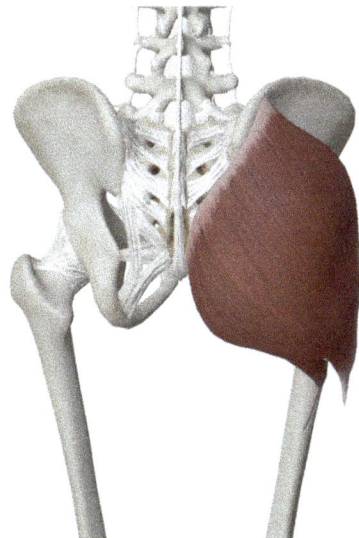

3) Gluteus Medius

Attachments

outer surface of ilium just below crest

lateral surface of greater trochanter

Action

abduction and medial rotation of femur

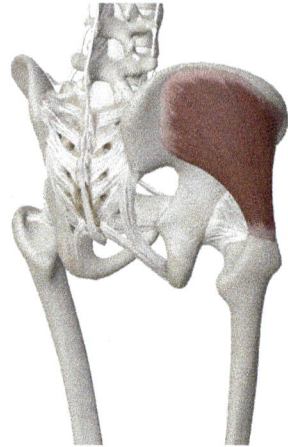

4) Gluteus Minimus

Attachments

outer surface of ilium just under crest

(under gluteus medius)

anterior surface of greater trochanter

Action

abduction and medial rotation of femur

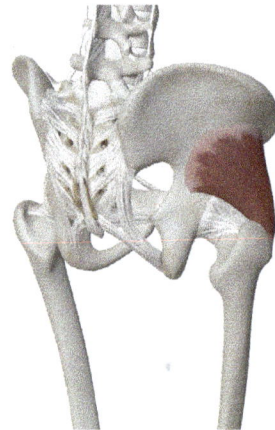

5) Piriformis

Attachments

anterior surface of sacrum

superior medial aspect of greater trochanter

Action

lateral rotation of femur

Note

one of the six deep lateral external rotators but only
one that attaches to sacrum. May be responsible
for sciatic pain due to 'pinching' the nerve

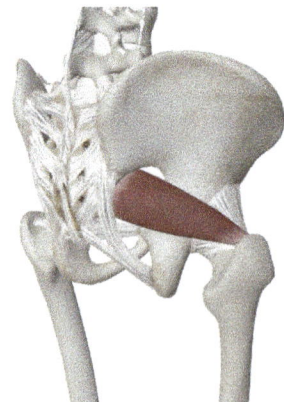

6) Gemellus Superior
Attachments
ischial spine
posterior surface of greater trochanter
Action
lateral rotation of femur

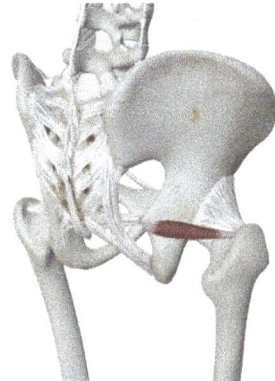

7) Obturator Internus
Attachments
covers the medial surface of obturator
foramen and runs posteriorly around the ischium in
the lesser sciatic notch.
posterior surface of greater trochanter
Action
lateral rotation of femur

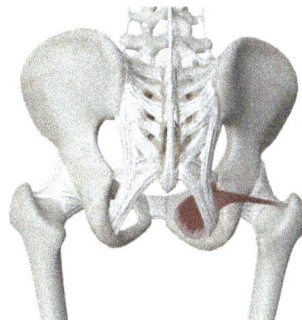

8) Gemellus Inferior
Attachments
superior border of ischial tuberosity
posterior surface of greater trochanter
Action
lateral rotation of femur

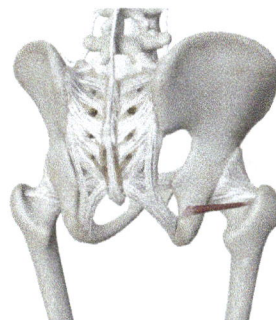

9) Obturator Externus
Attachments
lateral surface of obturator foramen
posterior surface of greater trochanter
Action
lateral rotation of femur

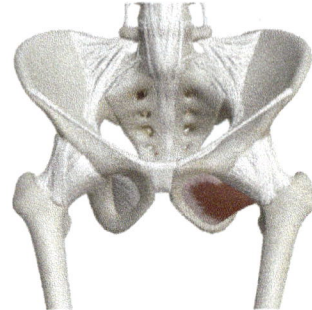

10) Quadratus Femoris
Attachments
ischial tuberosity
most inferior attachment of posterior surface of
greater trochanter
Action
lateral rotation of femur
Note
Piriformis, Gemellus Superior, Obturator
Internus, Gemellus Inferior, Obturator
Externus and Quadratus Femoris are
collectively known as the '6 deep hip rotators'

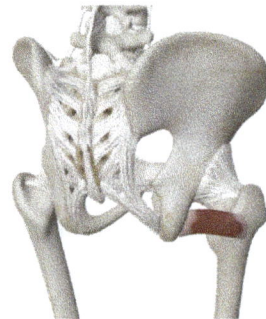

11) Sartorius
Attachments
ASIS
anterior medial surface of tibia via pes anserinus
Action
assists in flexion, abduction and lateral
rotation of femur as well as flexion and media
rotation of tibia
Note
(pes anserinus common tendon to Sartorius,
Gracilis and semitendinosus) longest muscle in body

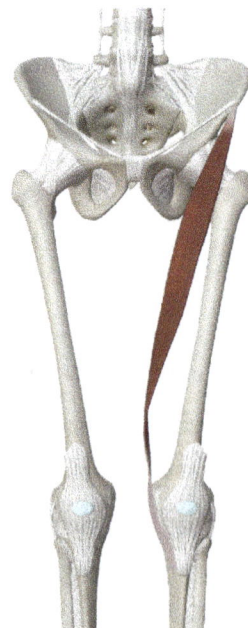

12) Rectus Femoris

Attachments

AIIS

tibial tuberosity via patella tendon

Action

extends knee, helps flex femur

Note

only one of the 4 quads which crosses hip joint

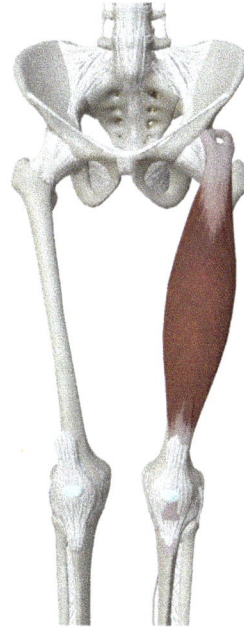

13) Vastus Intermedius

Attachments

anterior surface of proximal femur

tibial tuberosity via patella tendon

Action

extends tibia at knee

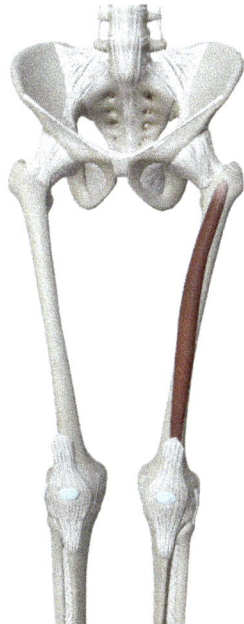

14) Vastus Lateralis

Attachments

lateral lip of linea aspera, gluteal tuberosity

tibial tuberosity via patella tendon

Action

extends knee

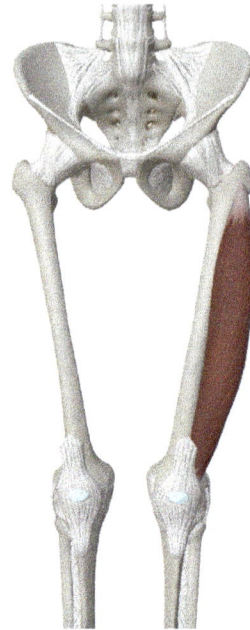

15) Vastus Medialis

Attachments

medial lip of linea aspera

tibial tuberosity via patella tendon

Action

extends knee

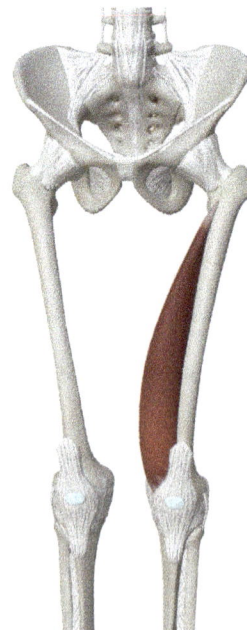

16) Pectineus
Attachments
anterior surface of superior pubic ramus
between lesser trochanter and linea aspera on
posterior femur
Action
adduction and flexion of femur. Assists
external rotation

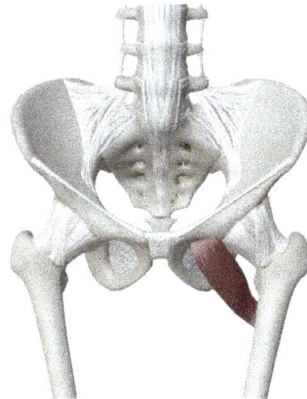

17) Adductor Longus
Attachments
pubic tubercle
middle third of linea aspera
Action
adduction of femur and assists in
flexion and medial rotation

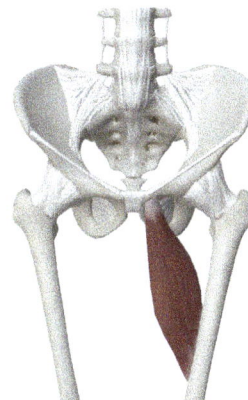

18) Adductor Brevis
Attachments
anterior surface of inferior surface of pubis just
below adductor longus
linea aspera just above adductor longus
Action
adduction of femur and assists in flexion and
medial rotation

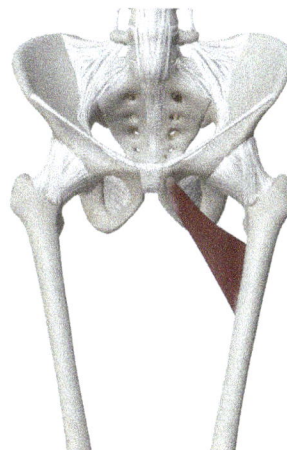

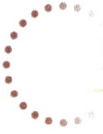

19) Adductor Magnus

Attachments

length of inferior pubic ramus to ischial
tuberosity

anterior portion : entire length of linea aspera

posterior portio: adductor tubercle of femur

Action

adduction and medial rotation of femur,
assists hip flexion and extension.

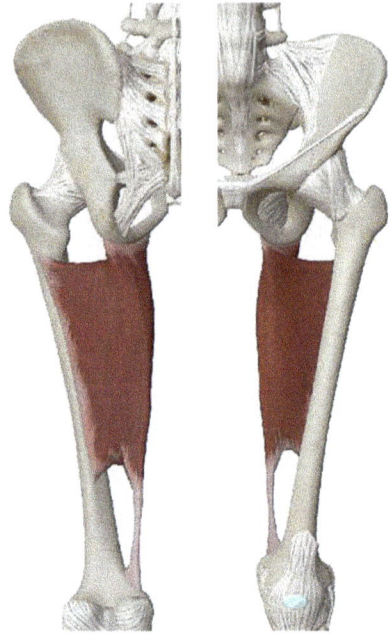

20) Gracilis

Attachments

medial margin of inferior ramus of pubis

anterior medial surface of tibia via pes anserinus

Action

adduction of femur and assists in flexion and
medial rotation of flexed knee

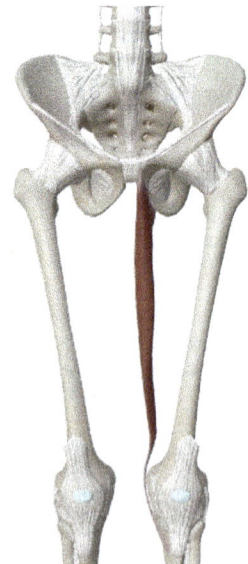

21) Biceps Femoris
Attachments
Long head - ischial tuberosity
Short head - middle portion of linea aspera of
femur
head of fibula
Action
flexion of tibia at knee, extension of femur at hip,
lateral rotation of tibia with bent knee

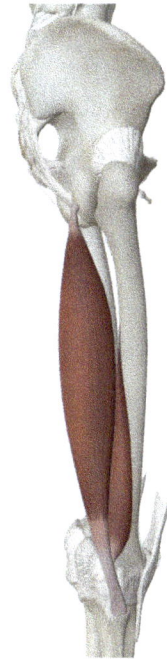

22) Semimembranosus
Attachments
ischial tuberosity
posterior medial tibial condyle
Action
flexion of tibia at knee, extension of femur at hip,
medial rotation of tibia with bent knee

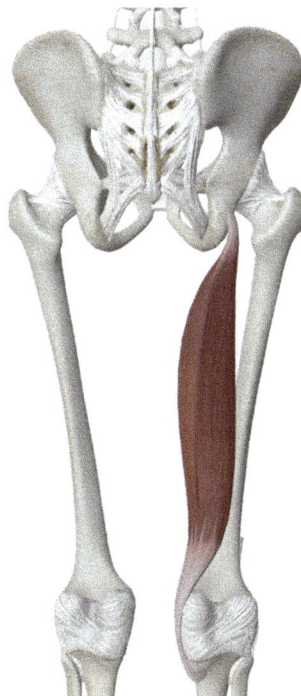

23) Semitendinosus

Attachments

ischial tuberosity

anterior medial surface of tibia via pes

anserinus

Action

flexion of tibia at knee, extension of femur at hip,

medial rotation of tibia with bent knee

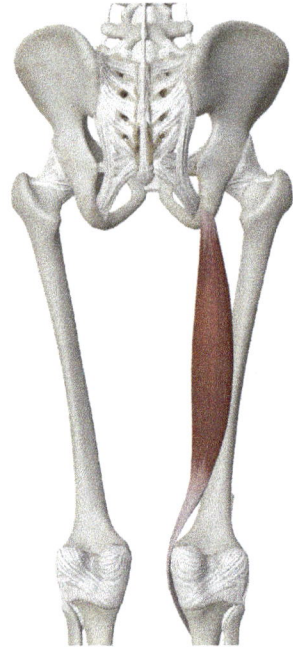

Hip Flexor Group

24) Psoas Major

Attachments

anterior surfaces of TP's and bodies of the lumbar

vertebrae lesser trochanter of femur

Action

flexion of femur and assists in adduction (assists

medial or lateral rotation of femur)

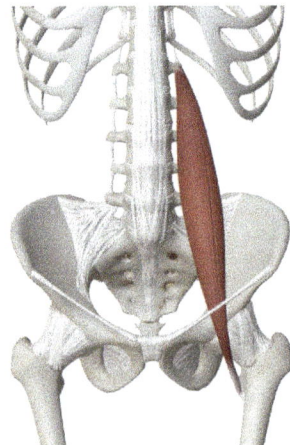

25) Psoas Minor

Attachments

body and transverse process of first lumbar vertebra

superior ramus of pubis

Action

assist lordotic curvature in lumbar spine.

Note

Present in approx 40% of population

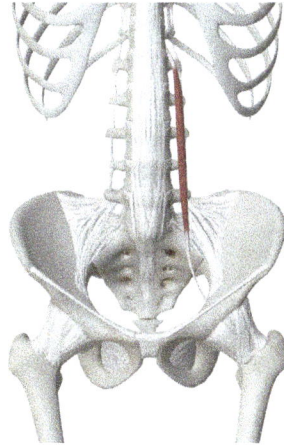

26) Iliacus

Attachments

inner surface of ilium

lesser trochanter of femur

flexion of femur and assists in adduction

(assists medial or lateral rotation of femur)

Note

Rectus Femoris is also a 'hip flexor' and often over used

Tension and shortening of the Psoas Major muscle is a major contribution to many back problems

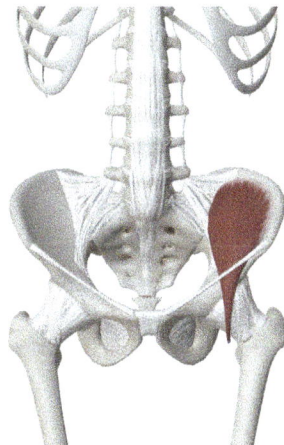

5.8 Ribcage & Abdomen

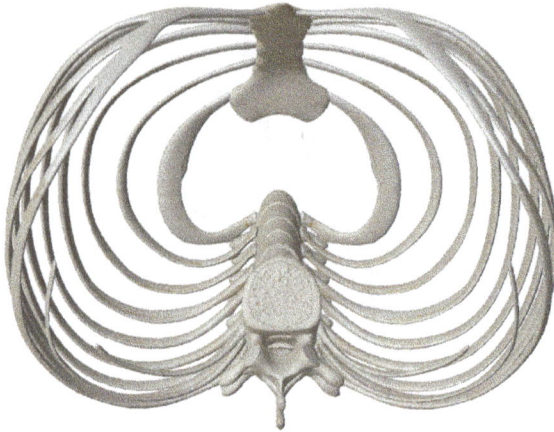

Bones:

1) Sternum
a. Manubrium (latin for handle of sword)
i) Upper portion
ii) Clavicular notches (sternoclavicular joint)
iii) Jugular notch
b. Body
sternal angle (angle of louis) - attachment for 2nd rib
c. Xiphoid process
inferior portion at bottom

2) Ribs
a. Head - vertebral end
b. Body –
i) main shaft of rib
ii) costal angle where rib is bent
iii) tubercle - lateral to head articulates with TP's of thoracic vertebrae
c. Costal cartilage - connects the rib to the sternum
3) Thoracic (rib) cage
a. includes ribs, thoracic vertebrae, sternum and

costal cartilages
b. first 7 pairs called True Ribs
c. remaining 5 pairs called False Ribs
d. last 2 pairs called Floating ribs - no costal attachment

4) Thoracic inlet
a. opening at top of rib cage also called Thoracic Outlet
b. functionally includes; clavicle, scalene muscles, hyoid muscles, brachial plexus, brachiocephalic arteries, esophagus and trachea
c. many 'carpal tunnel' problems are actually thoracic outlet problems

Joints and Ligaments

1) Ribs 2-9 each have 3 articulations in the back; the tubercle with the TP of its vertebra and the head with the demifacets of its vertebra and the vertebra above. This arrangement reduces the amount of spinal rotation between T2-T9.
2) Ribs 1, 10, 11 and 12 have 2 attachments ; the tubercle with TP of its vertebra and the head with its vertebra.
3) The sternum is attached to the spine via a wall of connective tissue attaching to the ALL
4) Scapulothoracic (ST) joint - is not a true joint as such but is the myofascial attachment of where the scapula articulates around the ribcage in the upper back.

The Ribcage

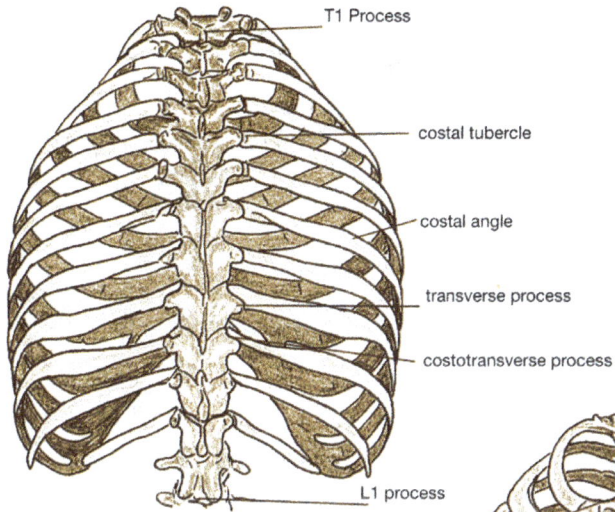

T1 Process

costal tubercle

costal angle

transverse process

costotransverse process

L1 process

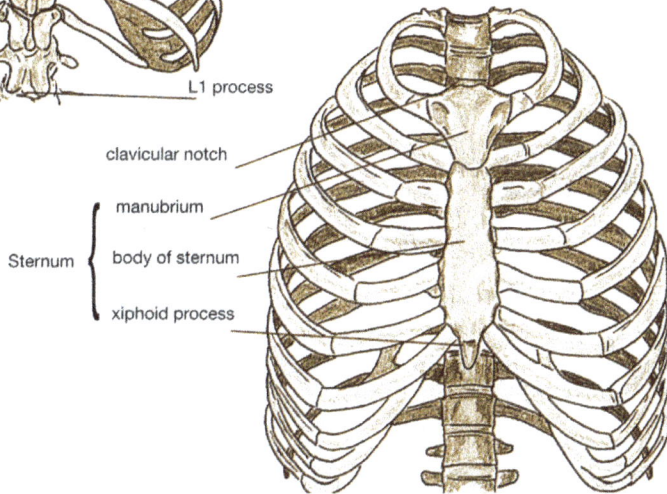

clavicular notch

manubrium

body of sternum

xiphoid process

Sternum

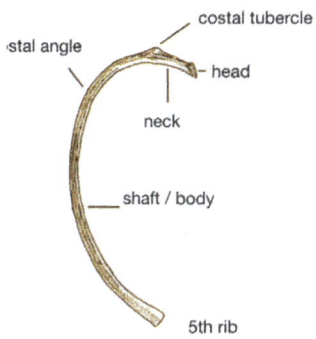

costal tubercle

stal angle

head

neck

shaft / body

5th rib

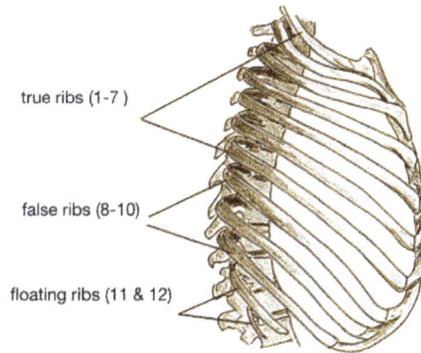

true ribs (1-7)

false ribs (8-10)

floating ribs (11 & 12)

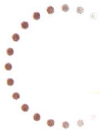

Abdominal Cross Section - Viewed from Above

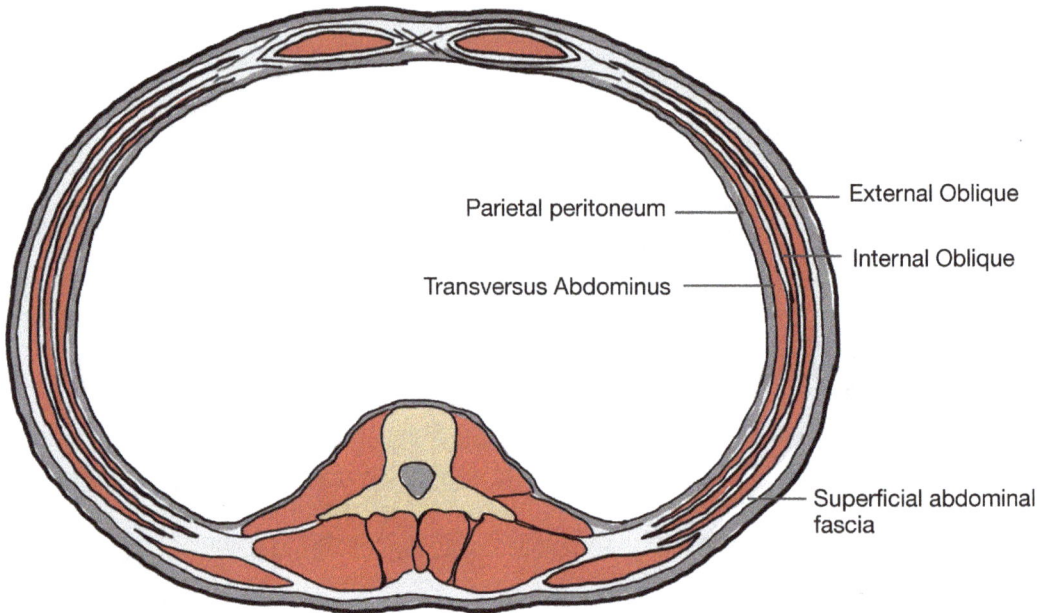

Parietal peritoneum ———————

Transversus Abdominus ———————

——— External Oblique

— Internal Oblique

—— Superficial abdominal fascia

Muscles (and fascia)

1) Abdominal Aponeurosis

   a. thick sheet of tendon covering the
whole of the abdominal wall.
At the bottom it is rolled up to form the
inguinal ligament

   b. composed of connective tissue of 3
abdominal muscles

   c. Linea Alba - vertical thickening of the
aponeurosis which runs from xiphoid
process to the pubic symphysis.

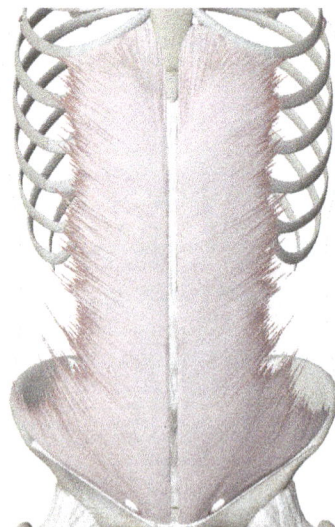

2) External Oblique

Attachments

outside surface of lowest 8 ribs and
interdigitate with serratus anterior and
latissmus dorsi

anterior iliac and abdominal aponeurosis to
linea alba

Action

bilaterally - flexion of trunk and compression
of abdominal contents

unilaterally - lateral flexion and contralateral
rotation of trunk.

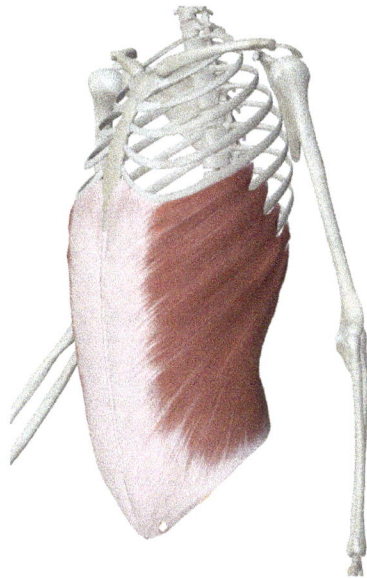

3) Internal Oblique

Attachments

lateral inguinal ligament, iliac crest and
thoracolumbar fascia

costal cartilages of lowest 4 ribs and
abdominal aponeurosis to linea alba

Action

bilaterally - flexion of trunk and compression
of abdominal contents

unilaterally - ipsilateral rotation of trunk

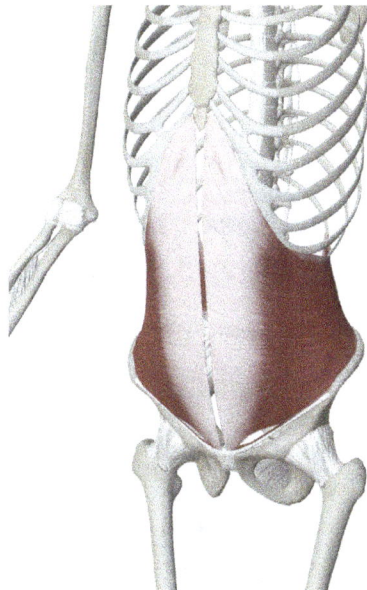

4) Transverse Abdominis

Attachments

lateral inguinal ligament, iliac crest,
thoracolumbar aponeurosis and lower margin of
rib cage (interdigitates with diaphragm).
abdominal aponeurosis to linea alba

Action

compression of abdominal contents

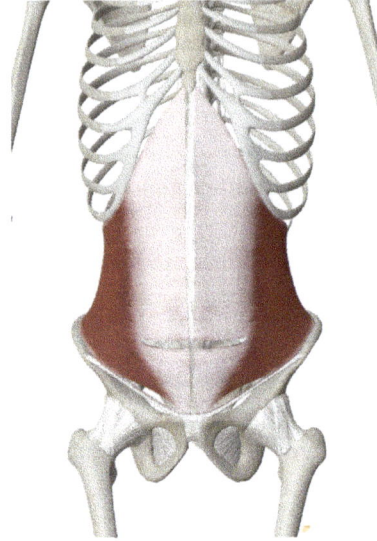

5) Rectus Abdominis

Attachments

crest of pubis and pubic symphysis
xiphoid process and costal cartilages of ribs 5,
6, and 7

Action

flexion of vertebral column and compression of
abdominal Contents

Note

important muscle to stabilize and the spine in
extension.

Intercostal Muscles: run between adjacent ribs

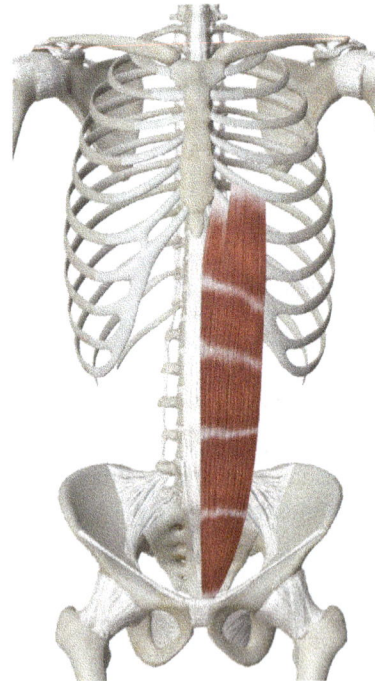

6) External Intercostals
   a. outermost set
   b. fibers run same direction as external oblique
   c. elevates ribs

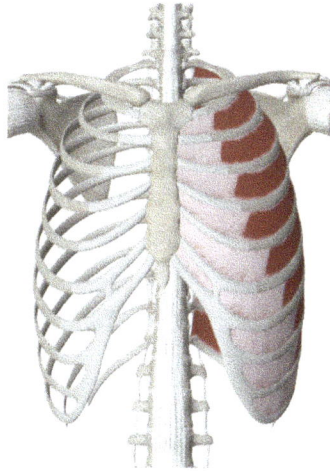

7) Internal Intercostals
   a. middle layer
   b. fibers run in line with internal oblique
   c. depresses ribs

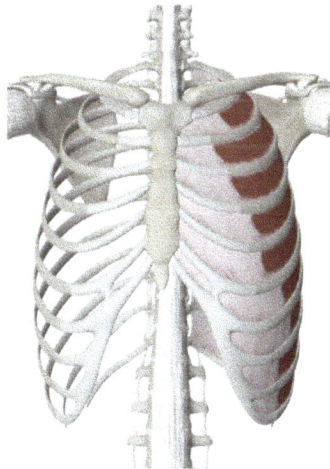

8) Innermost Intercostals
   a. deepest layer
   b. actually 3 sets of muscles
      i) Transversus thoracis -
         attaches to sternum and goes
         up to ribs 2-6 shaped like fan.
         Helps depress costal cartilages
         in expiration
      ii) Intercostals intimi - underneath
          main rib body aids in depressing ribs
      iii) Subcostalis - underneath rib angle
           also aids in depressing ribs.

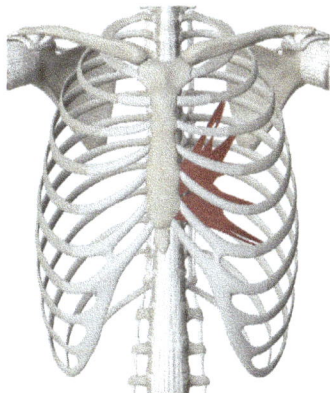

9) Respiratory Diaphragm

Attachments

costal arch, xiphoid process, anterior bodies of
upper 3 lumbar vertebra and ribs 11 and 12
central tendon of diaphragm.

Action

flattens central tendon thereby increasing the
volume of thoracic cavityinspiration. Primary
muscle for inspiration

Note

separates abdominal and thoracic cavity
Important spinal stabilizer

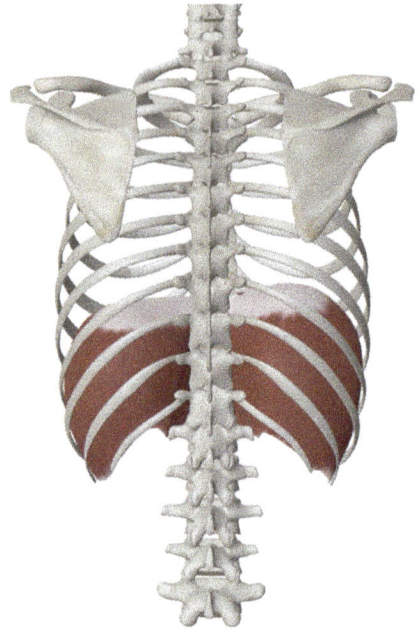

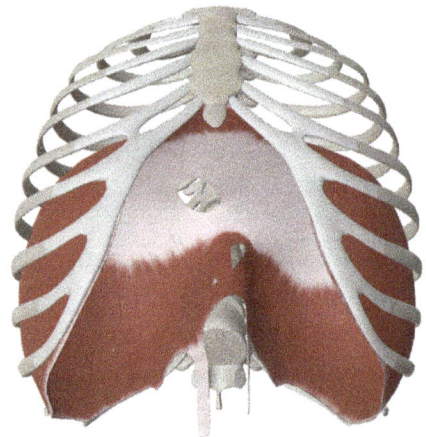

10) Serratus Posterior Superior

Attachments

spinous processes of C7 and T1 - T5

ribs 2 to 5

Action

elevation of ribs - aids respiration

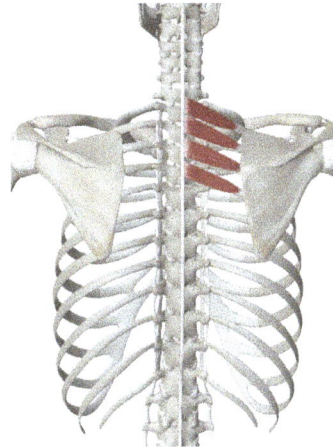

11) Serratus Posterior Inferior

Attachments

spinous processes T11 - L5

ribs 9 to 12

Action

depression of ribs - aids respiration

Note

Serratus posterior superior and inferior may
both be seen to be a retinaculae of the erector
spinae

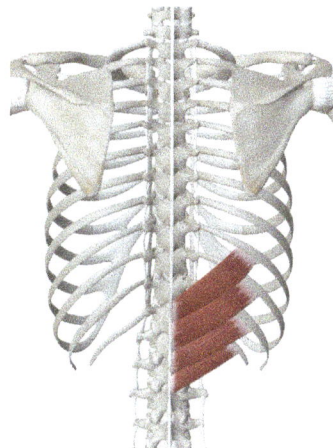

12) Levatores costales

Attachments

TP's of C7 to T11

rib directly below (brevis) or two below (longus)

Action

possible elevation of ribs in inspiration and/or
contralateral rotation and lateral flexion of spine.

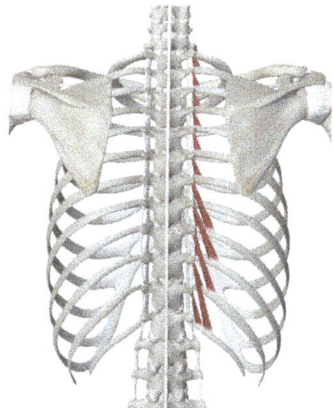

5.9 The Spinal Column

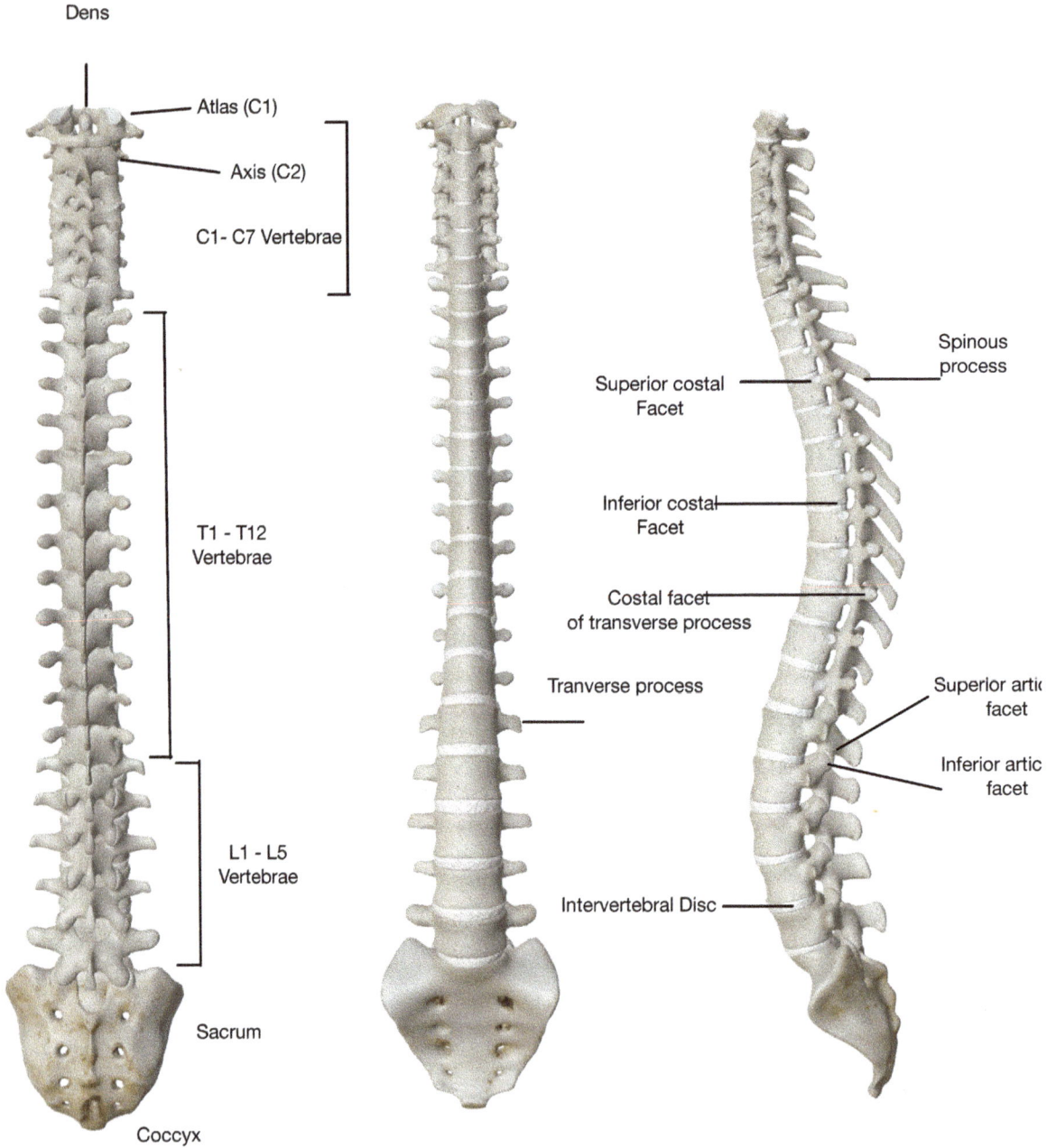

Dens

Atlas (C1)

Axis (C2)

C1- C7 Vertebrae

T1 - T12
Vertebrae

L1 - L5
Vertebrae

Sacrum

Coccyx

Spinous
process

Superior costal
Facet

Inferior costal
Facet

Costal facet
of transverse process

Tranverse process

Superior artic
facet

Inferior artic
facet

Intervertebral Disc

Bones:

1. Cervical vertebrae (7): C1 to C7. Short spinous processes allow good range of movement in extension whilst the transverse processes limit sidebending. C1 to C7 has a foramen in the each TP's to allow the passage of the vertebral artery and vein.

C1 is known as the Atlas
C2 is known as the Axis

Flexion / extension of the skull is primarily through skull articulating with the atlas (O/A joint)
Rotation of the skull is achieved through the rotation of the atlas on the axis (A/A joint)
2. Thoracic vertebrae (12) : names T1 to T12. Each vertebra has a pair of ribs attached to it. Allows for rotation, flexion, extension and side bending however the SP's are long and run inferiorly to limit extension
Lumbar vertebrae (5) : named L1 to L5 the largest to support overlying weight and allow for flexion, extension and sidebending whilst limiting rotation.

The Vertebrae

1. Body: main rounded section stacked on intervertebral discs
2. Vertebral / Neural Arch: posterior to the body where the processes are attached
3. Vertebral Foramen : formed by the body and arch of the vertebra and where the spinal cord runs.
4. Spinous Process (SP): 'sticky out thing' on the back of the vertebra
5. Transverse Process (TP); 'sticky out thing' on the sides of the vertebra
6. Transverse Foramen : only on the cervical vertebrae where the vertebral artery and vein passes.

7. Lamina: space or groove between the TPs and SP. The paravertebral muscles run through here.
8. Vertebral notch - archway in the pedicle where the spinal nerves run.
The intervertebral foramen is formed by the superior and inferior notches
9. Pedicle: the junction of the Vertebral Arch and Body
10. Articular Facet: processes with flat surfaces to articulate with adjacent vertebrae.Each vertebra has 2 pairs - superior and inferior
Demifacets - found in the thoracic vertebrae only to articulate with ribs.
11. Intervertebral Disc: shock absorber between superior and inferior body of vertebrae.

• *Annulus Fibrosis - the fibrocartilaginous outer ring, (dough of the doughnut)*
• *Nucleus Pulposus - the 'pulpy' centre (jam of the doughnut)*

Compressive forces on the discs make us shorter at the end of the day than in the morning.

Spinal Curve

1. Primary curve – Kyphosis
a. kyphosis is a curve which is convex posteriorly
b. curve of the spine a baby has in the uterus
c. thoracic and sacral curve

2. Secondary curve – Lordosis
  a. curve which is concave posteriorly
  b. is formed after birth
  c. cervical curve is formed when baby starts lifting its head and the lumbar curve when the baby starts crawling and walking.

3. Scoliosis

a. sideways curving of the spine

b. always involves spinal rotation

c. if in the thoracic region there will be some rib rotation

Joints and Ligaments

1. Supraspinous Ligament - Connects posterior ends of SP's of the thoracic and lumbar vertebrae. Resists flexion

2. Interspinous Ligaments - Connect adjacent SP's of the thoracic and lumbar vertebrae filling in the space. Resists flexion.

3. Nuchal Liagament - The 'Sail Ligament' is extension of interspinous and supraspinous ligaments from C7 up to base of occiput.

4. Intertransverse Ligaments - Connect adjacent TP's. Resist lateral flexion (sidebending) to opposite side

5. Anterior Longitudal Ligament (ALL) - Runs entire length of the anterior surface of vertebrae bodies from occiput to sacrum

6. Posterior Longitudal Ligament (PLL) - Runs length of posterior surface of vertebrae bodies inside the vertebral foramen. Firmly attached to intervertebral discs and narrows as it gets down to the lumbar area making the lumbar area more prone to herniations

7. Ligament Flavum
'Yellow Ligament' , connects the lamina of contiguous vertebrae

The Neck

Bones

1) Cervical vertebra

a. C1 or Atlas

Has no body - is all arch

has a small spinous process called the spinous tubercle

b. C2 or Axis

The dens of axis protrudes upwards to articulate with C1

Dens acts as body of C1

c. All seven vertebra have transverse foramen for the vertebral artery to pass through.

2) Occiput

a. The bone forming the posterior 'bottom' of the cranium.

b. Foramen magnum - hole in the base of the occiput where the spinal cord passes through

c. Occipital condyles - 2 convex surfaces either side of foramen magnum which articulate with the atlas

d. Occipital protuberance - the process on posterior centre of occiput

3) Hyoid bone

a. bone in the throat

b. free floating and attachment for muscles of tongue, mouth and neck.

Joints & Ligaments

1) Occipito - atlantal (O/A) joint

a. Joint between occiput and atlas

b. no intervertebral disc

c. ellipsoid joint

d. allows flexion and extension

Vertebra comparisons

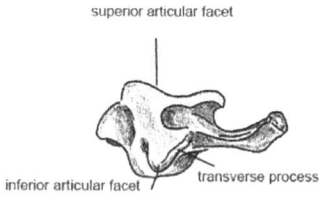

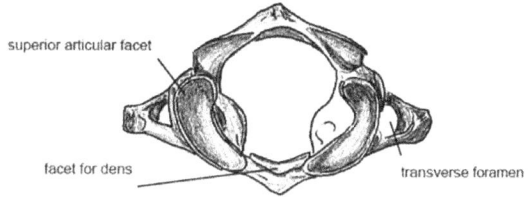

superior articular facet

inferior articular facet transverse process

Atlas (C1) left lateral view

superior articular facet

facet for dens transverse foramen

Atlas superior view

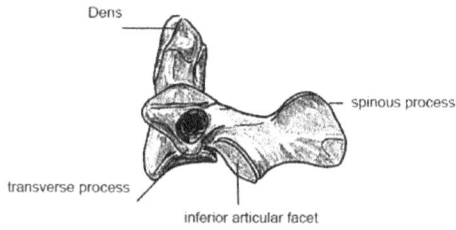

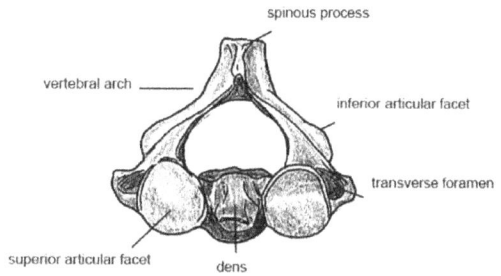

Dens

spinous process

transverse process

inferior articular facet

Axis (C2) left lateral view

spinous process

vertebral arch

inferior articular facet

transverse foramen

superior articular facet dens

Axis superior view

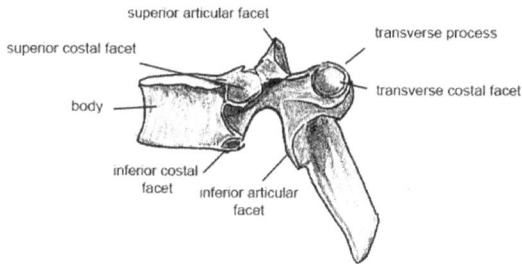

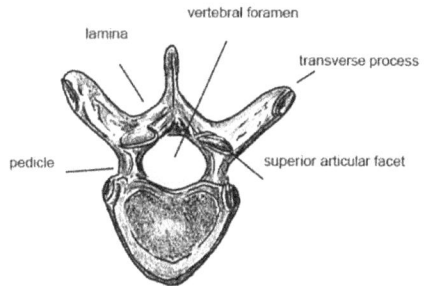

superior articular facet

superior costal facet

transverse process

body

transverse costal facet

inferior costal facet

inferior articular facet

T 6 left lateral view

vertebral foramen

lamina

transverse process

pedicle

superior articular facet

T6 superior view

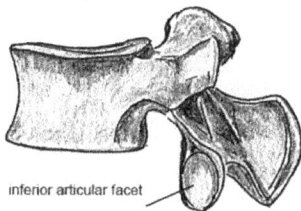

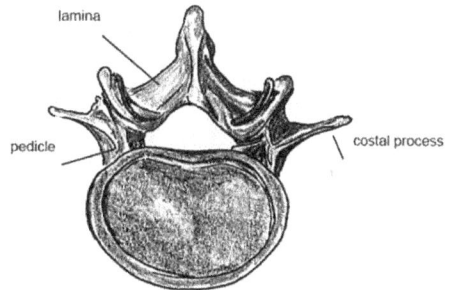

inferior articular facet

L2 left lateral view

lamina

pedicle

costal process

L2 superior view

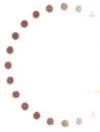

2) Atlanto-axial (A/A) joint
   a. joint between atlas and axis
   b. dens of axis sticks through the ring of atlas
   c. allows for rotation

3) Nuchal ligament (ligamentum nuchae)
   a. The sail ligament
   b. runs from occipital protruberance to sp of C7
   c. continuation of supraspinous and interspinous
ligaments

Muscles of the Neck

Posterior compartment

Superficial layer

1) Trapezius
Attachments
occiput, nuchal ligament and SP's of C7 to T12.
Upper Traps: lateral clavicle and acromium
Middle Traps: Spine of scapula
Lower Traps: root of spine of scapula
Action
Upper Traps: Elevation and upward rotation of
scapula
Middle Traps: Retraction of scapula
Lower Traps: depression and upwards rotation of
scapula
Note
Also works to stabilize scapulae and act as neutralizer.
Cause of many tension headaches and
severely affected by improper posture such
as sitting for prolonged periods.

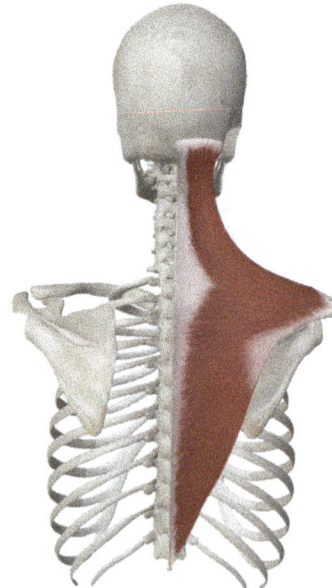

2) Levator Scapula
Attachments
TP's of C1 to C4
superior angle of scapula
Action
elevation and downward rotation of scapula

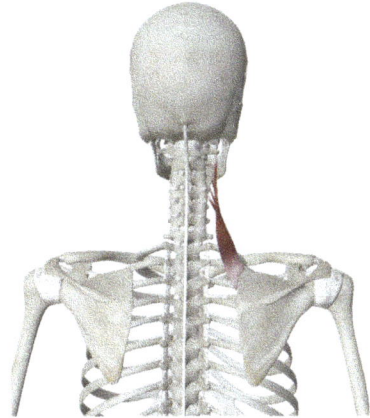

Intermediate Layer

3) Splenius
a. Capitis
Attachments
nuchal ligamnet and SP's of C7 to T3
mastoid process (under SCM) and occiput
Action
bilaterally - extension of neck
unilaterally - ipsilateral rotation of head

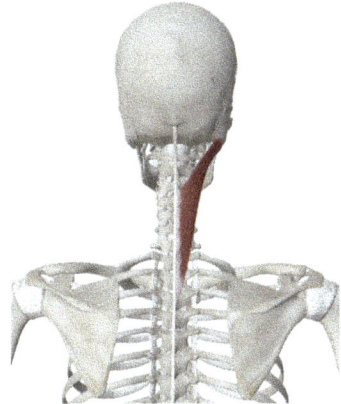

b. Cervicis
Attachments
Sp's of T3 to T6
TP's of C1 to C3
Action
bilaterally - extend neck
unilaterally - ipsilateral rotation of head
Note
the cervicis wrap around the upper erectors (the
'pony tail' muscles)

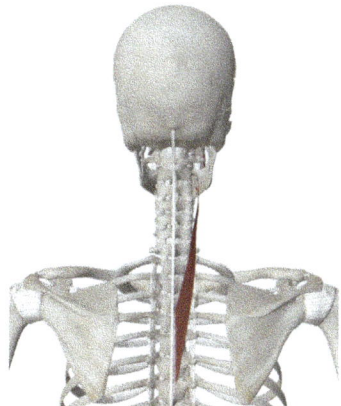

4) Longissimus
a. Capitis
Attachments
TPs of T5 to C4
mastoid process deep to the splenius muscle
Action
bilaterally - extends head
unilaterally - ipsilateral rotation of head

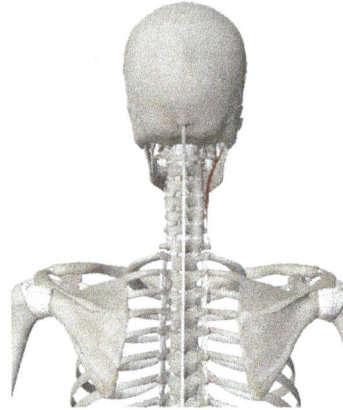

b. Cervicis
Attachments
TPs of T4 to T1
TPs of C1 - C6
Action
bilaterally - extension of neck
unilaterally - lateral flexion of neck

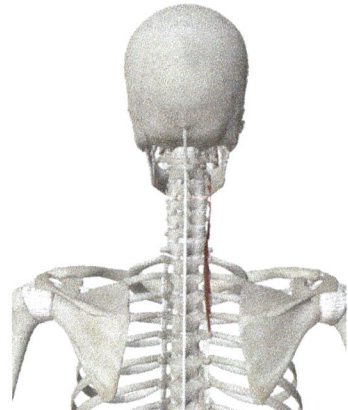

Deep Layer

5) Transversospinalis group
Run from TP's to Sp's (obiquely upwards) with the
deeper muscles spanning 1 or 2 vertebrae and the
not so deep ones more vertebrae.
When looked at bilaterally arranged like a christmas
tree with the muscles running in the lamina groove.

Semispinalis

a. Capitis
Attachments
TPs of C4 to T6
occiput beneath trapezius
Action
bilaterally - extends head
unilaterally - contralateral rotation of head

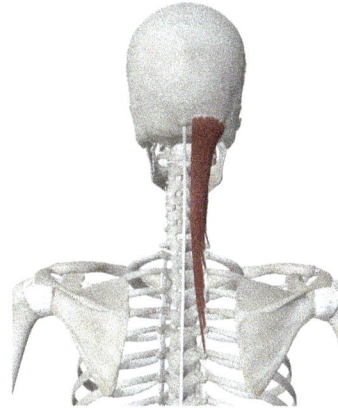

b. cervicis
Attachments
TPs of T1 to T6
SPs of C2 to C6
Action
bilaterally - extends neck
unilaterally - contralateral rotation of neck

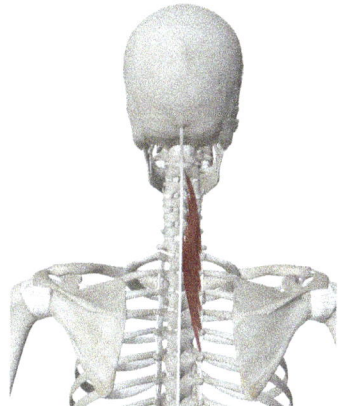

6) Rotatores and multifidi
a. These lie deep to the semispinales group
b. The muscles 'fill in' the lamina groove
c. Except for semispinales capitis the rotators,
multifidi and semispinales cervicis can be seen to
be arranged like a Christmas tree when looked at
from behind.

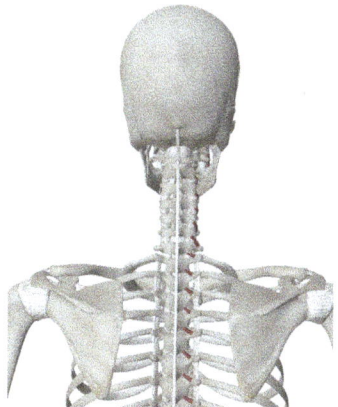

By looking at the splenius, longissimus and semispinalis muscles "the neck" can be seen to extend well into the mid thoracic region

multifidi are important for spinal stabilization and becomes weak when inhibited one of the 'Local Core Control' muscles and crosses SI joint.

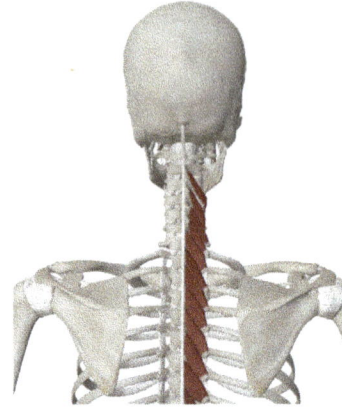

7) Suboccipital group
a. Rectus capitus posterior major
Attachments
SP of C2
base of occiput lateral to minors
Action
bilaterally - extends head unilaterally - ipsilateral rotation and sidebending of head

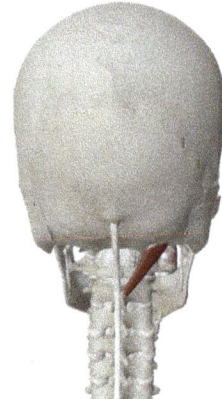

b. Rectus capitis posterior minor
Attachments
tubercle of C1
base of occiput medial to majors
Action
extension of head

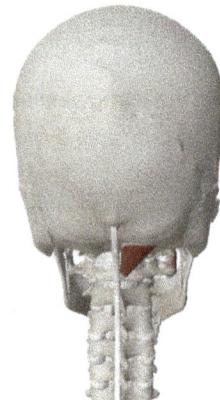

c. Obliquus capitis inferior

Attachments

SP of C2

TP of C1

Action

bilaterally - extension of head

unilaterally - ipsilateral sidebending of head and

ipsilateral rotation of C1 on C2

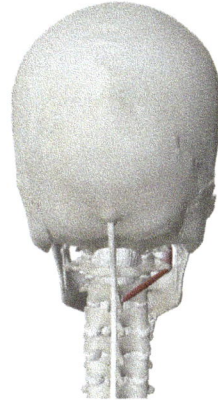

d. Obliquus capitis superior

Attachments

TP of C1

base of occiput, posterior to rectus capitis

posterior major

Action

bilaterally - extension of head

unilaterally - ipsilateral

sidebending of head

Except for obliquus capitis inferior the subocciptals

are more 'postural' muscles as opposed to prime

movers

The suboccipitals are 'hardwired' to the eyes and

lead the head and body

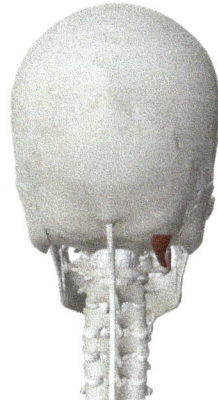

Lateral compartment of neck

Superfical layers

1) Platysma

Attachments

pectoralis fascia

inferior border of mandible

Action

draws down lower lip and angle of mouth

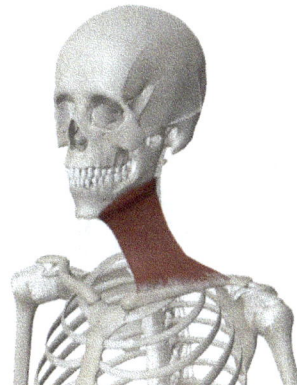

2) Sternocleidomastoid

Attachments

top of manubrium and medial clavicle

mastoid process of temporal bone

Action

unilaterally - contralateral rotation of head

bilaterally - flex or extends head depending on
other muscles working !

If prevertebral flexors are not working properly the
SCM will help extend the neck. If it works with
other neck flexors (ie longus coli) it flexes the head.

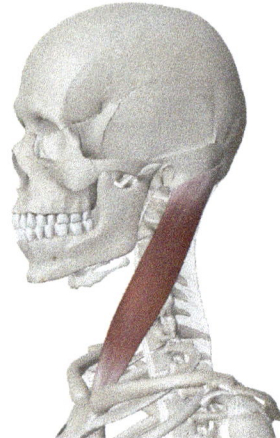

Intermediate layers

3) Scalenes - Anterior / Middle / Lateral

Attachments

anterior - anterior tubercle of transverse
process of C3 -C6

middle - posterior tubercle of transverse
process of C3 - C7

lateral - posterior tubercle of transverse
process of C5 – C7

anterior - scalene tubercle of 1st rib

middle - 1st rib

lateral - outer surface of 2nd rib

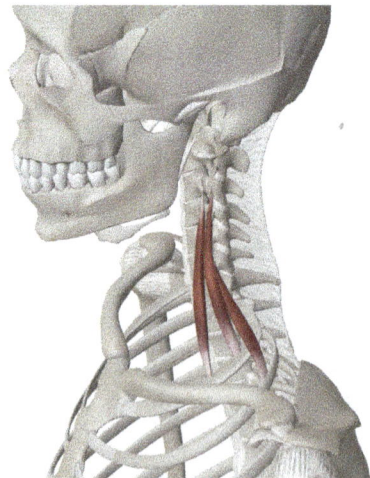

Action

raises upper ribs

unilaterally - flexes the neck

bilaterally - ipsilateral sidebending of cervical spine

Brachial plexus passes through the anterior and medial Scalenes.

They are wired to the "fight or flight" response.

Deep layer

1) Rectus capitis anterior

Attachments

Anterior surface of atlas

basilar portion of occiput anterior condyle

Action

flexion of head

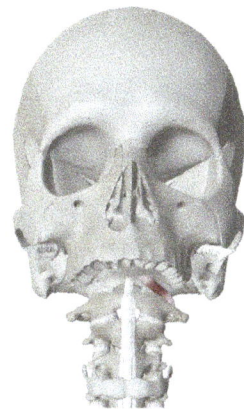

2) Rectus capitis lateralis

Attachments

TP of atlas

base of occiput lateral to occipital condyle

Action

ipsilateral sidebending of head and stabilizes head on occiput

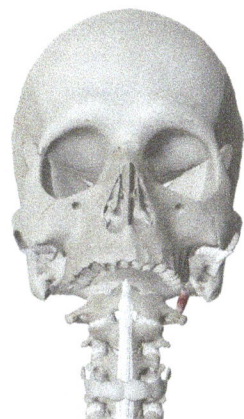

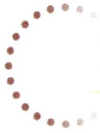

3) Longus capitus

Attachments

anterior surfaces of TP's C3 - C6

base of occiput anterior to foramen magnum

Action

stabilizes head,

bilaterally- flexion of cervical vertebrae and head.

unilaterally - ipsilateral sidebending of neck and
head

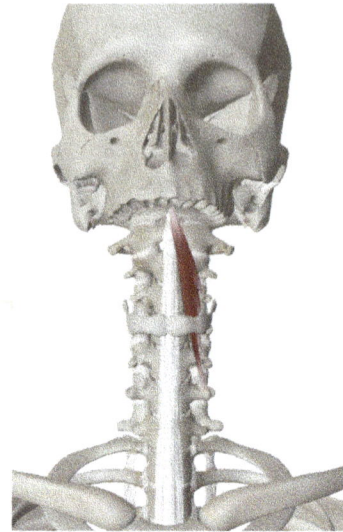

4) Longus coli

Attachments

anterolateral surface of cervical bodies and TP's

anterolateral surface of cervical bodies and TP's

Action

bilaterally - flexion of cervical vertebrae

unilaterally - ipsilateral sidebending and rotation of
neck

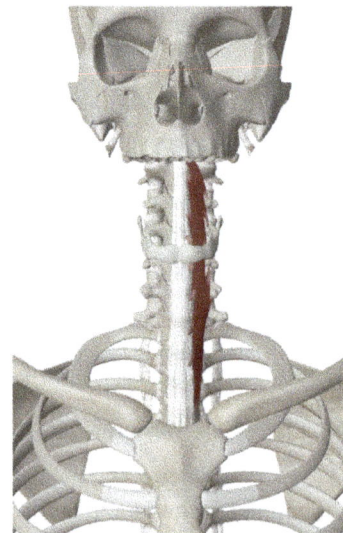

Muscles of Lower, Mid & Upper Spine

Most Superficial Layer

1) Latissimus Dorsi
Attachments
thoracolumbar aponeurosis from T7 to iliac crest
anterior proximal shaft of humerus
(in between teres major and pec major)
Action
extends, adducts and medially rotates humerus
Note
forms the posterior wall of the axillary cavity

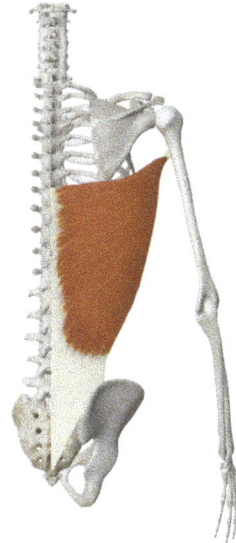

2) Trapezius
Attachments
occiput, nuchal ligament and SP's of C7 to T12.
Upper Traps: lateral clavicle and acromium
Middle Traps: Spine of scapula
Lower Traps: root of spine of scapula
Action
Upper Traps: Elevation and upward rotation of
scapula
Middle Traps: Retraction of scapula
Lower Traps: depression and upwards rotation of
scapula
Note
Also works to stabilize scapulae and act as
neutralizer.

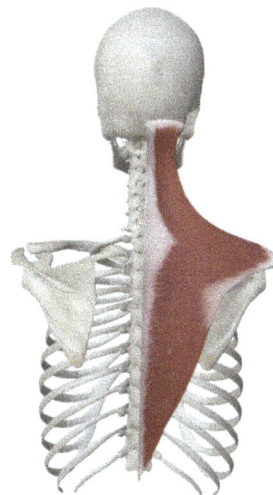

Superficial Layer

1) Rhomboid Major

Attachments

SP's of T2 to T5

medial border of scapula between the spine
and inferior angle of scapula.

Action

retraction and downward rotation of scapula

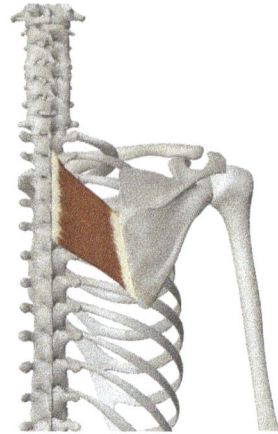

2) Rhomboid Minor

Attachments

SP's C7 to T1

upper portion of medial border of
scapula at level of spine of scapula.

Action

retraction and downward rotation of scapula

Note

lies under the trapezius and can become weak and
tight due to overuse of the traps due to improper
posture such as 'pulling back the shoulders'

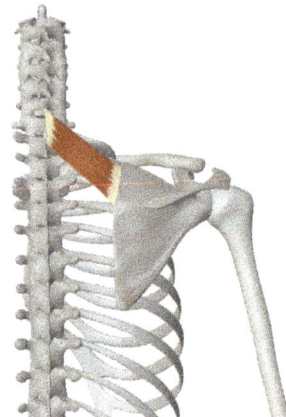

3) Levator Scapula

Attachments

TP's of C1 to C4

superior angle of scapula

Action

elevation and downward rotation of scapula

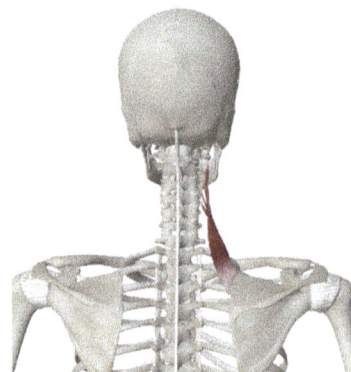

4) Serratus Posterior Superior
Attachments
spinous processes of C7 and T1 - T5
ribs 2 to 5
Action
elevation of ribs - aids respiration

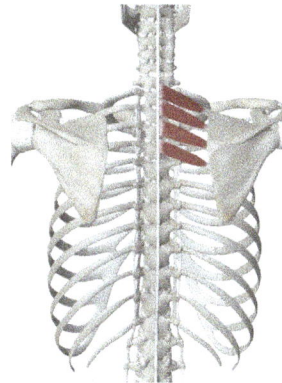

5) Serratus Posterior Inferior
Attachments
spinous processes T11 - L5
ribs 9 to 12
Action
depression of ribs - aids respiration

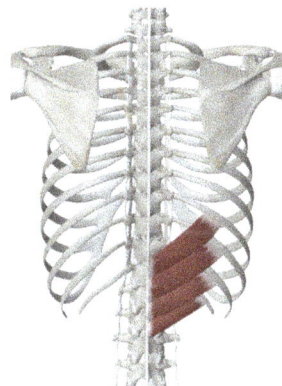

Intermediate Layer

1) Erector Spinae group (sacrospinalis muscles)
a. Illiocostalis lumborum, thoracis and cervicis
Attachments
thoracolumbar aponeurosis and posterior ribs
posterior ribs 1-12 and TP's of C4 to C6
Action
bilaterally - extends spine
unilaterally- sidebends spine
Note
Most lateral of erector spinae
b. Longissimus thoracis, cervicis, capitis

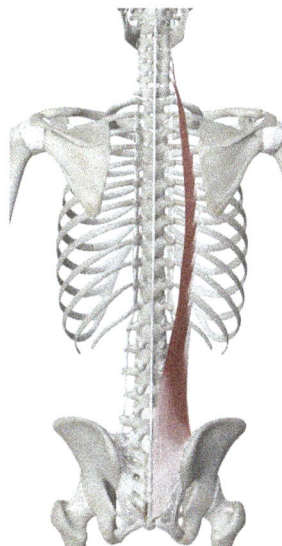

Attachments

thoracolumbar aponeurosis and thoracic TP's

cervical and thoracic TP's, mastoid process and
lower 9 ribs.

Action

bilaterally - extends spine and head unilaterally -
sidebends spine and head

Note

middle group of the erector spinae

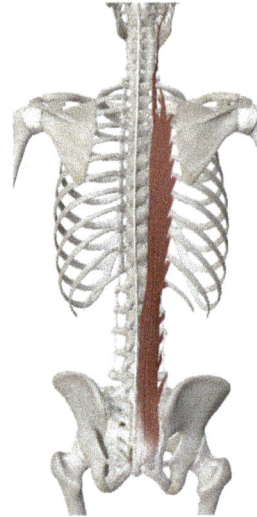

c. Spinalis thoracis, cervicis and capitis

Attachments

thoracic and upper lumbar SP's

cervical and thoracic SP's and occiput

Action

bilaterally - extension of spine

unilaterally - sidebending of spine

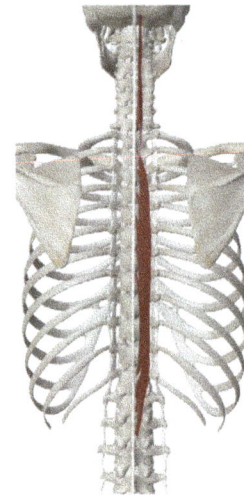

2) Splenius

a. Capitis

Attachments

nuchal ligamnet and SP's of C7 to T3

mastoid process (under SCM) and occiput

Action

bilaterally - extension of neck

unilaterally - ipsilateral rotation of head

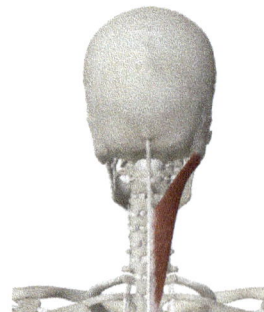

b. Cervicis

Attachments

Sp's of T3 to T6

TP's of C1 to C3

Action

bilaterally - extend neck

unilaterally - ipsilateral rotation of head

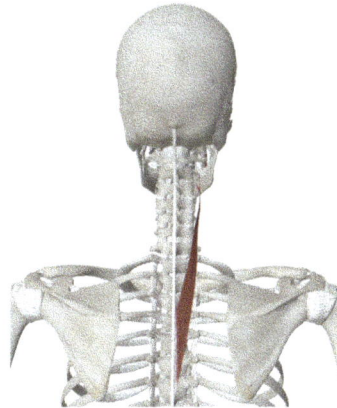

Deep Layer

1) Transversospinalis group

Run from TP's to Sp's (obiquely upwards) with the deeper muscles spanning 1 or 2 vertebrae and the not so deep ones more vertebrae.

a. Semispinalis thoracis, cervicis and capitis

Attachments

thoracic and cervical TP's

overlying SP's and occiput (3 -6 vertebrae)

Action

bilaterally - extends spine and head

unilaterally - contralateral rotation of head and spine

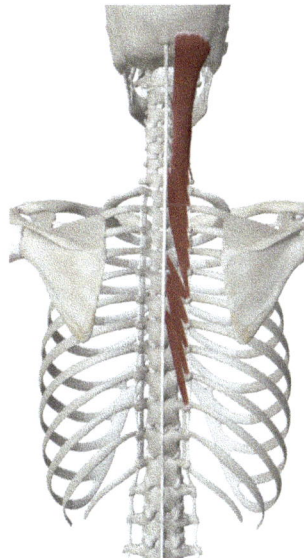

b. Multifidus

Attachments

sacrum and TP's of all vertebrae

SP's of overlying vertebrae (2 -4 span)

Action

bilaterally – extension

Unilaterally - contralateral rotation of spine

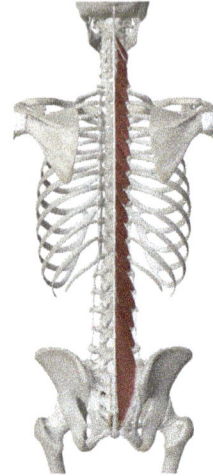

c. Rotatores

Attachments

TP's of all vertebrae

SP of overlying vertebrae

Action

contralateral rotation and extension of spine

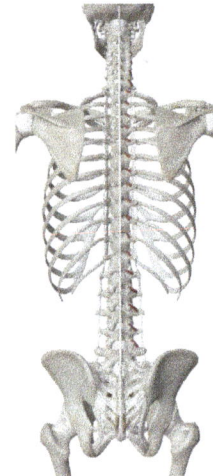

2) Intertransversarii

Attachments

TP's of cervical, lumbar and T10 - T12

TP's of vertebra directly above origin

Action

lateral flexion of spine

Note

These cross only one segment and run vertically

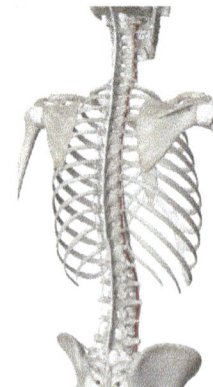

3) Interspinales

Attachments

SP's of cervical, lumbar and T1-T2 plus T11 to T12

SP's of vertebra directly above origin

Action

extension of spine

Note

cross only one segment

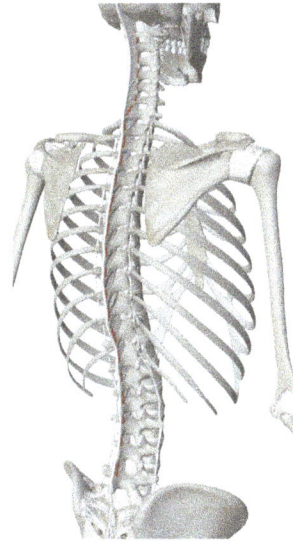

4) Levatores costales

Attachments

TP's of C7 to T11

rib directly below (brevis) or two below (longus)

Action

possible elevation of ribs in inspiration and/or

contralateral rotation and lateral flexion of spine.

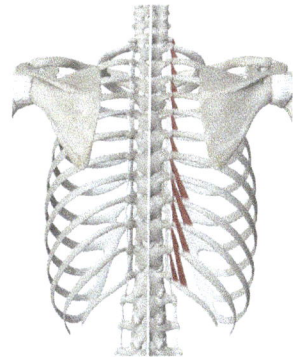

5) Quadratus Lumborum

Attachments

posterior iliac crest

12th rib and TP's of L1 - L4

Action

unilaterally - lateral flexion of trunk,

raises hip and stabilizes 12th rib during

inspiration.

Note

often involved in acute back pain

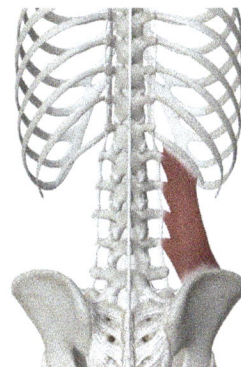

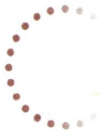

Notes:

1) The erector spinae ; splenii, transversospinales, intertransversarii, and interspinales are collectively known as the paraspinalis muscles.

2) The short deep muscles of multifidus, rotatores, interspinales, and intertransversarii are primarily used as spine / trunk stabilizers allowing other larger muscles to do most of the 'movement' work.

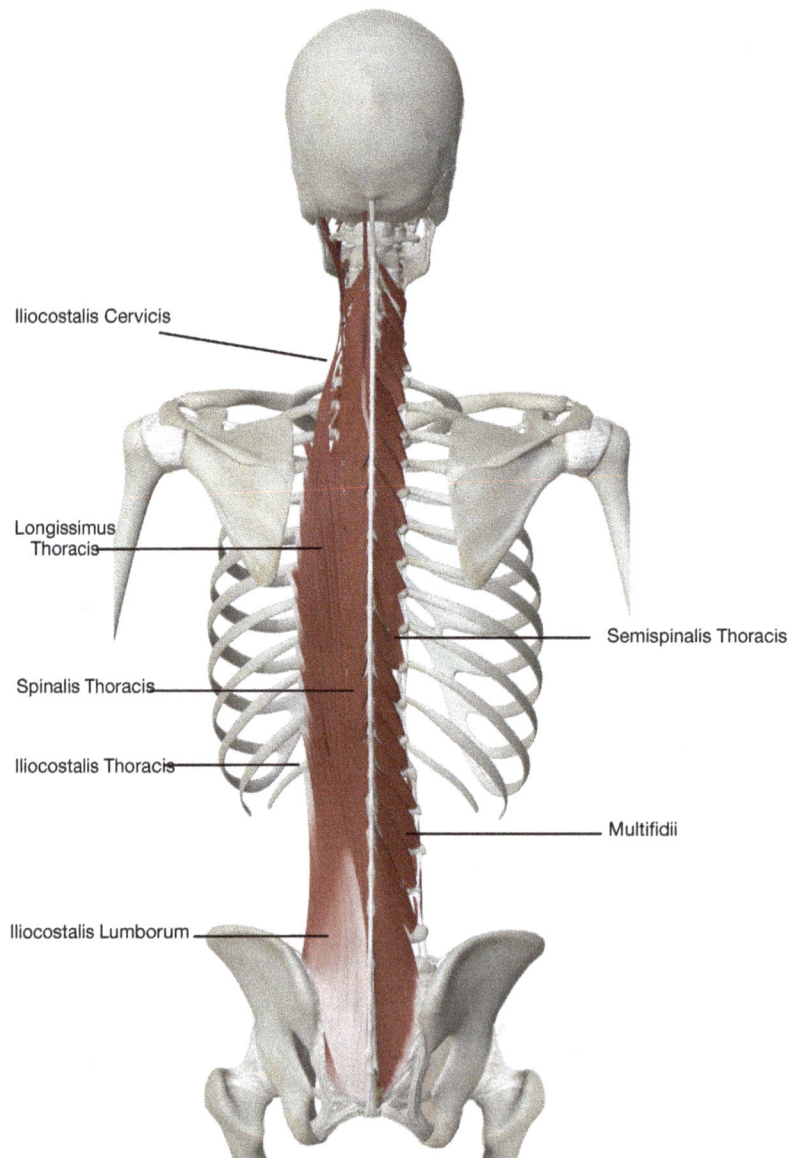

Iliocostalis Cervicis

Longissimus Thoracis

Semispinalis Thoracis

Spinalis Thoracis

Iliocostalis Thoracis

Multifidii

Iliocostalis Lumborum

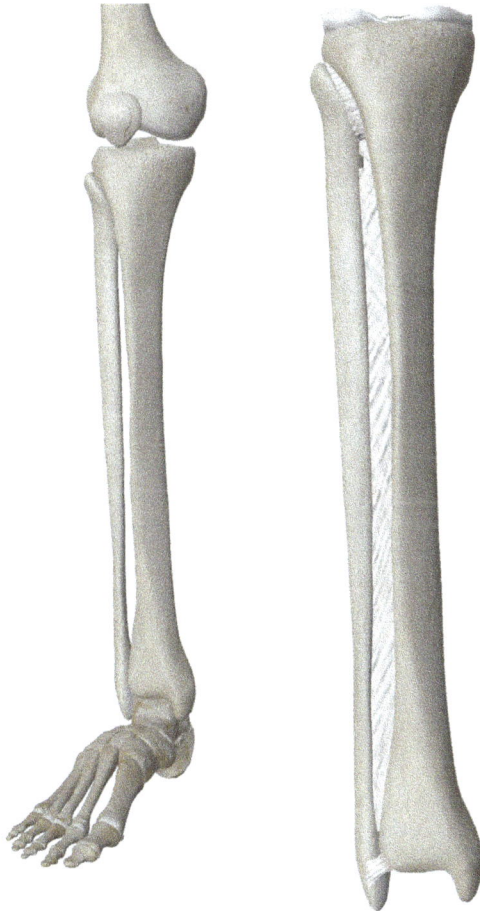

Anterior view of right lower leg

Lower Leg and Foot

Bones of lower leg

1. Tibia
a. shaft
b. tibial platform - (medial & lateral condyles, intercondyler tubercles)
c. tibial tuberosity
d. medial malleolus

2. Fibula
a. head
b. shaft
c. lateral malleolus

Foot

1. Tarsals
a. Calcaneus
b. Talus
c. Navicular
d. Cuneiforms - 1st, 2nd, and 3rd
e. Cuboid

2. Metatarsals
a. I to V (I is big toe)
b. base - proximal end of bone
c. head - distal end of bone
d. sesamoid bones - two small rounded bones under the surface of the first metatarsal to help distribute weight and act as groove for the tendon of flexor hallucis longus.

3. Phalanges
a. Hallux - big toe
b. Digits toes 2 to 5

Lateral View of Right Foot

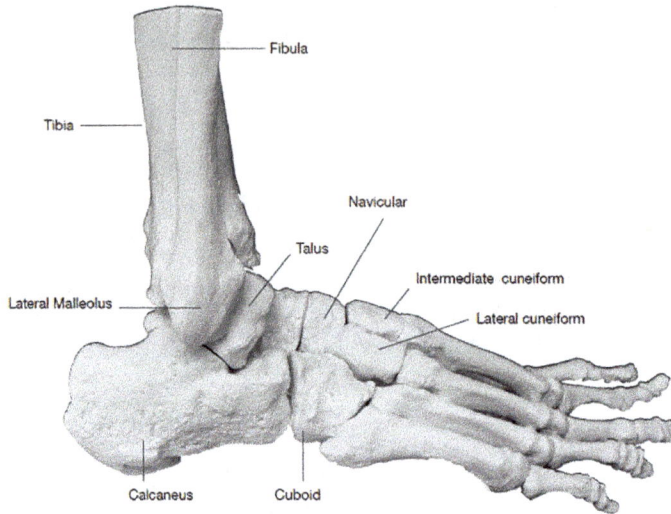

Fibula

Tibia

Navicular

Talus

Intermediate cuneiform

Lateral Malleolus

Lateral cuneiform

Calcaneus   Cuboid

Superior View of Left Foot

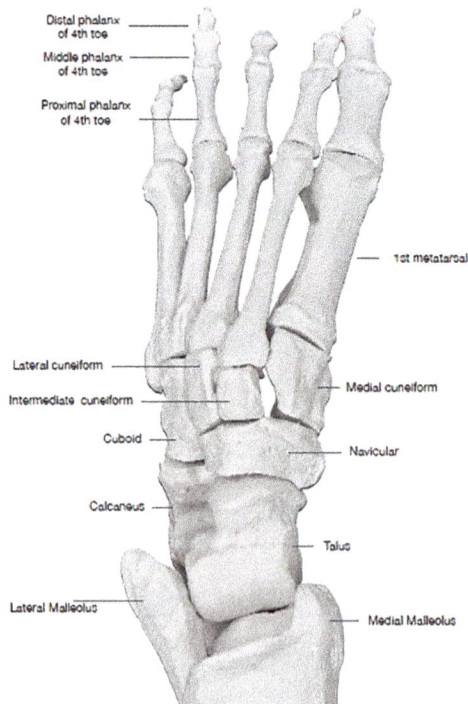

Distal phalanx
of 4th toe

Middle phalanx
of 4th toe

Proximal phalanx
of 4th toe

1st metatarsal

Lateral cuneiform

Medial cuneiform

Intermediate cuneiform

Cuboid

Navicular

Calcaneus

Talus

Lateral Malleolus

Medial Malleolus

Joints and Ligaments

1. Knee joint

femur articulates with the tibia

a. Patella (knee cap) - sesamoid bone articulates with the femur and lies in the tendon of the quadriceps femoris muscle

b. Lateral and Medial Menisci (2 meniscus) - 2 tangerine shaped fibrorocartilages between the condyles of the femur and tibia. Primarily act as shock absorbers and have attachments to the medial collateral ligaments and tendons of popliteus and semimembranosus

c. Medial & Lateral collateral ligaments - help to stabilize the knee by tightening in extension. They both slacken in medial rotation and tighten in lateral rotation. The lateral ligament is not part of the joint capsule.

d. Anterior and posterior cruciate ligaments - found outside the knee joint. The ACL resists anterior displacement of the tibia against the femur whilst the PCL resists posterior displacement of the tibia. Both ligaments slacken in lateral rotation and tense in medial rotation whilst remaining taut during flexion and extension.

2. Tibio-fibula joints

a. Superior joint is synovial which allows for little movement of the bones

b. Inferior joint is a fibrous one holding the 2 bones together

c. Interosseous membrane - sheet of connective tissue running between the tibia and fibula and also acts as attachment to tibialis anterior and posterior and extensor hallucis longus.

The Foot

The foot consists of 26 bones, 19 'large' muscles and more than 100 ligaments.

1. Three Arches :

a. Medial Longitudinal Arch – Calcaneus, talus, navicular, 3 cuneiforms, proximal end of the 3 medial metatarsals.

b. Lateral Longitudinal Arch – Calcaneus, cuboid, 4th & 5th metatarsals - support and propulsion

c. Transverse Arch – 3 cuneiforms and the cuboid - involved in shock absorbtion.

2. Tibiotalar joint

The articulation of the tibia and fibula with the superior surface of the talus.

3. Talocalcaneal & Talocalcaneonavicular (subtalar) joints

The talocalcaneal joint is where the talus rests on and articulates with the calcaneus. The talocalcaneonavicular joint is where the head of the talus articulates with the socket of the posterior surface of the navicular bone, the superior surface of the plantar calcaneonavicular ligament (spring ligament), the sustentataculum tali and the articular surface of the calcaneus.

This is essentially where inversion and eversion takes place.

4. Transverse or mid tarsal joint

a. Talonavicular joint.

b. Calcaneocuboid joint - an S shaped articulation of lateral surface of calcaneus and posterior surface of the cuboid.

Eversion - (abduction with dorsiflexion) at subtalar and transverse tarsal joints usually creates pronation

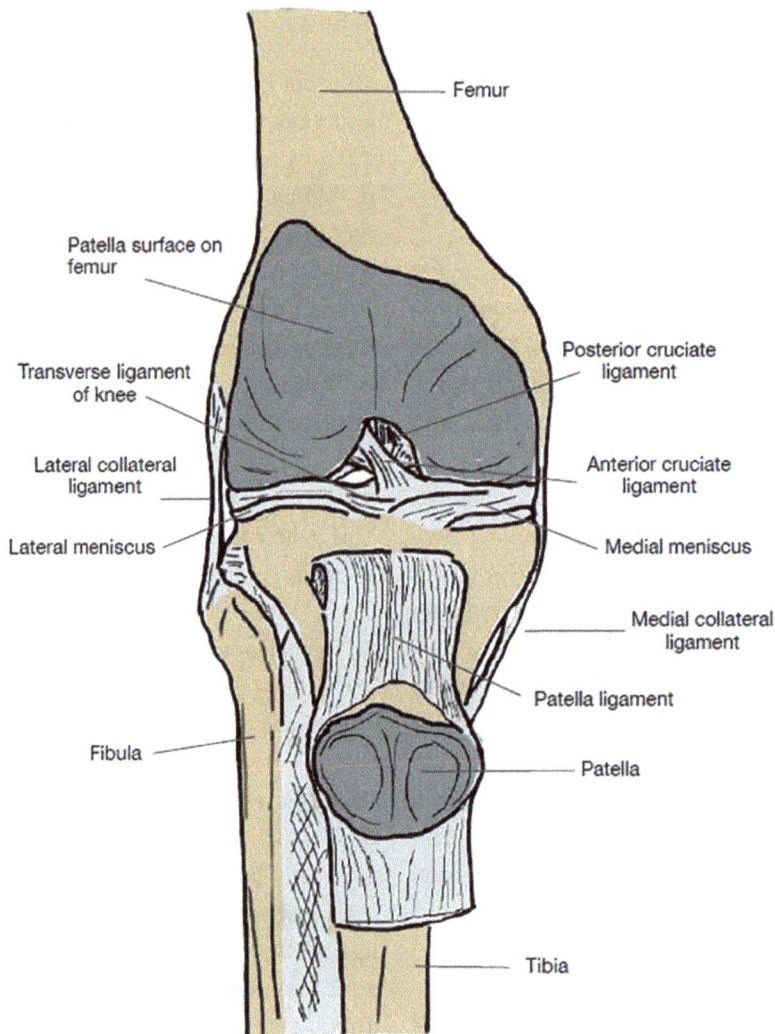

- Femur
- Patella surface on femur
- Posterior cruciate ligament
- Transverse ligament of knee
- Anterior cruciate ligament
- Lateral collateral ligament
- Lateral meniscus
- Medial meniscus
- Medial collateral ligament
- Patella ligament
- Fibula
- Patella
- Tibia

Inversion – (adduction with plantarflexion) at sub talar and transverse tarsal joints. Usually creates supination.

Supination – ankle plantar flexion, subtalar inversion, forefoot adduction, tightness of intrinsic foot muscles.

Pronation – (flat foot) ankle dorsiflexion, subtalar eversion, forefoot abduction.

5. Ligaments

a. Plantar calcaneonavicular liagament ; the 'spring' ligament. Runs from

b. Long plantar ligament runs from the bases of metatarsals II to V and helps support both longitudinal arches.

c. Short plantar ligament - from calcaneus to the cuboid.

Cross Section of Right Lower Leg - Viewed from Above

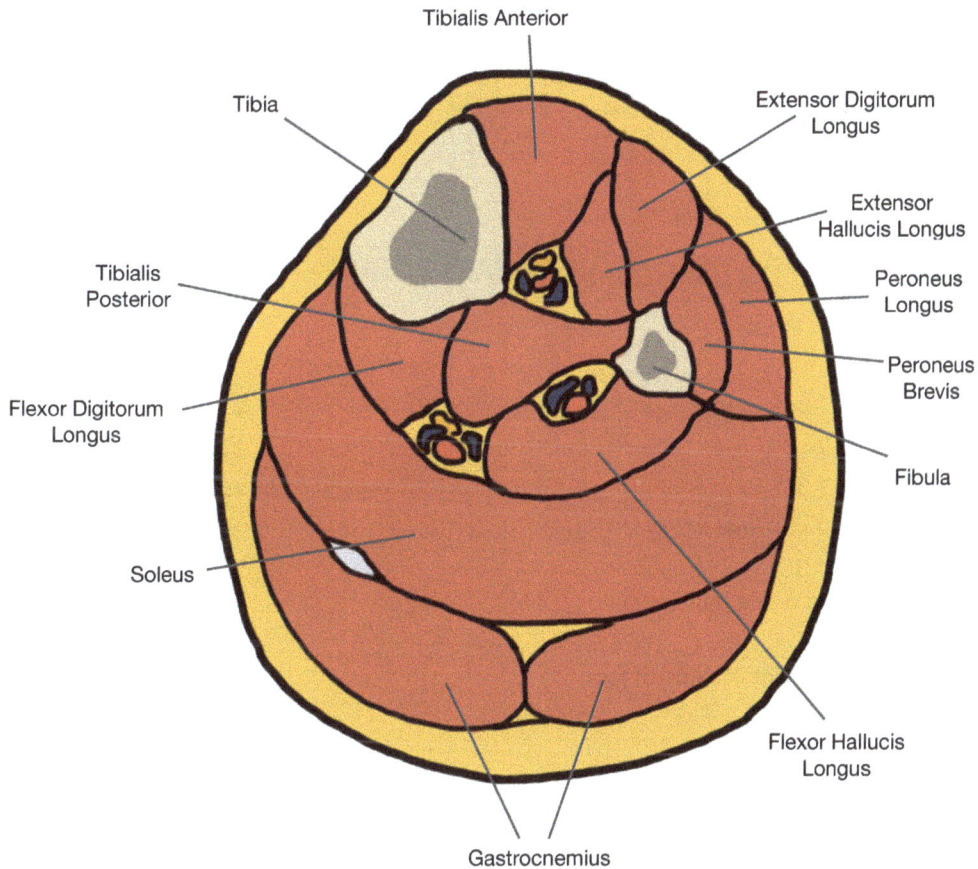

Tibialis Anterior

Tibia

Extensor Digitorum
Longus

Extensor
Hallucis Longus

Tibialis
Posterior

Peroneus
Longus

Peroneus
Brevis

Flexor Digitorum
Longus

Fibula

Soleus

Flexor Hallucis
Longus

Gastrocnemius

Muscles & Tissue

1. Crural fascia - deep or investing fascia of the lower leg, is a continuation of the fascia lata of the upper leg.

2. Intermuscular septa - continuation of the crural fascia deep into the leg and separates major muscle groups from each other.

3. Retinacula - (flexor,extensor, peroneal). Thickening of the crural fascia around the ankle joints and acts as a sheath for the tendons running under them.

4. Tendinous sheaths - structure which the tendons pass through to help the tendons slide easily under the retinacula

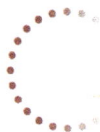

Anterior Compartment of Leg:

1) Tibialis anterior

Attachments

Lateral shaft of tibia and interosseus membrane

base of 1st metatarsal and 1st cuneiform

Action

dorsiflexion of foot and inversion. Helps maintain
medial arch

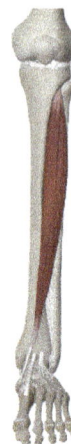

2) Extensor digitorum longus

Attachments

Lateral condyle of tibia and proximal 2/3 of
anterior shaft of fibula.

middle and distal phalanges of the four toes

Action

extension of toes and assists dorsiflexion of foot.
Helps maintain lateral arch.

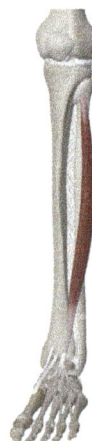

3) Extensor hallucis longus

Attachments

anterior shaft of the fibula and interosseous
membrane

superior base of distal phalanx of big toe.

Action

extension of big toe and assists dorsiflexion

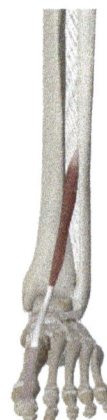

4) Peroneus tertius / Fibularis tertius
Attachments
anterior border of distal fibula
base of 5th metatarsal
Action
eversion, assists in dorsiflexion and supports
lateral arch

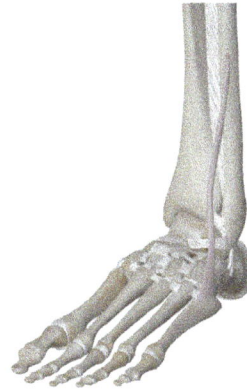

Lateral Compartment of Leg:

5) Peroneus longus
Attachments
Upper 2/3 of lateral shaft of fibula
plantar surface of base of 1st metatarsal and
1st cuneiform
Action
eversion and plantar flexion. Helps support
transverse arch

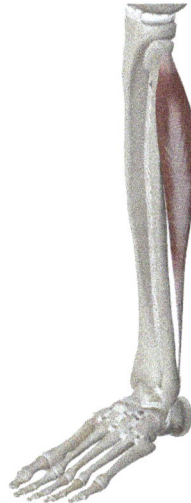

6) Peroneus brevis
Attachments
lower 2/3 of lateral shaft of fibula covered by
the longus
lateral tubercle of 5th metatarsal
Action
eversion and plantarflexion. Helps support
lateral arch

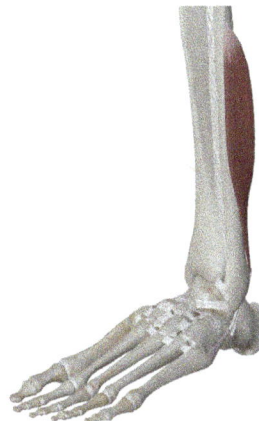

Posterior Compartment of Leg:

7) Gastrocnemius

Attachments

two heads; posterior surfaces of medial and
lateral epicondyles of femur
calcaneus via Achilles tendon

Action

plantar flexion or assists flexion of knee. 2 joint
muscle

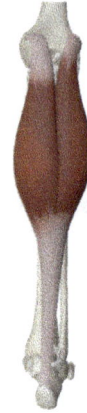

8) Soleus

Attachments

posterior proximal tibia and head and upper
shaft of fibula
calcaneus via Achilles tendon

Action

plantar flexion

Note

Gastocnemius and soleus are known together as
'triceps surae'.

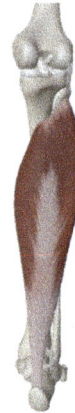

9) Popliteus

Attachments

lateral epicondyle of femur
medial condyle of tibia

Action

flexion of the knee joint and also medial
rotates to 'unlock' the knee

Note

deepest muscle in the back of the knee

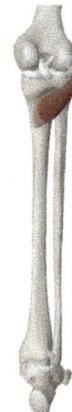

10) Plantaris

Attachments

lateral epicondyle of femur

calcaneus via Achilles tendon

Action

assists in plantarflexion and knee flexion

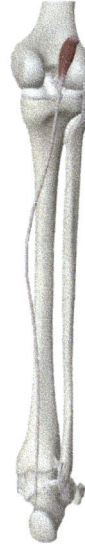

Deep Posterior Compartment of Leg:

11) Tibialis posterior

Attachments

posterior of tibia, fibula and interoseus
membrane

numerous bones of plantar surface of foot
including 3 middle metatarsals

Action

inversion and plantar flexion, helps maintain
medial transverse arches.

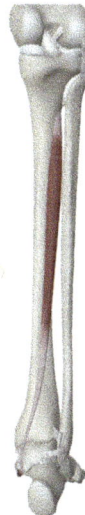

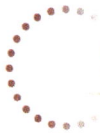

12) Flexor hallucis longus

Attachments

posterior shaft of tibia

distal phalanx of great toe

Action

flexion of great toe and assists plantar flexion

Note

tendon runs under the sustentaculum tali of
calcaneus making it crucial for support of medial
arch

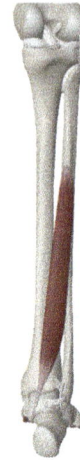

13) Flexor digitorum longus

Attachments

posterior shaft of tibia

plantar surface of distal phalanges of 4 toes

Action

flexion of toes and assists in plantar flexion, helps
maintain medial arch

Note.

Tibialis posterior, flexor digitorum longus and flexor
hallucis longus are collectively known as the Tom,
Dick & Harry muscles.

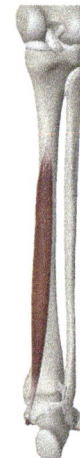

Important muscles of the lower leg :

1) The 'Ice Tongs"
Peroneus brevis & tibialis anterior - support lateral
and medial arches

2) The "Stirrup"
Peronues longus & tibialis anterior - support lateral,
medial and transverse arches

3) The "Sling"
Peroneus longus and tibialis posterior - Support
medial, lateral and transverse arches by squeezing
the cuneiforms and cuboid together.

Eight muscles pull down on the fibula :

1. Peroneus longus   2. Peroneus brevis
3. Tibialis posterior   4. Extensor hallucis longus
5. Extensor digitorum longus   6.soleus
7. Flexor hallucis longus   8. peroneus tertius

One muscle pulls upwards on fibula :

1. Biceps femoris

Levers

A lever may be thought of as a rigid bar with a fulcrum (or pivot point) which is used to move a fixed load by applying force or pressure at a given point.

The component parts of a lever in the body are :

1. Lever - nearly always the bone
2. Fulcrum - pivot point of the lever, which is usually the joint
3. Muscle Force - force that draws the opposite ends of the muscles together
4. Resistive Force - force generated by a factor external to the body (e.g. gravity, friction etc.) that acts against muscle force

5. Torque - the degree to which a force tends to rotate an object about a specified fulcrum
The majority of all muscles and joints in the body are Type 3 levers. It is important to understand the concepts of levers to obtain safe and effective training benefits.

First Class Lever

'The Catapult' - high mechanical advantage - low effort

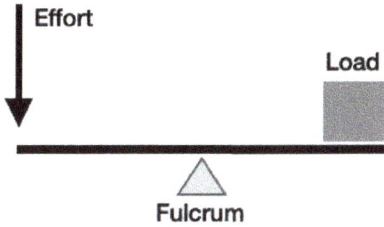

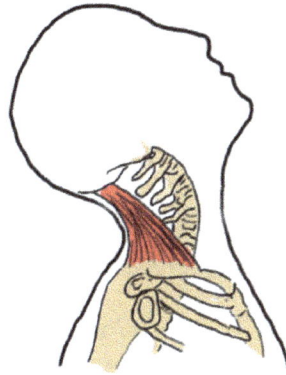

Second Class Lever

'The wheel barrow' - effort moves a large distance compared to load

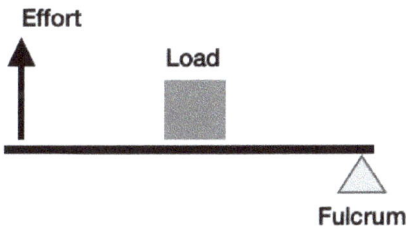

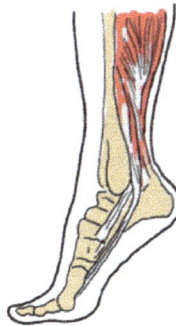

Third Class Lever

The 'Fishing rod' - low mechanical advantage - high speed.

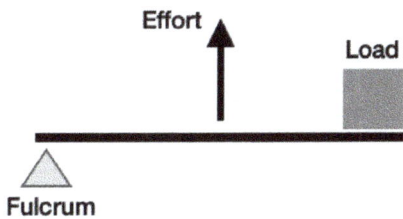

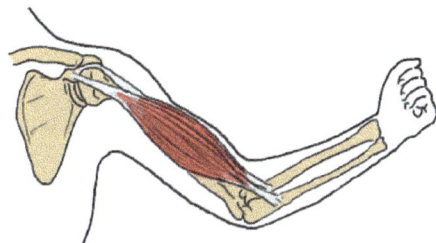

Form & Force Closure

Form Closure

The potential ability for 2 surfaces to adhere or 'close' upon each other. The shape of each surface would dictate the amount of force closure available. A good example of this is a 'key' stone used in an archway. In the body all joints have a certain amount of form closure available.

Force Closure

Force closure is ensured through the amount of force acting on the proximating surfaces. In the 'key' stone example of the arch it is supplied by gravity whilst in the body gravity and muscular effort exert the force needed. A major joint often affected through a disfunction of form and force closure are the sacral iliac joints which receive the forces from the upper body and the resulting force from the ground up through the legs.

CHAPTER

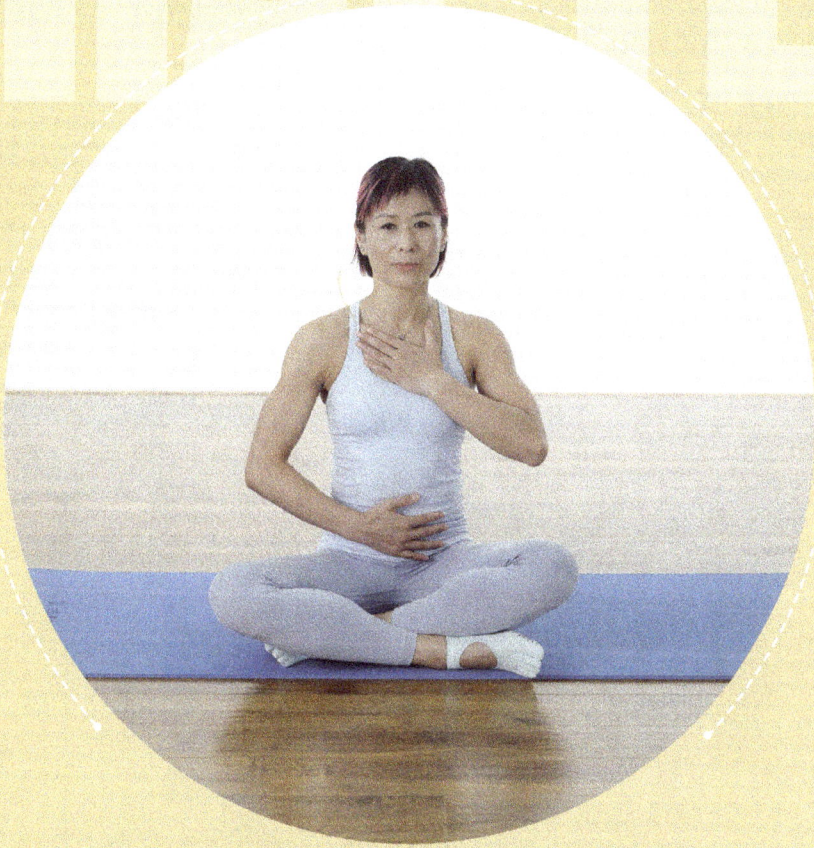

Six

Principles of Movement & Application to Training

6.1 Principles of Movement & Application to Training

Muscles move bones to produce locomotion. Optimum movement is dependent on a wide variety of environmental, emotional, and physical factors which integrates all systems of the body.

We may however simplify things to the extent that we are primarily concerned with 'Optimum Functional Movement' in relation to an 'optimum' synchronicity of local and global muscles and myofascia and related subsystems in terms of :

 • *Sequencing of muscle firing patterns (agonists, antagonists, synergists, stabilizers and neutralizers),*
 • *Balance of the fascial system,*
 • *Balance of gamma and alpha neuromuscular innovation,*
 • *Proprioceptive awareness of the individual*
 • *Structural integrity of the body in terms of potential for movement*

Movement training should take into account the above considerations as well as basic structural and movement principles to ensure efficient movement patterns. In doing so the body may be seen as operating as an integration of separate 'functional units'.

Let's start with an update or expansion on the six principles we already discovered as named by Romana Kryzanowska. If you remember these were

Functional Alignment	Lumbo Pelvic Hip Complex (LPHC)	Feet & Lower Limbs	Shoulder Girdle	Spinal Mobility / Stability
Breathing	Spinal Mobility	Ground reaction force	Upper Limb Mobility	Articulation
Hollowing	Spinal Stability	Stability / mobility	Upper Limb Stability	Core control
Core Control	Hip Differentiation	Force transmission	Upper Limb Integration	
	Core Control		Core Control	

Full Body Integration

concentration, control, centering, flow, precision and breathing.

To give a slightly different perspective on the above six principles we can add to them or rename them to give a variation in terminology. By giving them a different name we can view these principles in a slightly different manner.

Functional Unit Alignment

The alignment of the head, shoulder girdle & ribcage, pelvis, lower limbs and feet may be thought of as the alignment of 4 'functional units' through the placement of horizontal diaphragms which align and separate each unit whilst achieving and maintaining structural integrity. Misalignment of either unit will result in compensatory movements in the system above and below.

Head

The head controls the brain which is the central control system for the rest of the body. Position of the head has a direct effect on the eyes and vestibular system which along with the feet relate to total posture. Tension in the cranial bones and associated muscles have a profound effect on neck tension and posture. The head however as a 'functional unit' is outside the scope of practice for a 'Movement Therapist'.

Breathing

Breathing or respiration is the continual process of inspiration and expiration. Some common terminology for various 'types' of breathing are as follows :

1) Abdominal, belly, deep diaphragmatic, abdomino-diaphragmatic

3) Bucket handle
4) Pump handle, thoracic empowered
5) Posterio-thoracic
6) Constricted, shallow, accessory
7) Paradoxical (sympathetic)

Breathing is closely associated with the 'local core musculature' and therefore has a profound effect on the organization of the whole body. Breathing is also directly affected by and in turn affects our emotional state which will also effect performance.

It is considered essential to integrate good breathing patterns for effective, safe movement patterns.

As workload increases so must the need for stabilization and the need for a more forceful breath. Traditional Pilates teaches the application of 'Lateral - Posterior Breathing'

Focus is placed on drawing up the pelvic floor muscles whilst maintaining a narrow waist whilst placing an emphasis on breathing into the posterior lateral parts of the ribcage. This encourages the bucket handle movements of the lower ribs as well as the pump handle movements of the upper ribs.

When working under load an abdominal brace should be maintained on both inhalation and exhalation.

An abdominal brace involves activation of the the tranversus abdominus along with the pelvic floor, internal and external obliques and rectus abdominus muscles to ensure stability of the pelvis and spine.

Controlled breathing should use a muscular contraction on both inhalation and exhalation thus training the body to stabilize regardless of an inhalation or exhalation or motion.

The force of breath will determine which muscles are being used. On inhalation therefore the breath should

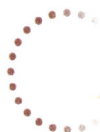

be slow and controlled without being too deep or too light. Too deep will stimulate belly or chest breathing. Breathing too light will not engage the diaphragm and other related local core muscles. Breathe in through the nose and out through the mouth.

Core Control

The Core

When we talk about the terminology of 'The Core' - we are usually referring to specific muscles and associated fascia around the waist however we can also define the core as falling into 3 categories :

- *Local core*
- *Global core*
- *Functional core*

Local Core

Local Core : These are mostly 'anticipatory' muscles and should contract before movement occurs to provide stabilization for the body.

Respiratory diaphragm
Multifidii
Pelvic floor
Transversus abdominus

Global Core

Global Core : These should contract after the Local Core muscles and help to stabilize the trunk and either initiate or prepare the body for movement.
As mentioned previously it should be noted that for most people with pain or a dysfunction it is not a problem with a 'weak core' but more often than not the inability for the musculature to sequence firing in

an appropriate manner.
The firing sequence between the local and global core musculature is realistically not possible to change through conscious effort however an understanding of how this may influence pain or dysfunctional movement is important when working with clients.

External Oblique
Internal Oblique
Rectus Abdominis
Psoas major
Gluteus Medius
Latisimus Dorsi

Functional Core

Any muscle that needs to pre contract to help stabilize a given movement

'Core' Basics'

As babies we have very little musculature and rely on neurological reflexes to help coordinate our bodies. The spine initially lacks a lordosis curve in the lower back and neck which only develops as a result of lifting our heads, crawling about and looking around our environment.
As a result of crawling an early reflex that develops is between the eyes, neck and spinal muscles. As we look around the muscles in the neck contract in relation to where we are looking. For this reason you may wish to include any manner of 'crawling' exercises into your routine although they are not included in this book.. In yoga for instance one of the fundamental principles for Asana practice is 'Dhristi' which refers to both looking outwardly and inwardly for awareness and proprioceptive feedback.

As we crawl and move around the system develops and the muscles supporting the spine also become stronger until all the muscles down the length of the spine contract. Eventually the muscles become strong enough not only to support the spine but also to help gross body movements.

Application of the 'Local Core' towards Training :
  • *Activation of the local core is dependent on correct breathing.*
  • *Increases intra-abdominal pressure and is responsible for segmental stabilization of the lumbar spine.*

Functional Movement

When functioning optimally the local core increases pressure in the peritoneum (similar to squeezing a balloon) creating a posterior force against the anterior surface of the lumbar spine. In addition to this increased intra-abdominal pressure, the thoracolumbar fascia provides added stability while the intrinsic muscles of the spine relay proprioceptive information back to the central nervous system to help maintain alignment of the lumbar vertebrae and discs.

It is possible that dysfunction of the local core may result in pain, dysfunction and injury such as sprains, strains, bulging disks, herniated disks, capsular damage, nerve impingement, arthritic changes, etc.

If the local core is functioning optimally it results in a stable lumbar spine and a stable Lumbo Pelvic Hip Complex (LPHC) capable of efficiently transferring force between lower and upper extremities.

This system however by itself IS NOT responsible for movement but creates stability enabling safe and optimal movement to occur. The activation of the local core helps increase stability of the LPHC, but no visible joint action. Optimal recruitment of this system is considered essential to the performance of the other lumbo pelvic hip complex myofascial slings and is thus considered of great importance for a number of Pilates exercises and especially for beginner starting out on a Pilates training program.

Notes on local core muscles

  • *They contract before movement occurs (anticipatorily)*
  • *Associated with eye and head movement*
  • *Have postural feedback*
  • *Connected to the breathing cycle*
  • *Related to walking*
  • *When the eyes move, the sub occipital muscles contract at the base of skull, thus transmitting neuro-myofascial feedback further down the kinetic chain of the spine and extremities.*
  • *The local core is interdependent on the integration of the lumbo pelvic hip complex*

Notes on global core muscles

It is very common for these muscles to become weak or under active due to actions of other muscles that do similar jobs.

Whilst local core muscles do not move or propel the body the global core muscles are used for both stability and mobility which makes them very vulnerable towards dysfunction

Lumbo Pelvic Hip Complex (LPHC)

Pelvis

The pelvis consists of the hip joints, sacrum, coccyx and right and left pelvic girdle bones of the ischium, pubis and ilium. The area inside the pelvis contains the center of gravity from which we express ourselves in space and also receives and transmits the upper and lower forces of gravity and ground reaction force.

As the transmission area of the lower extremities to the upper body dysfunction here will affect both upper and lower body dysfunction. The hips are an integral part of the pelvis and need to be able to be either mobile or stable depending on the demand imposed. The pelvic floor is an essential component of the mobile/stable demands for the hip joint.

The pelvis is directly physically connected to the lumbar spine and any movement in the lumbar spine is transmitted to the pelvis and visa versa. This is commonly referred to as the 'Lumbo Pelvic Hip Complex' . Together these muscles, tissues and joints act together to stabilize the spine and pelvis as well as absorbing and transmitting force to the upper and lower limbs.

Collectively this complex may also be referred to as the 'core' however this can be misleading as other referrals to the 'core musculature' quite often make reference to the four 'local core muscles' of the Tranversus Abdominus, Respiratory Diaphragm, Pelvic Floor and Multifidii muscles.

In classical Pilates this 'complex or system' of joints and muscles is simply referred to as the 'Powerhouse'.

Neutral Spine

The position at which the vertebrae and intervertebral discs create the optimum load transfer whilst maximising the natural curves of the spine and allowing maximum space through the intervertebral foramen for the peripheral nerves.

Neutral spine is a useful concept to bring awareness to the body when practicing stabilization of the pelvis and spine however it serves little practical purpose in functional movement patterns.

Feet and Lower Extremities

Due to gravity and the resulting ground reaction forces the feet become the first functional unit with which force is transmitted throughout the body in an erect standing position. The soles of the feet contain millions of receptors which (along with the temporal mandibular joint, vestibular system and eyes) constantly make use of a neurobiofeedback loop via the spine to the brain which helps the body arrange itself in gravity.

As a simple rule of thumb it should be remembered :

Feet and ankles = Mobility
Knees = Stability
Hips = Mobility
Sacral Iliac Joint & lumbar spine = Stability

If the feet become stiff and / or imbalanced then this can cause a knock on affect up the chain causing the knees to become the mobile element, the hips to become the stability element and the lower back to become the stability element thus leading to dysfunction and pain.

Shoulder Girdle Organization and Ribcage

Shoulder Girdle Mobility & Stability

The shoulder girdle consists of the clavicle and scapula bones including the sterno-clavicular, acromio-clavicular, gleno-humeral and scapulo-thoracic joints. Co ordination of these bones and joints is vital for the mobility and stability of these bones and joints for optimal movement.

The movement of the scapula is particularly important to integrate with the functions and movement of the upper limb. The position and stabilization of the scapula is thus extremely important for optimal force transmission between the upper limb and its connection through the scapula and ribcage to the core.

The shoulder girdle has a direct relationship to the ribcage and through to the hips. The shoulder girdle is largely reliant on the organization of the ribcage in relation to the head and pelvis and thus when looking at dysfunction of the shoulders the ribcage and its position can never be discounted. A common term I have often heard bandied around the Pilates studios is that of 'flared ribs'. I consider this to be an unhelpful term. What do we mean when we say 'flared ribs' ? Usually upon questioning a person about this it turns out that he or she is referring to the rib cage being 'open and stuck forward'. If a person wishes to lift his arms overhead such as when putting the luggage in an overhead locker then he or she must allow the ribcage to 'open' in order to facilitate functional movement of the shoulder girdle and arms. Failure to do so may quite often lead to injury or dysfunction of the shoulder joint. What is usually the case is that the problem has been 'misnamed'. In fact the ribcage has moved forwards in relation to

the pelvis and now puts excessive stress on the lower back and/or neck areas. So therefore we should be naming this problem as an 'anteriorly shifted ribcage in relation to the pelvis'. In this position the respiratory diaphragm is also unable to perform its job of stabilizing the spine and hence we now have a dysfunction of the lumbo pelvic hip complex. Note here that the issue is with the 'organization' of the tissues and not the so called 'core strength' of the individual.

The ribcage area also contains the muscles that directly transfer load from the upper extremities into the core musculature therefore good organization of the shoulder girdle and ribcage is essential for efficient and non problematic function of the upper body.

Spinal Stability / Mobility

The spine has the ability to flex, extend, rotate and sidebend. These movements have a direct and indirect affect on the head position, shoulder girdle, pelvis and lower extremities.

Breathing and Core Control are needed for safe and optimal spinal stability and mobility.

"The potential for Stability lies within the presence of Mobility and the Potential for Mobility lies within the presence of Stability"

Throughout the rest of the book I will try to adhere to the following pre mentioned principles to help the reader understand and achieve greater benefit from the exercises.

Functional unit alignment

Head, ribcage, pelvis and lower extremities of the legs and feet.

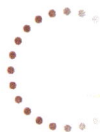

Breathing

Functional breathing patterns which maintain a certain amount of tension in the pelvic floor, torso and diaphragm in accordance to the imposed demand.

Hollowing

A technique used to 'isolate' the transversus abdominus muscle as much as possible.

Core Control

The integration of breathing and lumbo pelvic hip complex stability and mobility.

Lumbo Pelvic Hip Complex

The ability to be aware of the connection between the hip joints, pelvic bones, sacrum, coccyx and lumbar spine.

Feet & Lower Extremities

Ability to transmit and absorb ground reaction forces through the body system for stability, force transmission and propulsion.

Spinal Mobility & Stability

Awareness and ability to move and stabilize segments of the spine

Shoulder Girdle

Awareness and ability to stabilize, mobilize and integrate the upper extremities (arms & shoulder blades) into the ribcage for movement and support.

Integrated Movement

Putting it all together in an efficient and effective manner.

Myofascial Slings

Also known as 'myofascial tracks', 'myofascial kinetic chains', myofascial slings consist of groups or systems of muscles and fascia which act in series to help balance and stabilize the pelvis and axial skeleton thus producing required stability, the stability needed for functional movement or the movement itself.

Thomas Myers – Anatomy Trains

These myofascial tracks were conceived by Thomas Myers who expanded and systematically mapped the conceptual ideas of Ida Rolf and Structural Integration. These lines or myofascial tracks are now popular with both movement and structural therapists alike.

Deep Front Line
Superficial Front Line
Back Line
Front Functional Line
Back Functional Line
Lateral Line
Spiral Line
Deep Front Arm Line
Superficial Front Arm Line
Deep Back Arm Line
Superficial Back Arm Line

Andre Vleeming (Diane Lee)

These slings originate very much from a functional perspective as they are seen to be extremely important in the role of stabilizing the pelvis and spine in movement and having a significant effect on the sacro iliac joint.

Local Core
Anterior Oblique Sling (AOS)
Posterior Oblique Sling (POS)
Lateral Sling
Deep Longitudinal Sling

Muscle and Movement Terminology

This book is not aimed at teaching the reader functional anatomy however a basic understanding of some common movement terms would be of great use to maximize the benefit from the exercises that follow.

Concentric contraction

If a person lifts an object such as a glass / cup of water towards his or her mouth then the muscles of front of the upper arm (biceps muscle) will contract and shorten to bring the glass closer to the persons mouth.

Eccentric contraction

If the person now lowers the glass towards the table with control the muscle fibers of the biceps are still contracting. However this time they are lengthening as they contract because the load (weight of the glass) is greater than the muscular effort being exerted. Hence the muscle lengthens and contracts at the same time. If the weight were to be heavy such as when lowering oneself into a seated position (here the muscles on the front of the thigh would be contracting and lengthening) then the amount of work performed by the lengthening muscle would be sufficient enough to both lengthen and strengthen the muscle.

Important Note

As a general rule when practicing the exercises in this book try to not just think about the muscles that are shortening but inversely see if you can visualize or concentrate on the muscles that are lengthening or 'resisting / decelerating' the movement.
Many Pilates exercises are concerned with the eccentric phase of the movement as opposed to the concentric.

How to do the exercises

Many of the exercises in this book have a QR code printed next to them. If you see this code you can simply scan the code with your phone or mobile device and watch the exercise being performed.
The biggest mistake I consider the beginner makes with Pilates is to try too hard.
Yep for you lazy people out there it sounds too good to be true. A constant rule of thumb I give my students is to give an exercise a score on a scale of one to ten. A score of one equals basically zero effort and a score of ten equals more than eighty percent of maximum effort.
Technically speaking in fact the true score we want to achieve is only a five. This is because good breathing and movement technique should only involve approximately twenty to thirty percent of effort ! However the problem I have found with this approach is that the lack of some intensity in an exercise actually serves to make the exercise uninteresting and the person becomes bored. Conversely if the extensive is too intense then it becomes too difficult reducing the ability to focus on the elements needed in the exercise and there is a lack of achievement felt by the participant.

Therefore I suggest in a balanced forty minute routine the practitioner strives for the following :

• *Begin with breathing exercises*
• *Introduce gentle movement*
• *Practice a repertoire of movements that include all the principles of movement.*
• *Gradually increase the intensity of exercises to a level of seven or eight for approximately fifteen to twenty minutes.*
• *Finish with a cool down, stretching and breathing exercises.*

Remember the the exercises should NOT leave you in a state of exhaustion.
All the moments should be repeated five to eight times.
Focus is on HOW the movement is accomplished and not how far, how much, how many etc.
We are concerned with quality of movement and not quantity.
Whilst many exercises may look very simple and easy to perform it is the work being produced by the individual inside that counts and not how it looks on the outside to the observer. Pilates Master instructor Michael King commonly refers to "Show me your Pilates face" ! Where he refers to the look of ease on the outside but considerable amount of work being produced on the inside to hold or perform a particular movement.

A further note

If there is a left and right side component to the exercise you will see the exercises are described and performed only on one side. There is no preference as to which side to practice first and you should perform the exercises on both sides.

Just a few more useful things to know before we begin

You are probably getting impatient to start exercising right now but please bear with me as there are a few essential things to wrap our heads around first.
It is really worth the while to take a few minutes to learn and palpate some important landmarks on the pelvis. Trust me when I say this will really help gain much more benefit from the exercises that follow.

Anterior Superior Iliac Spine (ASIS) (image no. 1)

In a supine (lying down face up) position place the palms of your hands over the pelvis and gently rub up/down/forwards and backwards. You will notice there are two identical 'bumps' on the left and right

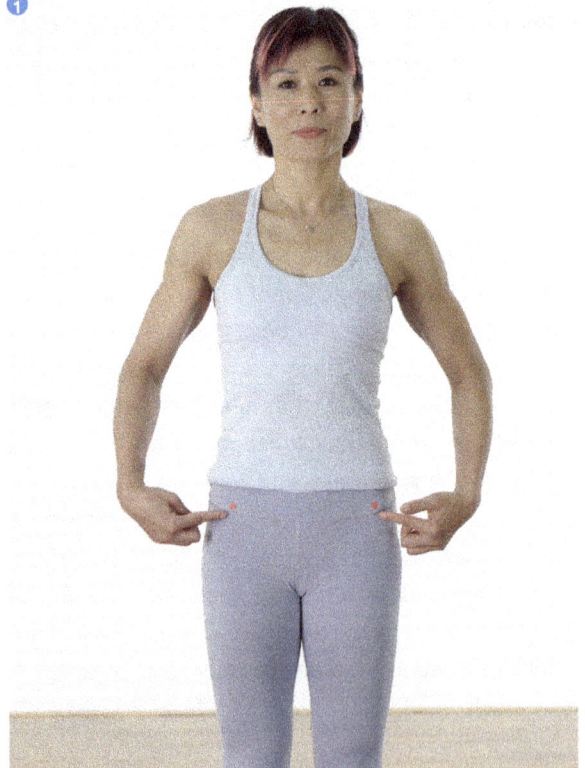

side of the pelvis that are easy to find and stick up into the palm of the hands. Refine your touch by using the fingers of each hand and then refine the touch even further to reduce your sense of touch to your finger tips. Congratulations you just found the left and right ASIS on each side of the pelvis.

Posterior Superior Iliac Spine (image no. 2)

These are the two 'lumpy bits' at the back of the pelvis. To find them come to a standing position and imagine you have a 'sore back'. Place your hands on the ridge of each pelvic side as though you want to press your thumbs into the area that gets sore in your lower back. As you bring your thumbs towards each other you will find a feeling similar to the lumpy bits of the ASIS you just found at the front. You can refine your touch to using your fingers. Congratulations you just found your left and right PSIS.

Pubic bones (image no. 3)

The left and right pubic bones come together at the pubic symphysis at the front of the pelvis. Lie on your back with the legs outstretched straight. Bring your right hand (or left hand if you so wish) to rest flat on your belly with the palm down and the thumb pointing towards your head. Slide the hand slowly towards the groin area applying a flat even pressure. At the place the two legs come together you should feel the edge of the hand meet a bony structure that runs in the center of the groin area from one side to another. With gentle touch you may find this structure to be shaped like a 'wooden dowel'. Great you just found your pubic bone.

Hip joints (image no's 3-5)

Do you know where your hip joints are ? Most people do not. Try standing with feet 'hip width apart' and perform a couple of sitting or squat movements. Bring your attention to where you feel are your hip joints.

Hold your hands as shown in the picture with thumbs pointed towards each other and resting along the length of the pubic bone. In the image you will see a little coloured dot placed at the 'junction' of the thumb and forefinger. Immediately under this point is your hip joint !

Now place your first and second finger over this point and repeat the previous exercise of sitting or

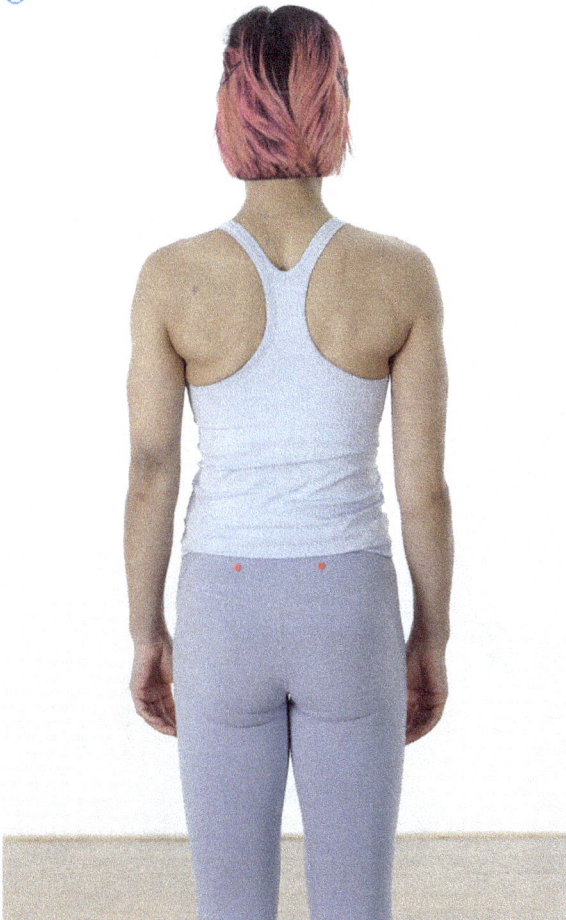

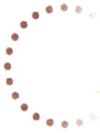

performing a squat. You should now get a sense of the fingers sinking into the joint as you squat and have a sense of the end of the femur (thigh bone) being just like a ball in a hole rotating as you move up and down. This feeling and sense of where is the hip joint will be very important for later exercises.

For instance the 'ball end' of the femur bone needs to rotate as freely as possible in the socket or hole of the hip joint. If the ball is stuck or can not move freely then something somewhere further up the kinetic chain will have to do the movement instead. This is usually the lower back ! Hence now when you walk there is a good chance that excessive tension and pressure is being used by the lower back because the hip joint is not free to move. In other words it is just like your legs are attached to lower spine instead

of your pelvis which is not going to be good news when you start moving.

Performing some of the exercises such as the Femur Arcs although seemingly quite 'boring' in nature are in fact extremely therapeutic as you will learn to stabilize the lower spine and pelvis whilst allowing the hip joints to move as freely as possible thus taking a lot of tension and stress away from the lower back.

This would be a great example of how Pilates can be 'therapeutic' over 'functional' in nature. Of course the next logical step would be to now incorporate this new found therapeutic movement into a functional setting such as walking, running etc.

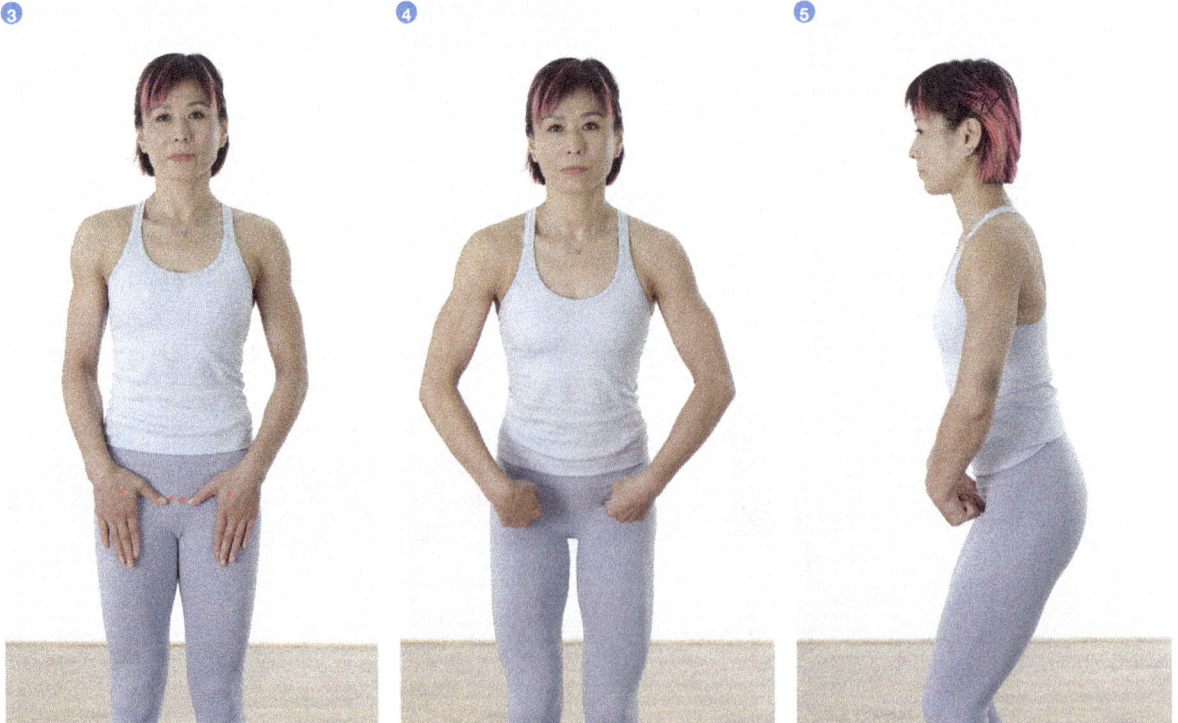

Teaching Skills - Cues

Every teacher needs to communicate with the student to achieve some sort of result. A teacher may refer to any or all of the following cues to achieve this :

Verbal Cue

Verbal cues can be very powerful ways to adjust or change an exercise or movement pattern.

Compare the following :

"Sit up straight" vs "Imagine a giant balloon attached to the top of your head slowly floating upwards and gently lifting the head, neck and spine into one line"
A good teacher will have numerous 'imagery' cues to help achieve the movement required. One teacher is known to connect her clients to an ultrasound machine before going through a list of 20 imagery cues to activate the pelvic floor muscles. Different clients respond to different cues but when one is found that works then all the client has to do is imagine what is verbally cued to 'switch on' her pelvic floor. This kind of cueing is invaluable for both during exercise as well as helping the clients during their daily lives.
Care must be taken however to ensure a verbal imagery cue is one that a client can use from his or her personal experience. A popular story to illustrate this is when teaching someone the bridge exercise and you want them to 'slide' the pelvis from left to right and visa versa. One might say "imagine your pelvis is a typewriter carriage that has to go from side to side". If the student has never used or seen a typewriter the verbal cue is of no use.
Another example is when I mistakenly tried to teach the mechanics of the occipito- atlanto joint on a course by referring the students to the gears of a car. I was receiving blank expressions as all the students whom could drive had only ever driven an automatic or electric car !

Tactile cue

Depending on where you are based in the world the tactile cue is one to avoid or use very often. It depends on the quality of your touch and whether or not you are 'legally entitled' to touch someone at a particular area. In the USA and Europe for instance a tactile cue is commonly preceeded with the words "Do you mind if I touch you here" ?
An example I will commonly use in class is to ask someone if they can flex forward from T4 in the spine which of course they will find impossible to do. However simply touching them very lightly on the spinous process of T4 with your finger tip is enough to give them some proprioceptive awareness of where they should be moving from. Another simple tactile cue is to use a tennis ball (or similar) roll it down the spinous processes as the client performs a standing rolldown.

Tactile cues can be seen as being :

- *Instructive / guided*
- *Assisted*
- *Resisted*

Instructive / Guided

An example of an instructive or guided tactile cue could be the instructor using the hands to illustrate the desired movement of the shoulder blade in a certain movement

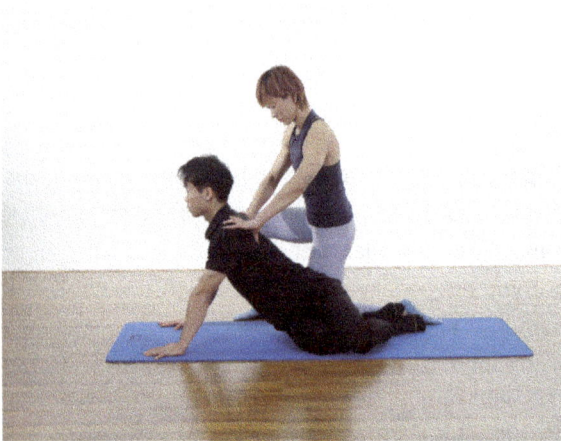

Resisted

For a resisted cue the instructor will provide added resistance giving the client something to push against in order to help perform the exercise. And example of this may be the teaser exercise where instead of helping to lift the legs the teacher presses against the soles of the feet enabling the client to find the correct muscles to perform the movement.

Assisted

In an assisted cue the teacher aids the movement by giving the client support or assistance. And example maybe when performing a Criss Cross exercise and the teacher helps assist the rotation component of the upper body whilst also holding the leg.

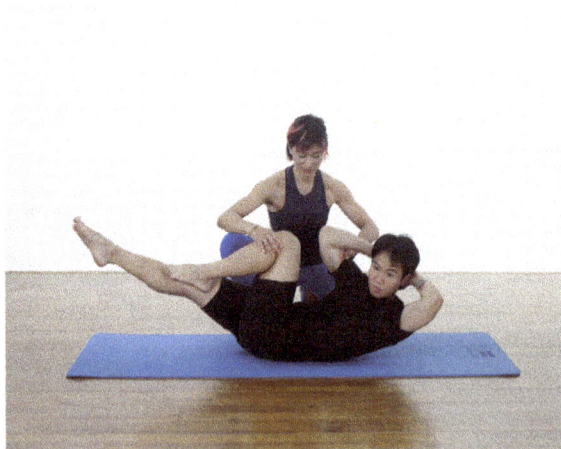

Common Tactile Movement and Stability Cues

Below you will find some safe and effective tactile cues to use with a friend or client. The principles behind the cues remain the same and are not restricted to just the exercises listed below. For instance any exercise that requires a principle of 'spinal flexion' may be helped using the 'Spinal Flexion' cue etc.

Bear in mind that a tactile should always be preceeded with a verbal cue so that the client understands what is required and why you, the instructor, are touching them in this manner. Also remember that the cue is used to enhance the benefit of the movement and should therefore meet the

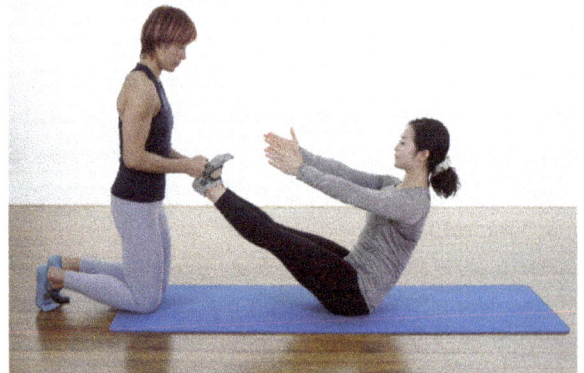

following criteria :

1 *Be safe*
2 *Increase the clients proprioceptive awareness*
3 *Help improve performance of the movement*

Spinal Flexion (top down)

Sit or stand behind the client and gently wrap the hands around each side of the ribcage with your thumbs on the posterior aspect of the ribcage over the twelve rib area. Ask your client to begin to flex down the spine from the head downwards. As you feel the movement reach the 12th rib / vertebra use a gentle scooping movement with the hands to help signal the ribs at the back to lift and move upwards whilst the ribs at the front move downwards and inwards.

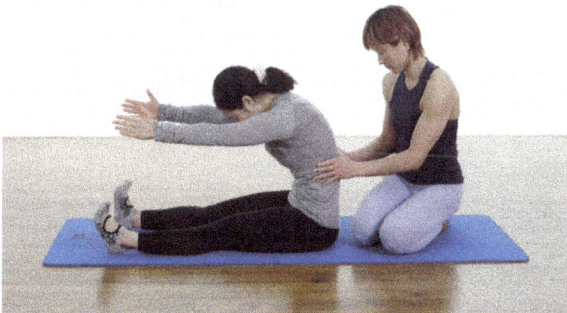

Spinal Extension (top down)

This can be performed in a prone or sitting or standing position.
Use the tips of the fingers on one hand to gently cue the clavicles and sternum to lift and 'move upwards' whilst the fingers of the other hand walk down the vertebra one at a time to encourage the sensation of 'dropping inwards and downwards' .

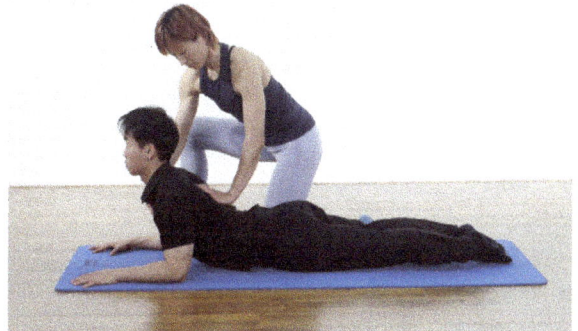

Flexion from Supine Position

Resisted, Assisted or Instructional cues can be used depending on the client.

Because the movement goes against gravity one of the desired outcomes of the movement is to encourage an abdominal hollowing so that the rectus abdominus muscle is not the dominant muscle for the movement. You should experiment with each one to see which one works for which type of client. For instance you may find that the action of holding the ankles works very well on clients with overactive rectus femoris muscles.

Resistance cue by stabilizing the ankles as the client rolls upwards or downwards during the movement
Assisted cue by helping to pull / lift the client from

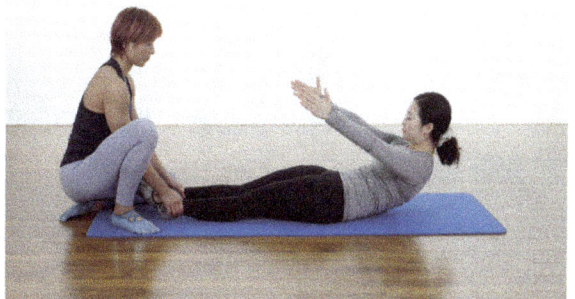

the mat as he or she initiates the rolling up movement.

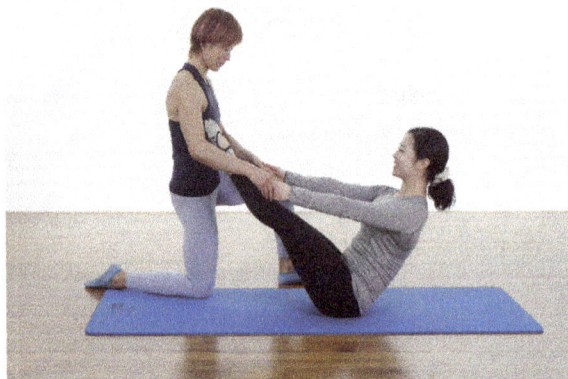

Spinal Rotation

An instructive cue where the instructor places a flat hand on the back of the ribcage and the other hand flat on the front of the ribs. As the client initiates a rotation the hands guide and slide the ribcage in the required direction.

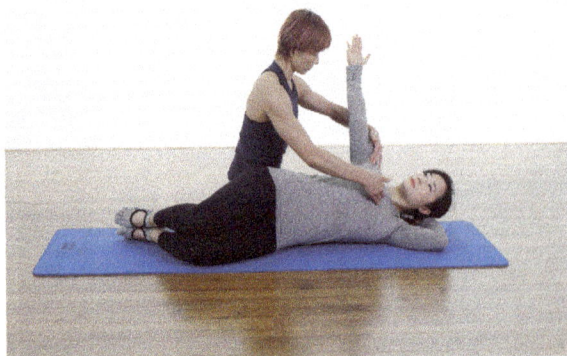

Lumbo-Pelvis Stabilization

A classic cue to use when teaching dead bug or similar exercise. One hand is placed gently against the lumbar vertebrae (especially L2,L3,L4) and the other hand lies gently on the lower belly. The hand placement gives the client proprioceptive feedback as to what is happening in his or her lower back and pelvis as the hips flex and extend.

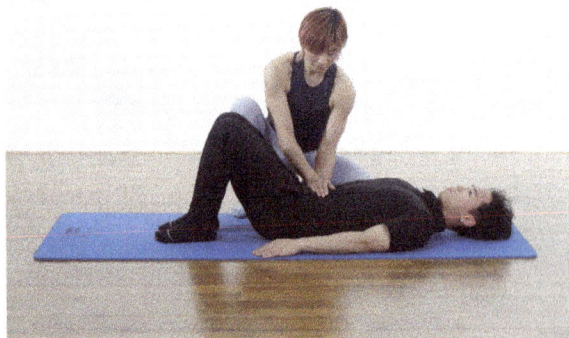

Gluteus Maximus Activation

Another classic cue. Because the gluteus Maximus muscle is such an important and often dysfunctional muscle it is good to have a simple quick test to see if it indeed is 'switched on'. The client performs a bridge and the instructor tries to lift the foot from the floor by pulling in a vertical direction. If the gluteus Maximus muscle is being activated optimally the foot will stay on the floor however if the client is using too much lower back muscles (thinking it is the glute max) then it will be easy to lift from the floor.

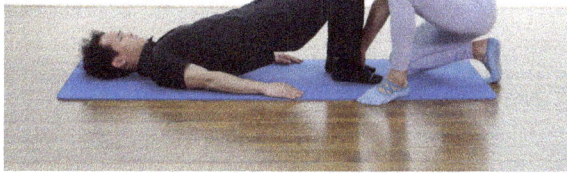

Almost ready to begin .... Breathing

Whats the very first thing you do and the very last thing you do in your life ?

Breathe in .... breathe out...........

Why choose breathing as the first exercise ?

If I had to pick only one of the principles and only practice that one I would most definitely choose breathing. Traditionally Pilates utilizes a type of breathing referred to as 'lateral posterior breathing'. What this means is that the practitioner maximises the use of the lower ribs to lift and expand sideways and 'backwards' to help create more space in the back of the ribs for the lungs to expand. If you were to open the chest wall on a body and look down on the lungs you will find that they sit very nicely in two 'cavities' at the back of the ribcage. There is no such space of cavity at the front of the ribcage meaning that we are designed to breath into the back of the ribs and not be lifting the front such as when you see the 'anterior' ribcage pattern. In essence when we breathe there

should be three parts :

The diaphragm lowers and increases the pressure in the abdominal cavity and the abdomen wall 'eccentrically resists' this pressure ie: it expands with tension.

As the diaphragm finishes moving down the central part of the diaphragm now becomes fixed and the begins to pull on the outer attachments connected to the ribcage. Along with the expansion of the lungs and recruitment of other associated respiratory muscles this causes the lower ribs of ten, nine, eight, seven and six to lift up to the sides whilst pivoting on the vertebral attachments and increase the volume of the ribcage especially towards the back.

As the inhalation continues the ribs five, four, three, two and one move is a slightly different orientation with ribs three, two and one having an emphasis on lifting from the front.

The attachment of the ribs at the spine forms a series of complex joints essential to the health of the spine. The movement of the ribs creates a pumping movement to help replenish the intervertebral discs with hydration and thus keep the spine mobile. If the discs were to lose hydration the vertebral joints would become compressed and cause a loss of mobility. This loss of mobility would now mean that the ribcage can not expand optimally and the individual would simply not be able to breathe properly ! This resultant loss of respiration potential would now create more loss of mobility in the spine and so on in a vicious cycle.

So now think about the number of times a day an individual breathes (or attempts to breathe). Somewhere in the region of fifteen thousand to twenty thousand times a day !

Your typical office worker is going to benefit immensely just from practicing good breathing exercises fifteen to twenty minutes every day !

The following exercises are designed to help improve your natural breathing. Please note that these exercises are breathing exercises and not necessarily how you should be breathing all day. The exercises are designed to help promote improved breathing during the day when you are not thinking about it !

Common Terms

Here's some common terms you will come across in the instructions on practicing the exercises :

Supine

Lying on your back face up

Prone

Lying face down

Sidelying

Lying on one side of the body

Triple Flexed Position

Lying supine with the hips, knees and ankles flexed so that the soles of the feet are on the floor and knees bent.

ASIS

Anterior Superior Iliac Spine (the bumpy bits at the front of your pelvis as described above) see page 140

PSIS

Posterior Superior Iliac Spine (the bumpy bits at the back of your pelvis as described above) see page

141

Dorsi Flexion

Positioning the foot by moving the ankle joint so that the top of the foot moves towards the leg

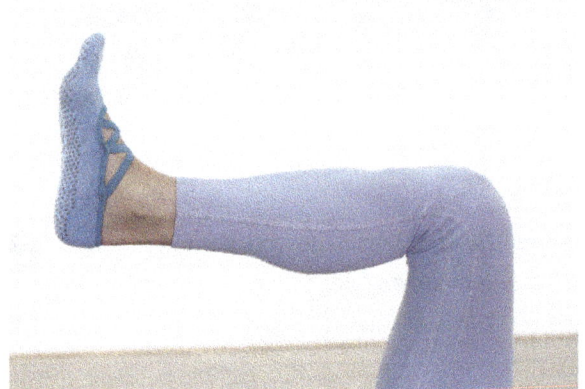

Plantar Flexion

Positioning the foot by moving the ankle joint so that the top of the foot moves away from the leg - also commonly referred to as 'pointing the foot',

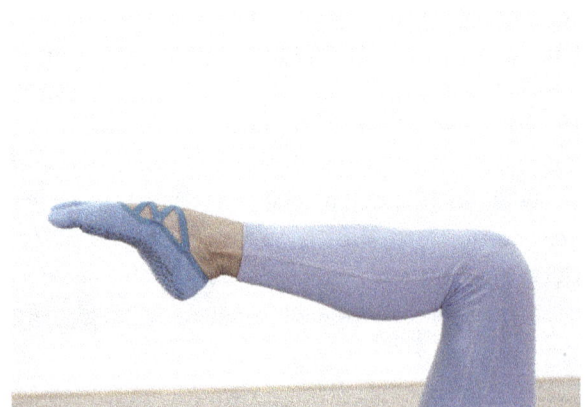

Vacuum

The act of drawing the belly button into the spine and 'up into the ribcage'

Apnea

A period of time with no inhalation (ie holding your breath).

Neutral Spine

A position of all the vertebrae in the spine whereas each one is optimally stacked on the one below to maximize distribution of load through the spine and allow maximum space between each vertebra for the nerves. In a 'neutral spine' position there should be naturals curves of the spine when looked at from the side.

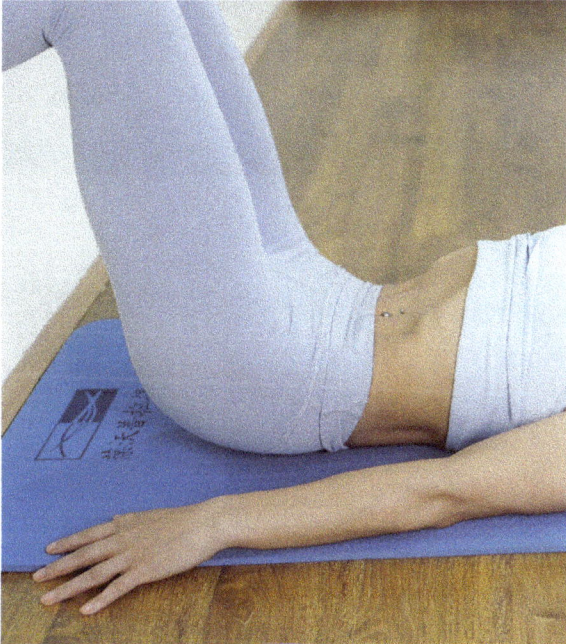

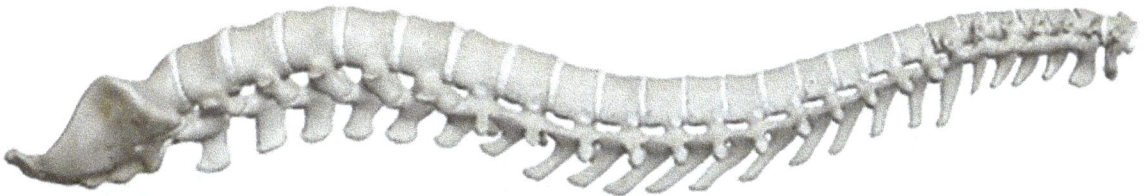

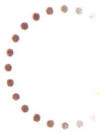

Breathing-01

Crocodile Breathing

Benefits

Improve diaphragm function and reduce tension
in the lower back
Helps reduce sympathetic tone.

Contraindications & Precautions

Pregnancy

Principles

Breathing

Cues

Verbal : Feel the belly pressing to the floor and
the lower back lengthen (between my hands)
Tactile : One hand on the sacrum and other
hand over T12/L1

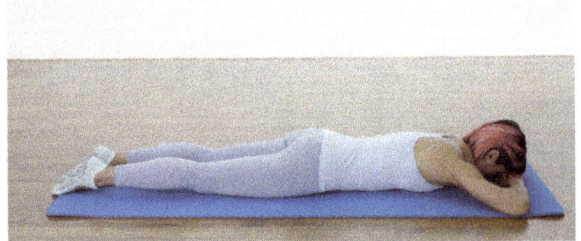

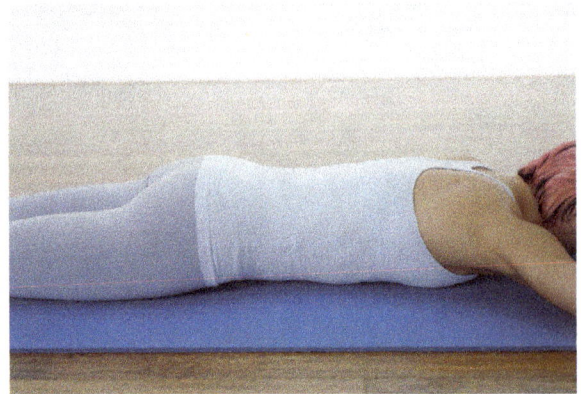

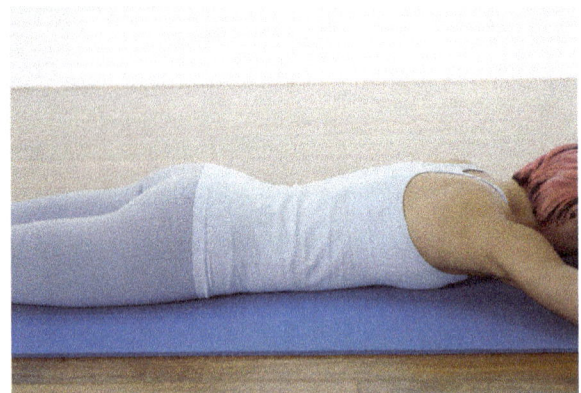

Set Up & Movement

Lie on belly with hands under the forehead. Focus on the inhalation part of the breath. Feel how when you inhale the belly presses into the floor and in turn causes the pelvis to 'rock backwards' making the lower back flatten out and stretch the lower back muscles. This process also helps to strengthen the diaphragm muscle and reduce stress on the kidneys which in Chinese medicine are considered a prime source of energy and vitality.

Continue for approximately ten minutes or longer if so wished.

Do you feel the belly or chest press into the floor first ?

Breathing - 02

Supine Breathing

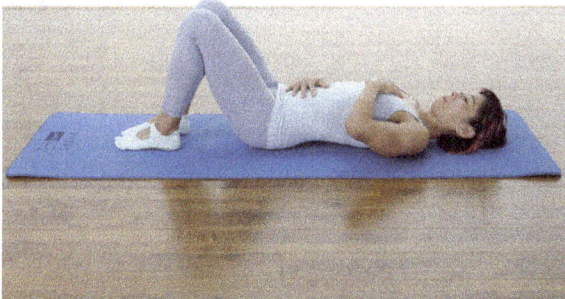

Contraindications & Precautions

Do not stay too long in this position after 2nd trimester of pregnancy.

Set Up

Lie on your back with the legs in the triple flexed position hip width apart. Place your right hand over the belly and the left hand over the chest.

Movement

Take a gentle inhalation and observe which hand 'moves first'. Gently exhale and observe which hands moves first on the exhalation.

Continue breathing whilst using a count of :

Inhalation for 4 counts

Hold the breath for 4 counts

Exhalation for 6 counts

Hold the breath for 4 counts.

You can count to yourself something like this …. "IN 2,3,4 - HOLD 2,3,4 - OUT 2,3,4,5,6 HOLD 2,3,4 - IN, 2,3,4" etc…

Principles

Breathing

Whilst breathing in this manner observe how the sides and back of the lower ribs expand outwards and backwards into the floor on the inhalation. If you don't feel this movement then possibly you are restricted in this area of breathing or maybe you are not 'kinesthetically aware' of this movement. Remember one of the goals of Pilates is help increase an awareness of oneself internally and externally within space.

Secondly, on the inhalation observe how the

Inhalation

Exhalation

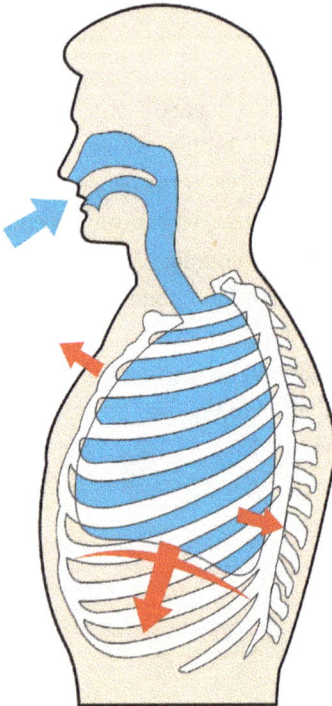

Diaphragm moves downwards
Upper ribs expand upwards
Lower ribs expand outwards and backwards

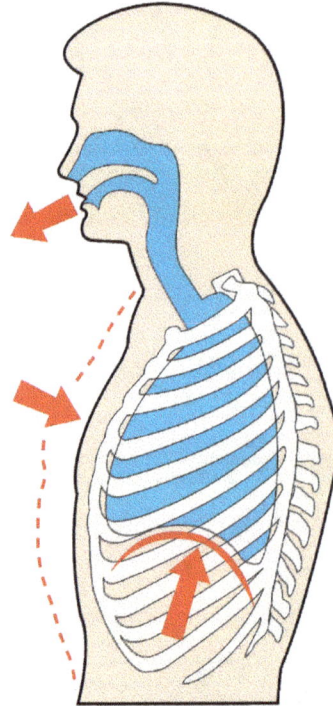

Diaphragm moves upwards
Ribs relax downwards and inwards

movement of the ribs changes so that the upper ribs move upwards as the thoracic spine flattens out as a continuation of the lower rib movement.

Spend 3 - 5 minutes in this position observing your breath but using a natural, gentle amount of effort.

Supine Breathing to Lower and Upper Ribs

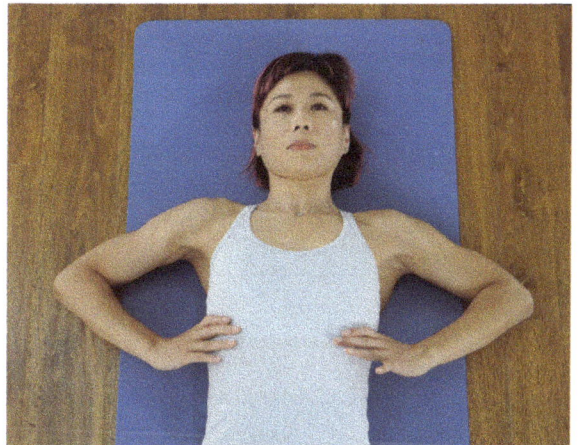

Benefits

Improve awareness of natural breathing pattern
Prepare for breathing exercises
Release tension in mid back area
Help reduce sympathetic tone

Cues

Verbal : Self count period for inhalation - hold - exhalation - hold

Tactile : One hand over the belly and the other hand over the chest

Which hand moves first on the inhalation ?
Can you feel the movement of the belly - lower ribs and upper ribs ?

On the Exhalation which hand moves first ?
You may determine that the hand over the abdomen moves first if you are using the abdominal muscles to push the air out however see if you can find the difference between the 'chest hand' and the 'abdominal hand' moving first on the exhalation. How does that make you feel ?

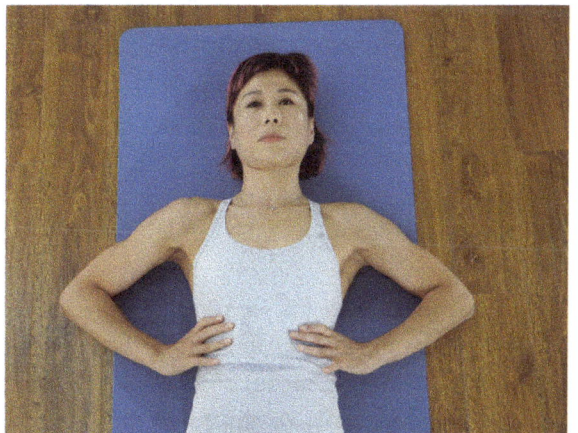

Contraindications & Precautions

Do not stay too long in this position after 2nd trimester of pregnancy.

Benefits

Improves posterior thoracic breathing pattern
Helps activate the intercostal breathing muscles
May help with neck and back pain

Principles

Breathing

Cues

Verbal : Imagine your ribs like Venetian blinds opening and closing.

Tactile : Place the hands on the sides of ribs or alternatively see if you can place your fingers along the spaces between the ribs.

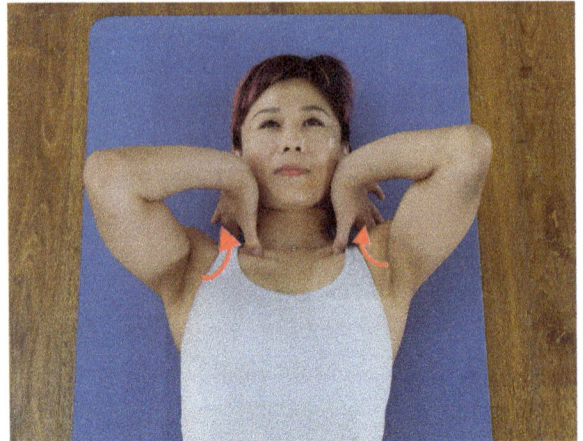

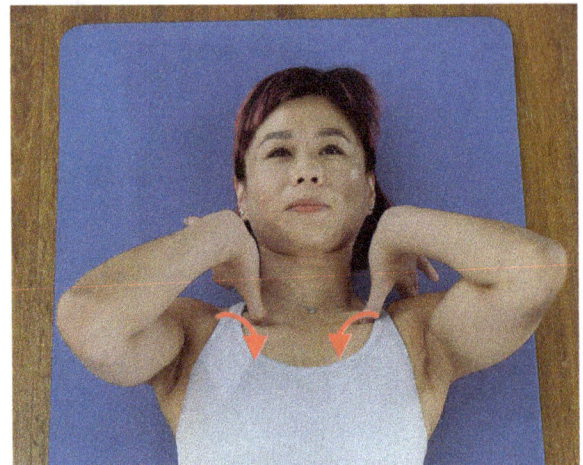

Lie on your back with the legs in the triple flexed position. Place the palms of your hands over the sides of the lower ribcage and apply a gentle 'pressing pressure' towards the center of the body from each hand.

Inhale and observe how the ribs expand outwards into the hands and backwards into the floor.

Exhale and observe how the ribs relax away from the hands.

Now change your hand positions so that the palms face upwards and the thumbs gently 'hook' into the under part of the collar bone (clavicle) .

Observe now the movement (if any) of the clavicle (collar bone) in the last stage of the inhalation. The clavicle should rotate and lift upwards around the fulcrum of the sternoclavicular joint (where the clavicle attaches to the sternum).

On the exhalation the clavicle will lower and rotate downwards.

Summary of Exercises 1 & 2

After completing exercises 1 and 2 it is hoped you will be able to determine the different stages of a 'complete breath' beginning with an inhalation :

• *Diaphragm moves downwards*
• *Abdomen expands in 4 directions - front, left, right, backwards*
• *Lower ribs lift sideways and expand backwards (bucket handle movement)*
• *Upper ribs lift upwards (pump handle movement)*
• *Clavicle rotates upwards and elevates*

All of the above happens on the Inhalation. However note that these movements are also happening together - they do not exist by themselves one by one. It's probably better to think of the sequence as 'a tendency for one part to lead the others' as opposed to isolated movements.
Now - do the following listed in the yellow box below

Try exhaling with different amounts of effort.
Try an open mouth with relaxed jaw.
Make different sounds as you exhale : sshhhh or maybe aaaaahhhh or a psshhh.
Imagine you are blowing up a balloon.

What happens to your abdominal muscles on the various exhalations ?

Can you feel how the sounds engage the abdominal muscles in different ways ?
We are looking for the sound that helps engage the Tranversus abdominus and oblique muscle groups
When these muscles engage the waist will narrow and the front of the abdomen will 'hollow' somewhat so that they help to push the air out of the lungs.

Breathing - 04

Breathing in Sitting

Practice the same breathing exercise as before in a sitting position either cross legged on the floor or sitting on a chair.
There are a couple of things to be aware of in the sitting position :

1) Gravity
Gravity has changed. Meaning that the abdominal, back and other postural muscles need to be engaged in the upright position.

2) Awareness
The upright position means there is no proprioceptive awareness of your spine in relation to the floor which makes it harder to determine the position of the spine.
The change in gravity and spinal awareness may produce a considerable change in the way you breathe. Observe how this compares to the supine position in the different stages of the breathing cycle.

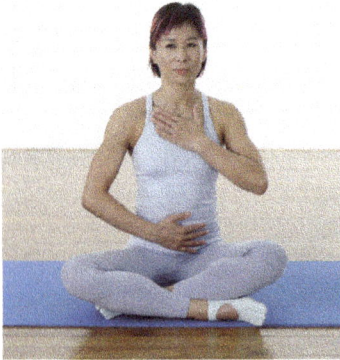

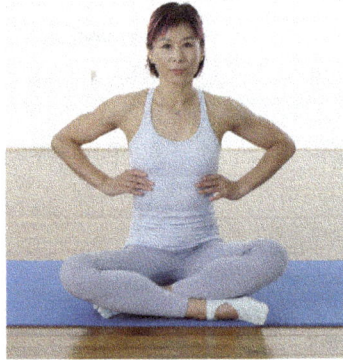

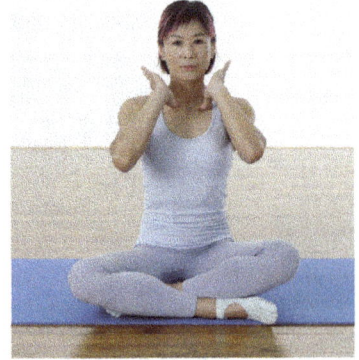

Breathing - 05

90 - 90 Supine Breathing with Pelvic Curl

Lie supine with feet against the wall and hips at 90

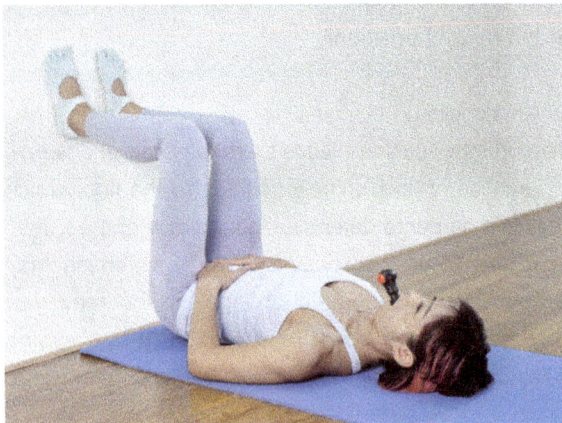

Contraindications & Precautions

Pregnant women and persons with high or low blood pressure should not hold their breath

degrees. Place a straw, balloon or breathing apparatus in the mouth to create some tension on the exhalation.

Inhale to the lower and mid rib cage and exhale through the straw, balloon or breathing apparatus. On the exhalation focus on :

• *The spaces between the ribs on the sides of the ribcage gently closing.*
• *The waist narrows*
• *The abdominals 'hollow'*
• *The area under the hands on the pelvis 'shrinks and tightens'*

Perform 8 - 10 repetitions.

Now on the exhalation roll the pelvis backward towards your chest so that your butt gently lifts from the floor and your lower back rounds slightly. Stop lifting and rounding the spine when you reach the point of contact of the ribcage on the floor.

Now perform an inhalation with focus on the breath coming to the posterior lateral part of the ribcage.

Exhale again in this position and hold the breath.

Whilst holding the breath roll the spine and pelvis

back to the Start position.

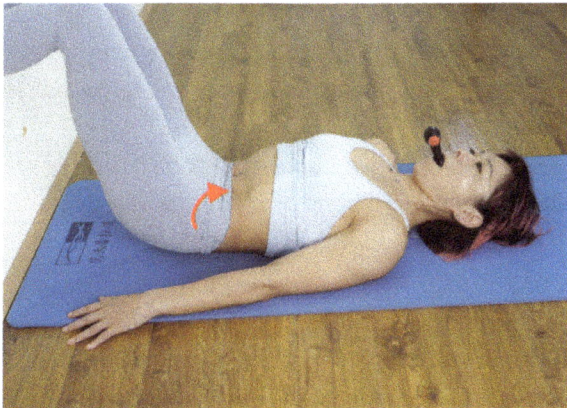

To recap :

Move on the first exhalation
Hold position on the first inhalation
Hold position on the second exhalation
Hold the breath to roll back down
Second inhalation is performed in start position.

Breathing - 06

90/90 Breathing with Breath Hold and Vacuum.

When performing the forced exhalation can you maintain length in the front of the abdomen so that the muscles 'close from the sides' instead of shortening from the front.

However if you have a contraindicated condition you should be able to perform the following exercises simply by leaving out the breath holding and vacuum part.

Again common sense is the number one rule to follow and if in doubt consult a qualified professional It should also be noted that the breathing exercises should be performed with 'relative comfort' meaning that you should use no more than 30 - 50 % effort. That means if you are instructed to exhale as much

Benefits

Improve diaphragm function, improve use of abdominal component of breathing, improve stabilization of lower back and pelvis, improve lateral posterior breathing, open the rib cage, release hyperpressive tension on the pelvic floor muscles and internal organs, release tension in mid and upper back, release tension in neck ...... and many more !

Principles

Breathing

air as possible you do so using only 30 - 50 % of effort to do so. Other muscles in our body respond well to maximal stimulus that is - if you wish to increase muscle size of your legs then performing weight exercises to failure is usually a good way to go. However do not confuse this rationale with what we are doing here.

The respiratory system does NOT respond well to maximal stimuli and if we were to do so we can have an adverse effect on many aspects of heathy body functions.

This exercise is essentially split into 3 parts :

Part 1 - Focuses on the exhalation phase and encourages you feel the contraction of the transversus abdominus and pelvic floor muscles.

Part 2 - Brings your attention to the inhalation phase

Part 3 - Involves a 'vacuum' or 'drawing in' of the abdominal wall whilst holding an Exhalation.

Part 1 : 90/90 Exhalation

Perform the 90 / 90 Breathing exercise as listed above for 5 - 8 repetitions with the feet against the wall and hips at 90 degrees. Place the hands either by your sides or make a triangle with the hands and place on the pelvis.

Preferably use a straw, balloon or breathing apparatus in the mouth to create some tension on the exhalation. Inhale to the lower and mid rib cage and exhale through the straw, balloon or breathing apparatus. On the exhalation focus on :

The spaces between the ribs on the sides of the ribcage gently closing.
The waist narrows
The abdominals 'hollow'

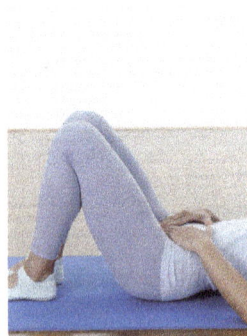

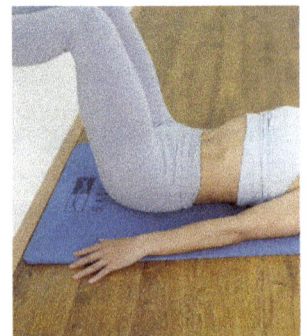

The area under the hands on the pelvis 'shrinks and tightens'

Part 2 : 90/90 'Inhalation'

Continue with the exhalation part of the exercise but now mentally shift your focus to the inhalation phase. After an exhalation hold the breath for a five count

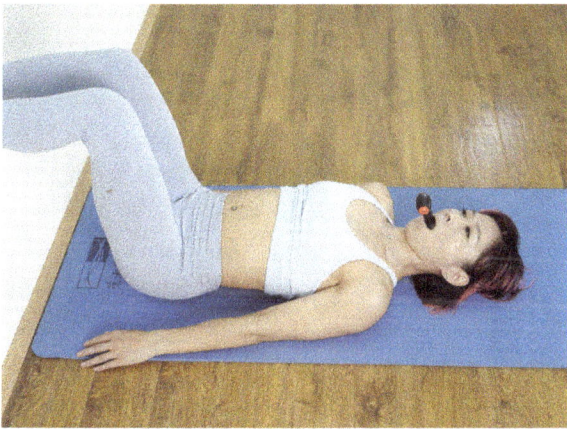

Inhalation - the abdominals and rib cage expands

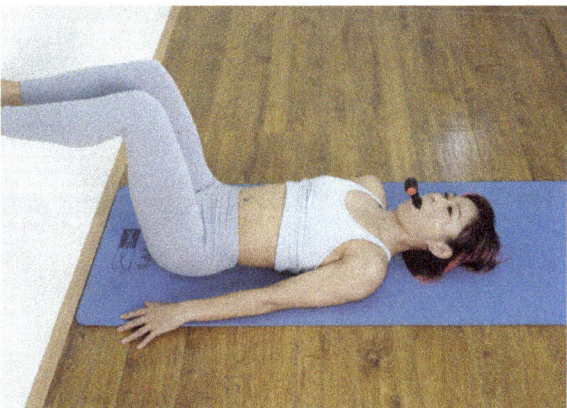

Exhalation - the ribcage contracts - abdominals contract and tighten / narrow

without letting any air in. On the inhalation focus on maintaining the tension of the pelvic area tissue as before but now bring your attention to the ability of the ribs to expand backwards and outwards (posteriorly and laterally) into the floor. Lying on your back on the floor allows you get wonderful feedback from the floor as to just how well the ribs are expanding in both directions. If you are a habitual chest breather the feeling of the ribs expanding into the floor and outwards will come as a comfortable surprise . The feeling is often described as though you are being pulled into the floor'.

Continue with the exhalation and inhalation as follows :

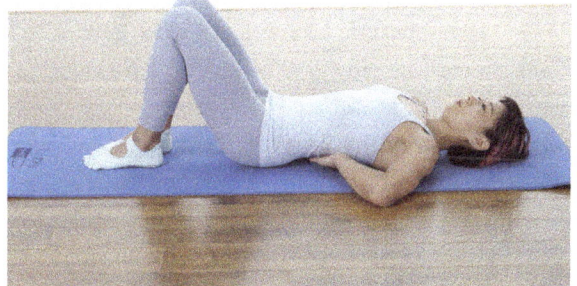

You can place the hands on the mat palms downwards to help feel the ribs expand

Inhalation : 5 counts
Breath hold : 3 - 4 counts
Exhalation : 5 counts
Breath hold : 3 - 4 counts

And so on for a total of 8 - 10 rounds / breaths.

Part 3 : 'Hollowing'

Now the focus will shift towards you being able to engage the tranversus abdominus (TA) muscle and the pelvic floor musculature. The TA is the muscle that wraps around your waist like a corset and is important for keeping the abdominal organs in place. If this muscle is dysfunctional then the muscles that lay over the top of it (oblique muscles) can not do their job properly to stabilize the torso.

Imagine you have a bag of jelly that needs to be wrapped up. If you try to wrap another bag around the jelly bag then you won't be able to make it very tight, the jelly will keep popping out everywhere. However if you were to get some cling film and wrap this around the jelly bag first it will enable you to wrap the whole thing up quite nicely using another bag on top. The TA is the cling film around the jelly bag !

In my studios in Shanghai we use a 'hypopressive' approach to 'switching on' the transverses abdominus muscle. This is different to the traditional Pilates approach but I have found this is a useful component of learning to access your 'core muscles' not just for Pilates but for every sport you can think of. It is also a fantastic exercise to use for post natal recovery. The reason for this is it reduces the pressure in the abdomen instead of increasing the pressure which is what most exercises do. The decrease in pressure helps to switch on the TA muscle without accidentally using the more dominant oblique muscles which lie immediately over the TA. Another benefit is that the reduction in pressure pulls the pelvic floor and diaphragm muscles as well as the abdominal organs in an upwards direction making it an invaluable tool for training the pelvic floor and maintaining the health of the abdominal organs which more often than not are in a unhealthy descended position in most people which in turn contribute to hundreds of pathologies and muscle skeletal dysfunctions.

I believe this one particular exercise so important that if I had to choose only one exercise to do the rest of my life and no other then I would most definitely choose this one ! Yoga practitioners may recognise this as learning to 'switch on' Uddiyana bandha.

To perform the exercise we begin with the exhalation and contraction of the tissue under our hands on the pelvis. Now instead of going straight on to the part for the ribcage inhalation we add another component.

Immediately after exhalation hold your breath and don't let any air come in. Cover your mouth with one hand and pinch your nose with the the thumb and fingers of the other hand. With your airways now blocked it should be impossible to breathe in any air. Now, relax your abdomen (this is important !) and 'try to breathe in' whilst keeping the airways covered. You will find that your belly starts to 'get sucked in and up' towards your chest. This 'sucking in' or 'drawing in' of the TA muscle is a vital component to also using the pelvic floor muscles.

Other cues to help you access the pelvic floor musculature are as follows :

Ok so now you know how to access your pelvic floor muscles along with the TA muscle we can continue the exercise.

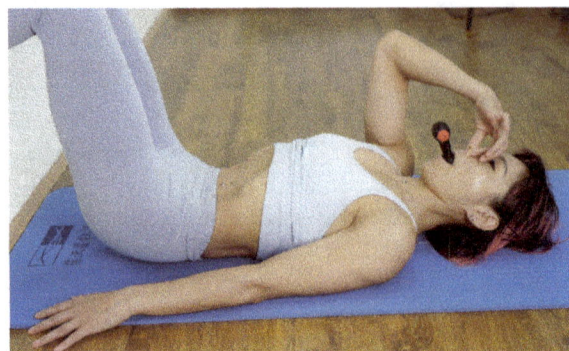

Hold this exhalation (with TA and pelvic floor contraction) position with one hand over the mouth (or in our case with the breathing apparatus in the mouth) and the other pinching the nose for a count of 5.

If you focus only on the vacuum without the hands covering the mouth and nose to begin with how does this change the exercise ?

For Guys :

Exhale and narrow your waist. Towards the end of the exhalation imagine you are putting on a tight pair of jeans and 'suck you nuts up' ! Yep - sorry ladies but I have found there is not a guy on the planet who can not follow that cue. So if you are a yoga or pilates teacher looking for a cue for the guys I suggest you either get used to saying this to your clients in an appropriate manner of just simply write it down and let the guy read it !

For the ladies :

Exhale and narrow your waist. Towards the end of the exhalation imagine you are putting on a tight pair of jeans and that you can 'suck a small ping pong ball up your vagina' that was conveniently placed between your legs at the start of the

exercise ! Now imaging the ball floating around in your pelvis and see if you can 'draw it up towards your belly button'. There are a couple of ways you can do this. The first is by using quick contractions and the second is by maintaining a constant slow and relatively gentle contraction. Experiment with both ideas and try to use each as often as possible.

This holding the breath for 5 counts is important to allow you to shift your mental focus to the next step whilst also allowing your body to build a tolerance towards carbon dioxide in the body which is excellent for the blood and calming the nerves.

After the 5 count take the hands to the side of the ribcage and focus on a deep but gentle inhalation whilst maintaining tension on the abdominal muscles and pelvic floor.

BUT - I hear you say, when you inhale the pelvic floor SHOULD go down ! Yes this is correct however you will find that in actual fact it WILL go down - it's just a case of whether it goes down all floppy or if it moves downwards in a controlled manner still under tension - remember the term 'eccentric contraction' ?

Repeat the exercise 5 - 10 times or even more if appropriate.

To summarize :

Inhale - count of 5
Hold your breath - count of 4
Exhale - count of 6
Hold your breath - count of 4 - 6
Whilst holding the breath :
Relax the abdomen
Draw the abdominal wall inwards and upwards
Inhale to the back of the ribs

You may most certainly spend your time practicing only the breathing exercises listed above for at least 4 - 8 weeks before embarking on the rest of the exercises. It is of great importance to spend time focusing on the basis for the exercises to obtain the maximum benefit.

You may also wish to practice the exercises in different positions. If you don't have a breathing

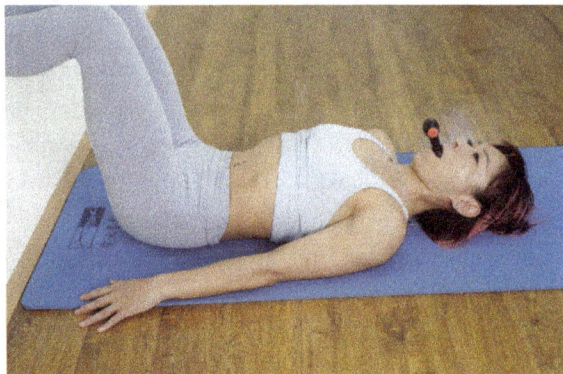

Inhale - Exhale

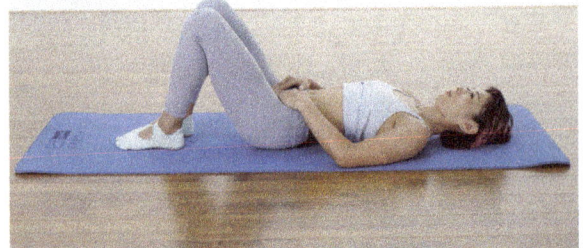

Inhale - count of 5
Hold the breath - count of 4

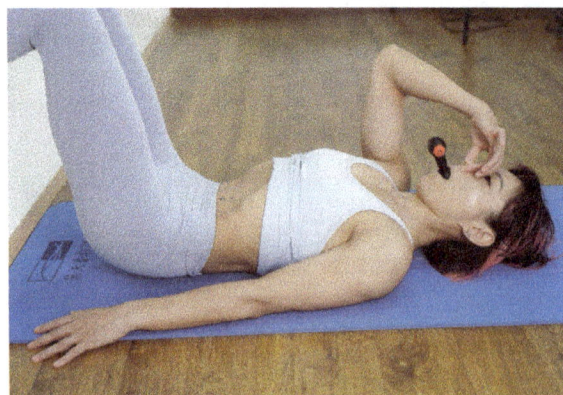

Hold the breath and relax the abdomen

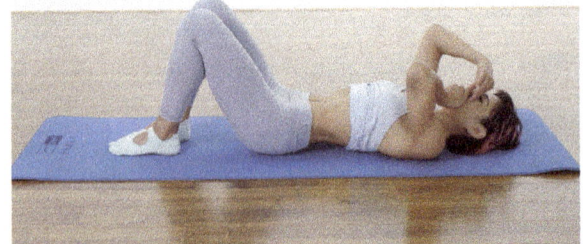

Exhale - count of 6
Hold the breath and relax the belly.'Hollow' the abdominal cavity drawing inwards and upwards.

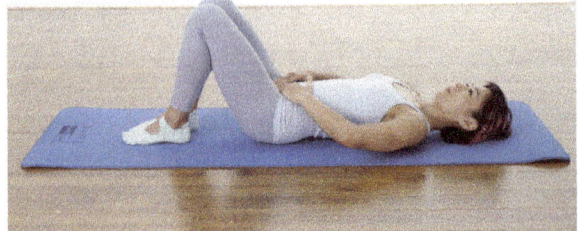

Cover the nose and mouth and hollow the abdominals whilst still holding the breath.

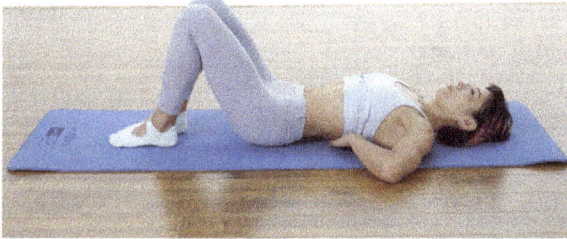

Inhale to the back of the ribs

trainer or straw handy you can simply practice without. You may also practice without using a wall with the hips and legs in the triple flexed position.

If you are coming into the exercises from a rehabilitative perspective due to chronic musculoskeletal dysfunction or pain you may well indeed be very pleasantly surprised just how much improvement can be obtained simply by practicing these breathing exercises themselves.

So what's next ?

After gaining some proficiency and some awareness of your breathing and core musculature it is now time to include these into the mat exercises. It is important to understand that your core muscles are basically your breathing muscles. For instance you will quite often see a 'Plank' exercise as being one to

Scan the QR code to view the exercise 90/90 with abdominal hollowing

train your core. This however is not the case as performing a plank will not improve your core. What it does do however is integrate the muscles of the upper and lower body into the core muscles which means that you need to have some semblance of core muscle activation BEFORE you attempt a plank. If you are not convinced I challenge you to perform the Plank before and after the breathing exercises listed above. You will almost undoubtably find that you have much better control and stability after you have learned to 'switch on' the core muscles related to your breathing than if you perform the exercise without this ability.

Exercise Progressively

There is no need to go all out and perform all the exercises in this book immediately after doing the breathing exercises. However feel free to go through the exercises at your discretion just so that you can have an awareness or baseline of how they feel for your body at the start of your exercise plan. In fact you may wish to practice the exercises BEFORE you have performed the breathing exercises just to gain an extra comparison.

A basic rule of thumb for a exercise sequence can be seen in the following chart. One should note that this sequence may occur in a single session or be broken up into multiple sessions depending on the individuals ability or if he or she is in need of rehabilitative or corrective exercise.

So now lets move onto the next sequence of exercises where we will attempt to bring in the other principles of movement as listed previously with regards to the spine, pelvis and linking the upper and lower extremities into the core. We can simply label these are being 'Preparation Mat Exercises'.

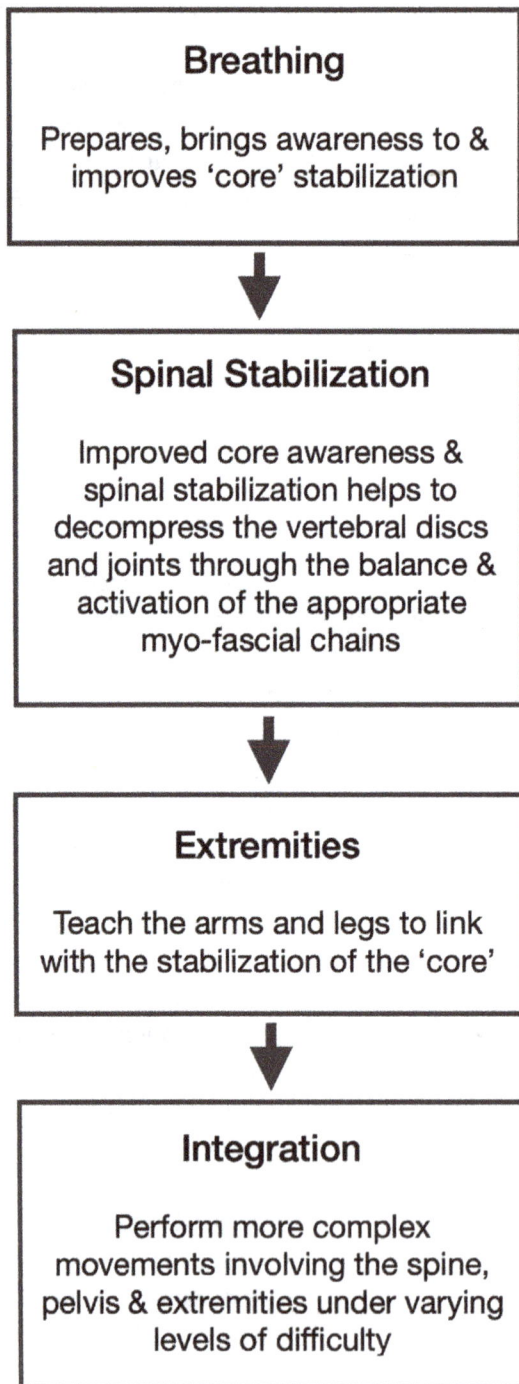

Breathing

Prepares, brings awareness to &
improves 'core' stabilization

⬇

Spinal Stabilization

Improved core awareness &
spinal stabilization helps to
decompress the vertebral discs
and joints through the balance &
activation of the appropriate
myo-fascial chains

⬇

Extremities

Teach the arms and legs to link
with the stabilization of the 'core'

⬇

Integration

Perform more complex
movements involving the spine,
pelvis & extremities under varying
levels of difficulty

CHAPTER

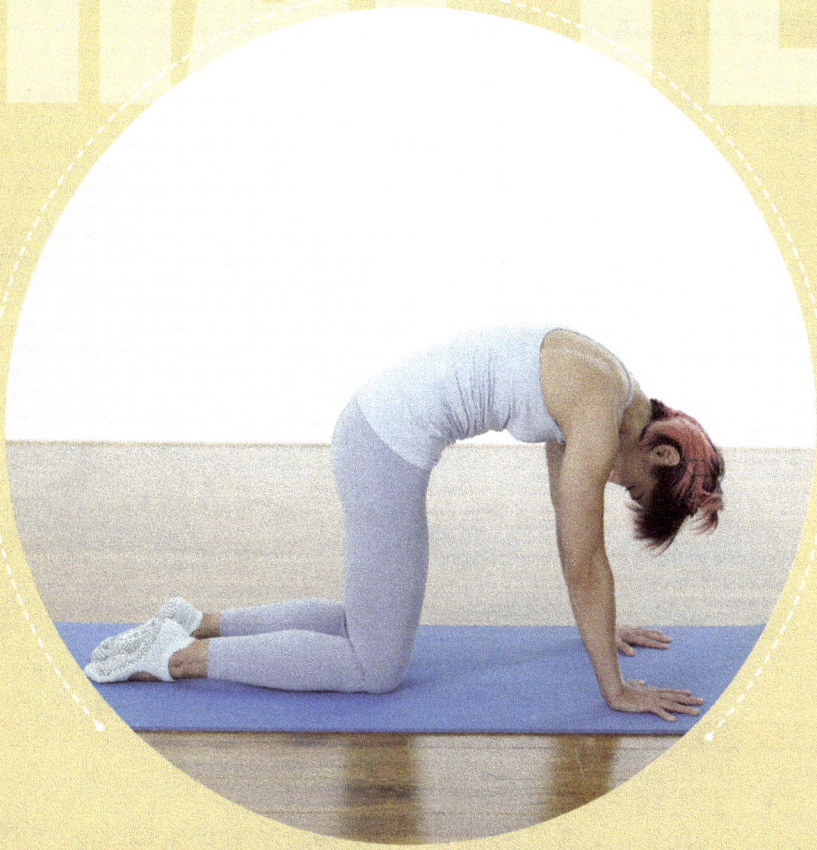

Seven

Preparation Mat Exercises (PM)

7.1 'Preparation Mat Exercises' (PM)

PM1 - Pelvic Clock

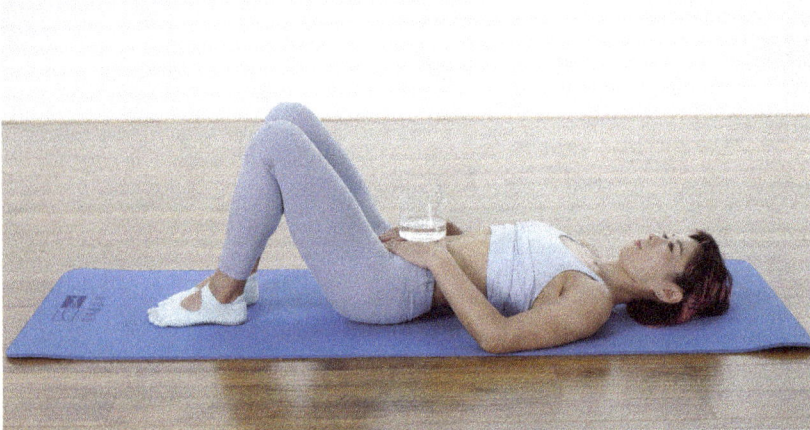

Contraindications & Precautions

There are no specific contraindications for the Pelvic Clock exercise however persons with low back pain and particularly those with a spondylolisthesis may find the extension movements uncomfortable if performed using the lower back muscles as the drivers.

Benefits

Release lower back tension
Improve movement of the hip joints
Improve spinal flexion and extension
Brings awareness to the lumbo pelvic hip complex
Increase awareness of lower abdominal muscles

Principles

Breathing
Lumbo Pelvic Hip Complex mobility
Core Control

Part 1- Anterior - Posterior

Set Up

Lie on your back with hips flexed in the 'triple flexed position'.

Bring the thumbs and tips of each forefinger together on each hand to from a triangle made from the border of the thumbs and forefingers. Now place the hands over the lower abdomen and pelvic area so that the tips of the middle fingers and / or forefingers are touching your pubic bone.

Movement

Close your eyes and imagine a glass of water on the hands resting over your pelvis. Is the water in the cup level or is the cup tilted ? Try moving your pelvis in a forwards movement to tilt the imaginary cup so that water would spill towards the feet (anterior tilt) and then try tilting the pelvis backwards so that the water would spill onto you belly (posterior tilt).

Continue this anterior and posterior tilting of the pelvis and then choose the position you consider to be exactly half way. The imaginary water should be level to the floor and your pelvis would now be in what we term a 'neutral pelvic position.

Note that in this neutral pelvic position :

• *The sacrum is 'heavy' in contact with the ground*
• *The bony landmarks of the pubis and left and right anterior superior iliac spine (ASIS's) are at the same height so that if you lay a book across the three points of contact the book would be horizontal to the floor.*
• *There should be space between the lower back and the floor. The lumbar spine vertebrae of the lower back make a gentle arch or shallow tunnel to the floor.*

It is very common for people to feel slightly uncomfortable in this position due to tension in the chest and/or lower back and hip flexors. If you are one of these people simply place a book or cushion approximately 1.5 - 2 cm in thickness under your head.

This will take away the tension caused by the tight chest area and allow the ribs to relax into the floor.

Most people will compensate for this discomfort by flattening their lower backs into the floor which is not a good strategy !

Flattening the lumbar spine into the floor is considered to :

• *Compress the vertebrae in a structurally unsupported manner*
• *Flatten the spine and push the intervertebral discs backwards which over time may lead to an impinged nerve.*
• *Tuck the sacrum and coccyx under you which pulls on the neck and shoulders, and stresses the hip joints as well as adding unwanted tension to the spinal cord.*

From this 'neutral pelvic' position tip the imaginary cup of water forwards and backwards as before but this time you have a reference point for the center or starting position.

For most people the posterior movement is easier than the anterior movement due to the anterior tilt being

> Which movement seems to take you further from the starting point, a posterior or anterior tilt ?

produced using the lower back muscles as the driver. Try again with a focus on initiating the movement using the Psoas muscle (deep hip flexor). If the spine is fixed the Psoas will flex the hip joint and move the femur however if the femur is fixed (as in this exercise) then the movement is created by drawing the spine towards the femur resulting in the anterior tilt.

If this movement is created well then the spine gets pulled towards the femur with each vertebra being daisy chained as it gets pulled along due to the movement of the vertebra below it - ie L5 pulls L4 which pulls L3 which pulls L2 etc. This is very different to the compressive shearing force produced on the vertebrae if the movement is initiated from the lower back muscles..

Now bring your attention to the 'posterior movement'.

For many persons the rectus abdominus muscle will shorten with the chest and pubic bone being pulled towards each other creating a posterior tilt. This

Which muscles are the likely candidates to lead this movement ?

would then produce a compressive force through each vertebra which is not what we wish to achieve in this exercise.

What if we could 'scoop the tail bone and sacrum from the floor upwards and towards the back of the knees" ?

This would help create a 'lengthening' of the posterior aspect of the vertebrae similar to lifting and pulling a bicycle chain (or string of pearls) from the floor.

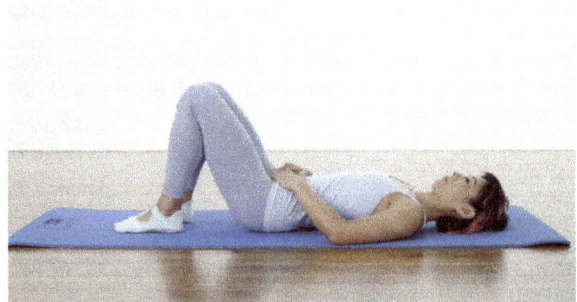

Pelvis is 'neutral'

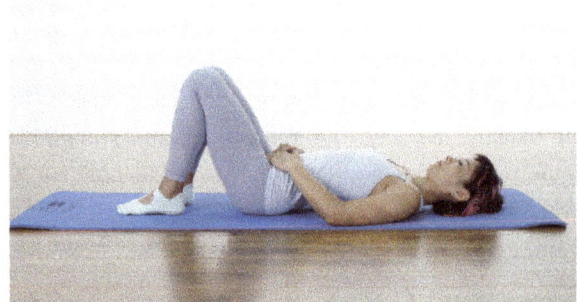

Pelvis moves anterior

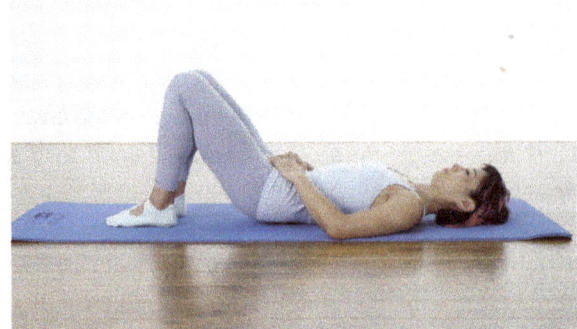

Pelvis moves posterior

Part 2- Side to Side

Return the pelvis to the neutral position.

Imagine a glass teapot on your pelvis and a cup placed on the mat next to your right hip and one next to your left hip. Can you tip the teapot to pour into the cup on the left side ? How about the right side ?

In these movements we wish again to move the pelvis on the femur as opposed to the femur on the pelvis. Therefore the femur should be a fixed point and should not drop out to the side with pelvis as it tilts right or left.

So now bring your attention to the left knee as you lower the pelvis to the left. Does the knee 'drop out' with the pelvis? Or does it stay relatively fixed ? In fact the knee will have to move due to the mechanics of the hip joint. But rather than move from side to side the left knee should travel towards the left hip and the right knee should move in the direction of the right foot as the pelvis tilts left. As the pelvis tilts right the right knee moves in the direction of the right hip and the left knee moves towards the left foot.

Now think about the diagonals and the points on a compass. North would be a point forwards between the two knees, south would be the belly button, west would be next to the left hip and east would be the right hip.

Move the pelvis from neutral towards the north-west followed by the south east direction.

Now move from neutral to the north-east followed by south-west.

Follow the directions of the compass around all the points first by moving to each point from neutral and then from a position for choice.

After completing the 'Pelvic Clock' exercise you should be able to :

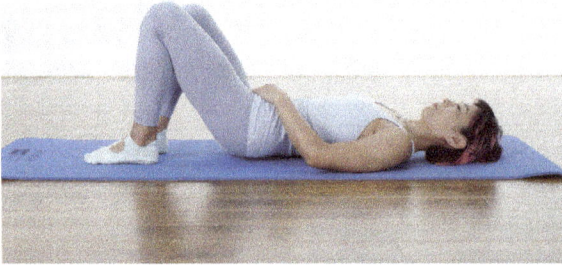

Pelvis tilts right

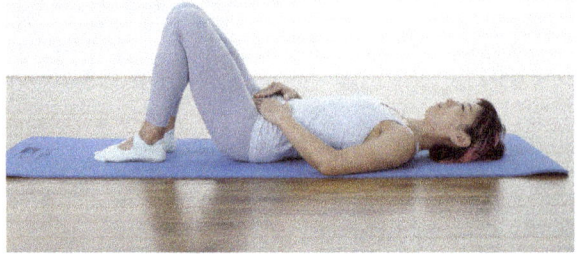

Pelvis tilts left

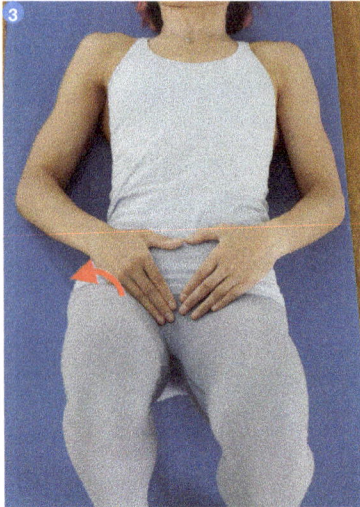

Pelvis tilts right

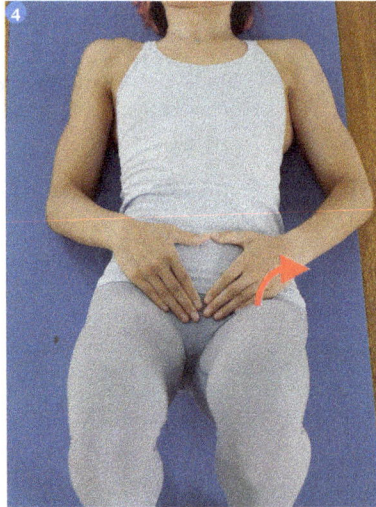

Pelvis tilts left

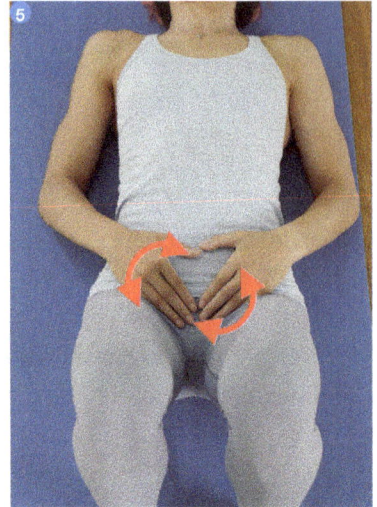

Pelvis rolls around the clock

Scan the QR code to view the exercise - Pelvic Clock

• Differentiate between pelvis on femur and femur on pelvis movements

• Differentiate the two pelvic halves

• Improve awareness of lumbar extension and flexion

• Improve awareness of how pelvic floor muscles affect the lumbar spine

• Improve awareness of how the core musculature is influenced and in turn influences the hips, pelvis and spine

• Improve awareness of hip flexion muscles

• Improve awareness of hip extension muscles

• Improve awareness of how the pelvis can drive the lumbar spine and the connection up through the thoracic and cervical spine to the head.

All of the above are important for efficient and optimal functional movement patterns.

PM2 - Sexy Cat

Contraindications & Precautions

Persons suffering from osteoporosis or stenosis should be cautious of the flexion & extension movements respectively.

Set up

Begin on all fours with the knees under the hips, hip width apart and the hands directly under the shoulders. The pelvis and spine are held in a 'neutral position' with the sit bones 'open'. If you were a dog imagine your tail is held out and away from the body.

The head is held in line with the spine and pelvis.

Movement

Curl your tail towards the back of you knees to initiate a curl of the pelvis. The abdominals hollow and the lower back rounds as the spine flexes.

Continue flexing through the spine to finish with the eyes looking towards the knees.

Now lift your eyes and nose and imagine holding a paint brush in your mouth to draw a line up the wall the ceiling to bring the spine and pelvis to an extended position.

Repeat this flexion - extension movement 8 times

In the extended position use your eyes to look towards your right foot as far as you can comfortably see. Now move into the flexion position allowing your head to lower to finish looking towards the left foot in the flexed position.

Perform the movement slowly paying attention to the quality of the flexion, extension and side bending of the spine.

As you begin to feel comfortable with the movement slightly increase the tempo to a slow fluid movement so that you can feel the head drawing an imaginary big circle in the air as the spine undulates in all 3 planes of movement for extension, flexion, side bending and rotation.

Repeat the movements to the other side so that you look left on extension and right on flexion.

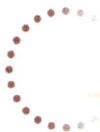

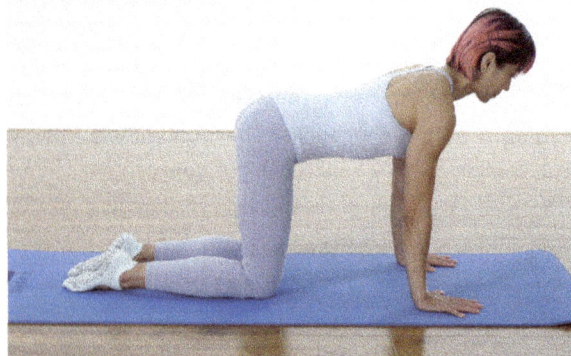

① Begin in neutral

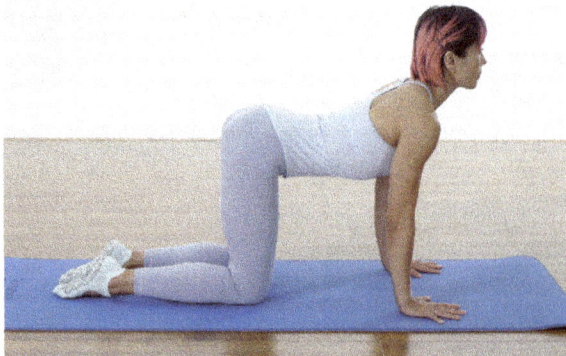

② Extend the spine

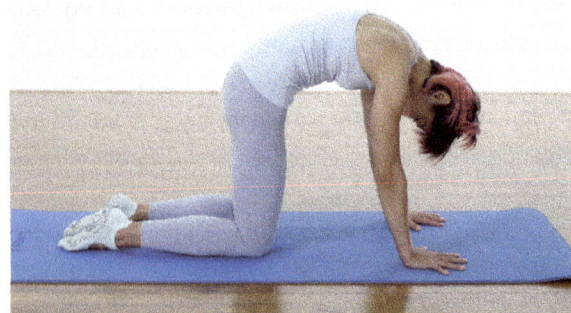

③ Curl the spine

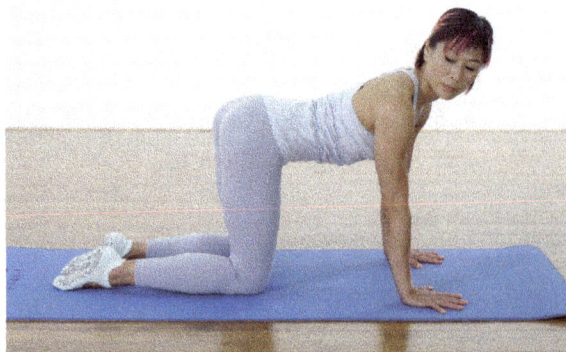

④ Look right - spine extended

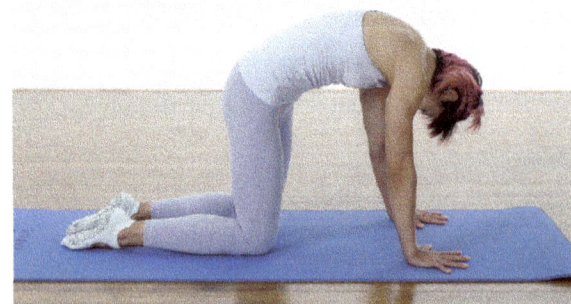

⑤ Look left - spine flexed

Benefits

Release lower, upper back and neck tension
Improve movement of the hip joints
Improve spinal flexibility in all 3 planes of movement
Brings particular awareness to lower spine
Improves mobility of ribcage

Cues

Verbal : Curl your tail towards your knees
Imagine you are a cat being picked up and stretched as you round your back
Imagine balloons attached to your lower, mid and upper back slowly lifting you towards the ceiling
Draw your ribcage away from your shoulder blades
What is the 'minimum effort' you can use to articulate the spine in all directions
Imagine lifting your tail to the ceiling for the extension movement

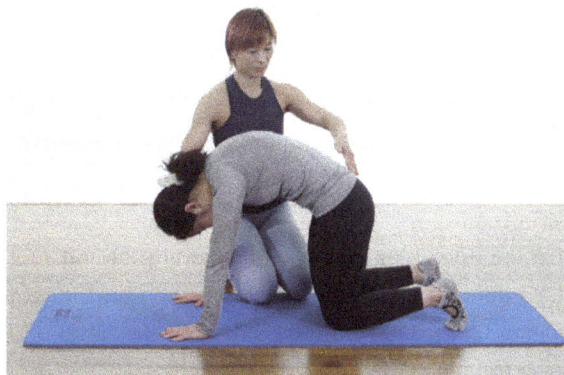

Teacher guided cue for Cat / Camel exercise

Scan the QR code to view the exercise - Sexy Cat

Perform the movement using different drivers :
Use the head to lead the flexion and extension.
Use the tail to lead the flexion and extension
Use the tail to lead the flexion and the head to lead the extension
Use the head to lead the flexion and the tail to lead the extension.
Use an exhalation for the flexion and an inhalation for the extension
Use an inhalation for the flexion and an extension for the extension.

How do all these movement combinations compare ?

Contraindications & Precautions

Persons with knee problems may find this difficult - try using padding under the knee.

PM3 - Dog Wags it's Tail

Set Up

Begin on all fours with the knees touching each other in the center line of the body and the hands directly under the shoulders. The pelvis and spine are held in a 'neutral position' with the sit bones 'open'. The head is held in line with the spine and pelvis.

Movement

Take the left knee over the outside of the right knee and place the left knee on the mat with the lower leg held off the floor so that the left foot points to the ceiling.

Use the knee as a pivot point to swing the left foot like a pendulum from side to side. Each time the foot swings to the left and right side turn the head and torso to look at the foot.

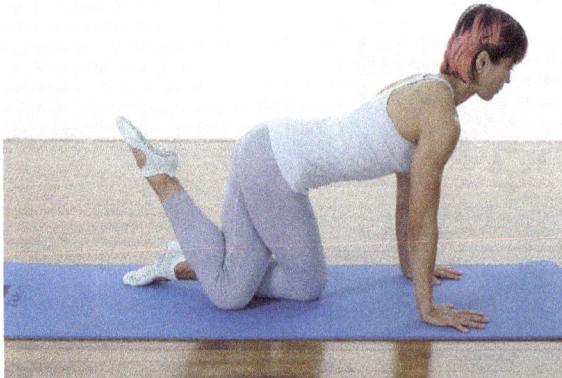

Leg swings left - look left

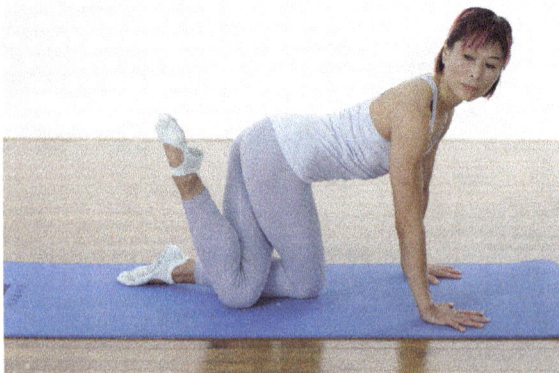

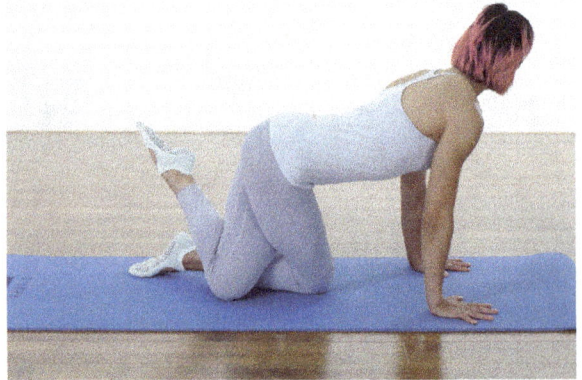

Leg swings right - look right

Principles

Breathing
Core Control
Spinal Articulation

Benefits

Release lower, upper back and neck tension
Improve movement of the hip joints

Cues

Verbal : Imagine your tail bone is the tail on a dog. Swing the tail to the left and right to move the leg.

Compare the tension in your lower back and neck before and after performing the exercise.

Scan the QR code to view the exercise - Dog Wags its' tail

PM4 - Thoracic Rotation (sitting / kneeling)

Set Up

Sit upright in a chair or in a 'high kneeling' position on a mat. Ensure the spine, ribcage and pelvis are held in alignment.

Place the left hand across the lower ribcage on the left side with the heel of the hand resting on the sides of the ribs and the fingers pointing towards the right ASIS. The right hand rests lightly over the left hand.

Movement

Use the right hand to gently slide the left hand towards the right ASIS. As you slide the hands rotate the the ribcage to the right at the same speed as the hands moving diagonally down and across the abdomen. Allow the head to turn with the torso so that you finish with the ribcage and head turned to the right.

The restraint in this movement is that the pelvis is NOT allowed to turn.

Repeat 3- 5 times and repeat the other side.

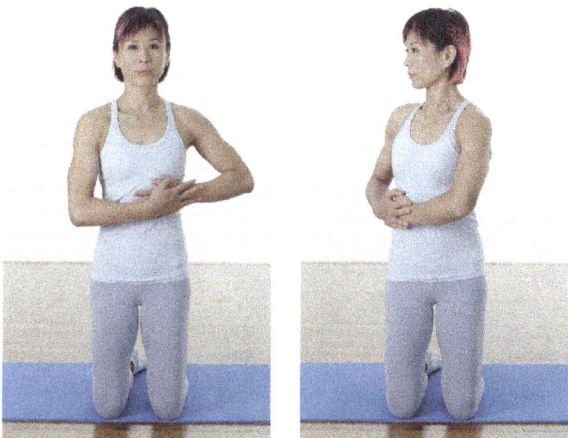

Principles

Spinal Articulation - in rotation

Benefits

Release low back tension
Helps improve mobility of the ribcage
Improves rotation

Cues

Tactile : Feel the directionality of the hand as it slides down and across the abdomen

Compare rotation to the left and right after completing ONE side of the exercise.

Contraindications & Precautions

There are no specific contraindications for the Dead Bug exercise however you be aware of any potential tension or stress in the lower back due to the weight of the legs pulling into the spine through the hip flexor muscles. Any pain or discomfort in the spine means that there is not enough stabilization of the pelvis and spine from the core musculature.

PM5 - Dead Bug

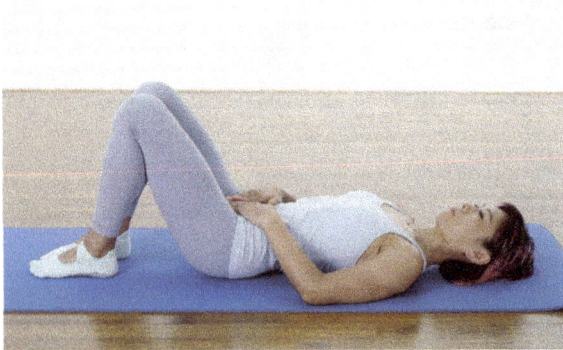

The dead bug exercise is a classic preparation exercise for the matwork in Pilates. Much of your preparation work with the breathing is important to perform this exercise well.

Setup

Lie in the supine position with your legs triple flexed and make a triangle with your hands placed over your pelvis. Begin with a few inhalations and exhalations to ensure that your core is stabilised and you are breathing into the back and sides of your ribs.

Use your hands and your own kinesthetic awareness to ensure the pelvis is stable and doesn't move throughout the exercise.

Slowly lift your left leg from the floor keeping the knee flexed. Observe if there is any movement in your pelvis or tension in your lower back. If there is tension in your lower back you will need to adjust your position or repeat the movement until there is no tension.

Float your right leg in the air to join your left leg so that the knees are slightly apart and pointing to the ceiling with the hips flexed at 90°. There should be 1 to 2 fist widths space between the knees and the inside pf your feet are pressed gently together. The position with your feet together and knees apart switches on your adductor and hip rotator muscles which all have an effect on your pelvic floor.

Ensure that your knees are relaxed and flexed. Now, slowly lower your right leg pivoting at the hip joint and see if you can just touch the paint on the mat with your right big toe. Return the leg to the up position and repeat the movement with the left leg. Now repeat the movement alternating between the right and left leg.

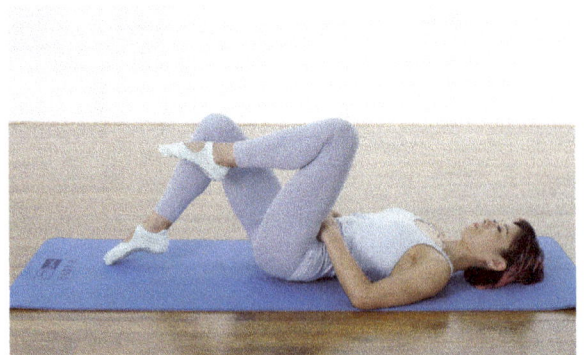

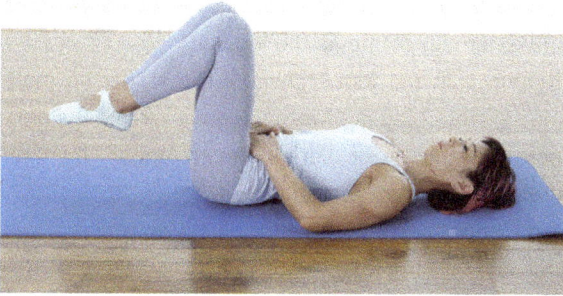

One leg moves at a time

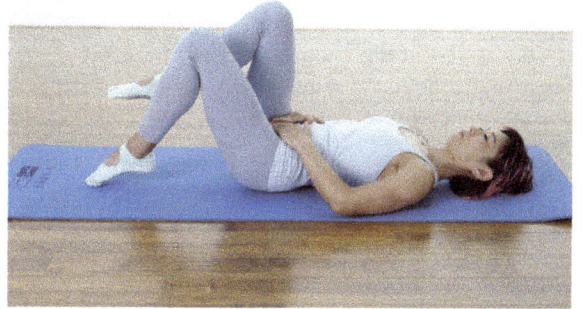

Alternating legs - as one leg moves downwards the other is moving upwards

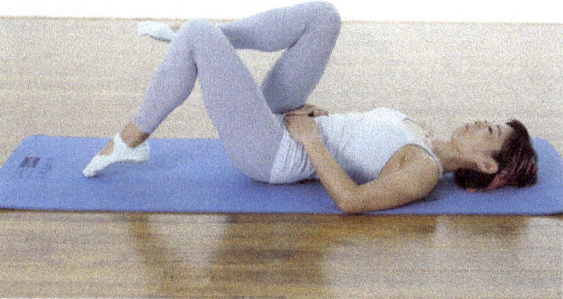

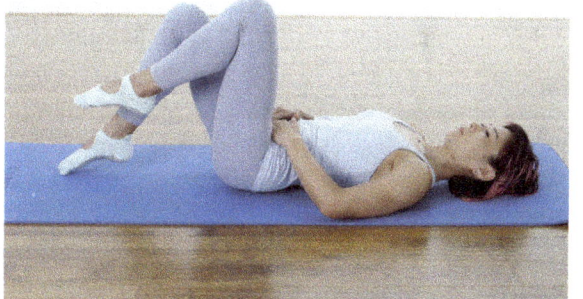

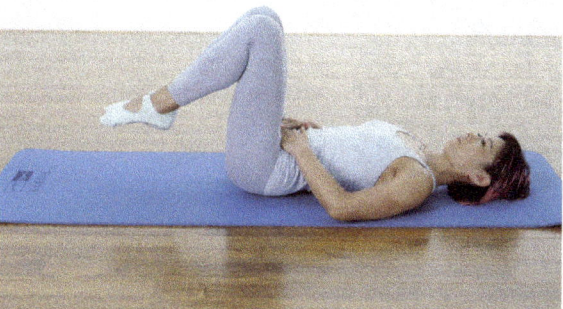

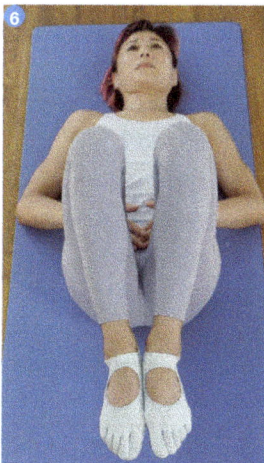

"Feet together - Knees apart and flexed"

Principles

Lumbo Pelvic Hip Complex stabilization with ability to differentiate the hip joints
Core control

Benefits

Improve stability of LPHC
Improve hip mobility

Cues

Verbal : Imagine oil in your hip joints lubricating the head of the femur in the acetabulum
Use the hands to help give you proprioceptive feedback on pelvis and spine stability.

Tactile : Teacher should place one hand under the lower back and the other over the abdomen to sense stability of spine and pelvis

Compare lifting a single left leg to lifting a single right leg. Is there a difference between the two ?
Use variations of the same exercise - can you determine the differences between a progression and a regression ?
How does the exercise change if the hands press into the floor by your sides ?

Variations :

One leg remains on the floor
Internally rotate the hips as legs move downwards and externally rotate as the legs lift.
Perform with the foot higher form the floor (ie more knee extension) to produce a longer lever into the hip.
Increase the lever length even more by half straightening the leg at the knee.
Place both hands on the floor palms downwards and pressing into the floor.

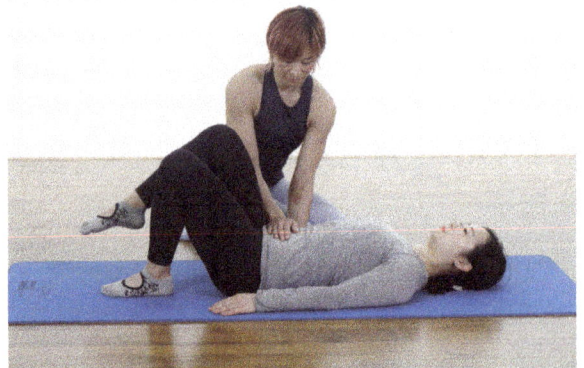

Teacher guided cue for Dead Bug exercise

Scan the QR code to view the exercise - Dead Bug

PM6 - Supine Rotation (Bottom Up)

Set Up

Supine position with the left leg in triple flexed position and right ankle placed across the top of the left thigh with the right hip flexed and externally rotated. The arms are placed out to the sides palm downwards at approximately 60 degrees.

Movement

In the pelvic clock exercise the pelvis moved on the femur (leg) however in this exercise the leg is rotating in the hip joint before pulling the pelvis along with it.
Begin by lowering the left and right legs to the left side. The left hip goes into external rotation and the right hip goes into internal rotation in relation to the pelvis.
Observe how this movement can be accomplished with minimal movement in the lumbar spine.
Now continue this movement through the pelvis and up the spine until the right foot reaches the floor. Can you place the right foot on the floor without the right shoulder lifting from the mat ?
Ensure the right knee does not 'drop' towards the floor during the movement and that upon the right foot reaching the floor the right knee is vertical over the right ankle.
From this position see if you can travel the right tibia (shin bone) over the right big toe. This action should engage the right gluteus maximus muscle.
Return to the start position by 'pulling' the right side of the ribcage towards the mat.
The start of the movement - bottom up driver.
The return to start position - top down driver.

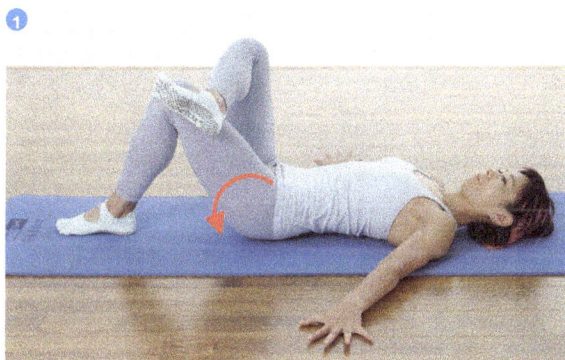

Pelvis remains still as legs move to the side

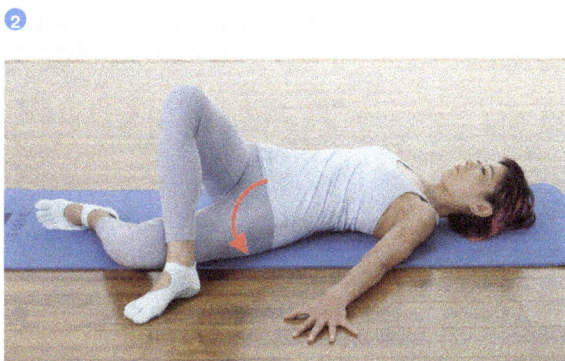

Pelvis and spine rotates

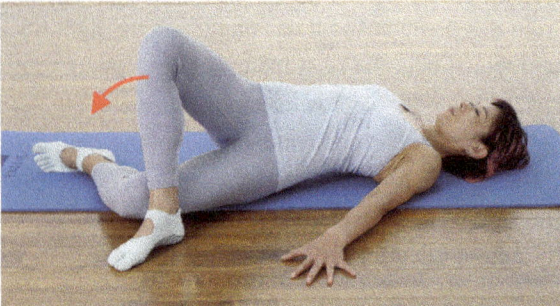

Right foot presses into floor as right shin bone moves over big toe

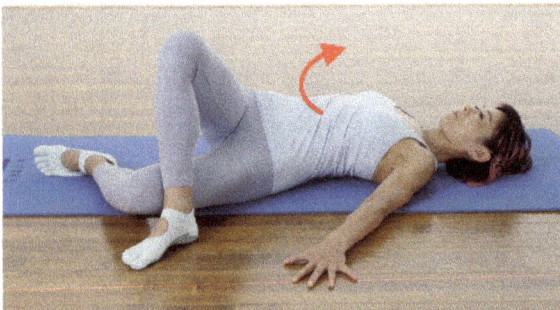

Movement to start position is initiated from the ribcage

Benefits

Improve organisation of pelvis, spine and ribcage

Release lower back, neck and shoulder tension

Improve rotation of thoracic spine (the mid to upper spine where all the ribs attach) - improve breathing and takes tension away from the lower back.

Helps mobility of the ribcage - improve breathing and takes tension away from the lower back.

Helps release tightness and shortness in front

of shoulder and upper chest - helps to bring the head back to a better position over the ribcage thus being very beneficial for the neck and shoulders.

Helps activate the gluteal muscles (your butt) - good for posture and taking tension away from the lower back.

Principles

Articulation in rotation

Organization of pelvis, spine and ribcage

Cues

Verbal : Press into the floor with the contralateral (opposite arm to direction moving) arm.

Imagine one vertebra moving away from the one above it one-by-one.

Maintain a gentle soft breath throughout the movement to keep the ribcage mobile.

Tactile : Teacher can place one finger / walk the fingers up at each spinal level to cue rotation.

Compare the movement by initiating the rotation from different positions (drivers). How does it feel if you lower the legs by moving the pelvis first instead of the femurs ?

How do your shoulders and neck feel during this movement ?

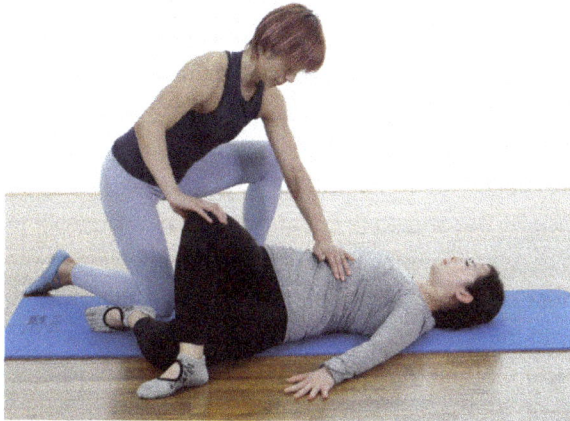

Teacher guided cue for Supine Rotation exercise

Scan the QR code to view the exercise - Supine Spinal Rotation

PM7 - Seated Arm Press (against wall)

Although a relatively simple looking exercise this is great for persons with excessive anterior tilting of the pelvis, anteriorly shifted ribcage, forward head posture, shoulder dysfunction and neck and shoulder issues

Set Up

Sit on a stall or chair facing the wall with the arms extended in front of you so that the palms of the hand are flat on the wall at shoulder height and shoulder width apart.

The pelvis should be upright with the spine, ribcage and head stacked appropriately over the pelvis.

Movement

Your goal is to 'wrap your shoulder blades' around the front and back of the rib cage as much as possible maintaining the 'fixed position' of the elbows - that is they are not allowed to either bend or straighten from their position.

We are usually adapt at moving our hands and arms around our body especially as this helps us to express ourselves and reach into the outside world. However many of us lack the ability to move the shoulder blades in a cohesive manner when there is a limitation of having to keep the hands fixed against the wall. Many of us will in fact bend the elbows in an effort to produce the required movement instead of actually moving at the shoulder blades.

The vast majority of shoulder and neck problems are actually either linked or caused by this inability to mobilize and stabilize the shoulder blades effectively against the ribcage. This results in compensatory movements down the arm at the elbows and wrists or further into the shoulder girdle at the shoulder joint itself (glenohumeral joint), acromioclavicular joint and or sternoclavicular joint resulting in any number aches, pains and dysfunctions of the upper body and limbs.

To produce the required movement begin by pulling or squeezing your shoulder blades together while keeping the hands fixed on the wall - no lifting the heel of the hands !

For this to happen the chest will have to move closer to the wall and it can only do this effectively if you keep your whole spine rigid and in fact pivot on your hip joints. If your knees are too high in relation to your hips you will not be able to accomplish this. The most common error in this movement is to allow the ribcage to 'shift anteriorly' meaning that the whole spine does not move towards the wall but the mid back is arched or extended in an effort to make the movement. This unwanted and dysfunctional movement is further enhanced because it happens at the exact point the spine changes direction from a convex curve to a concave curvature making it very difficult to stabilize at this point.

Now that you have managed to move the ribcage closer to the wall whilst retracting your shoulder blades without the dreaded 'anterior rib shift' you need to pull the whole ribcage away from the wall as far as possible without hunching the shoulders.

People with short upper shoulder and neck muscles will find this movement very difficult without 'hunching the shoulders' or excessive rounding the back.

The shoulder blades should have a feeling of 'sliding around the ribcage' towards the wall whilst the spine stays in an upright position.

Perform this exercise 15 - 20 times.

A special note about this exercise is that for maximum benefits you should in fact try to it as often as possible throughout the day. For those of you seated at a desk all day this is one of those exercises you should set your smartphone alarm to ring for every hour ! That's right - every hour. Set your alarm to ring and swing your chair around to the nearest wall and practice 15 to 20 of these movements before swinging the chair back around again and continuing your work.

Progression :

A progression of extra benefit from this exercise can be gained by adding some 'piano playing'. First wrap your shoulder blades back around the ribcage by bringing them together with the arms in the extended position and hands on the wall. Now lift the little finger of the right hand away from the wall and place

it back on the wall again. Repeat the same movement with the 4th, 3rd, 2nd finger and then the thumb and repeat the whole sequence two more times. After completion of the moving the thumb on the third round take a big inhalation followed by a full exhalation and consciously try to relax the right elbow. You should find that it drops and relaxes into a better aligned position. Compare the feeling of the right arm and left arm and then repeat the process with the left arm.

Now that you have completed the exercise on both arms do the same thing all over again but this time but this time with the shoulder blades in the fully protracted position. You may be surprised how much more difficult this exercise is with the shoulder blades protracted as opposed to being in the retracted position.

Principles

Organization of the shoulder girdle
Core control
Integration of the upper extremity into the core

Cues

Verbal : Imagine pinching a pencil between the shoulder blades
Imagine a very hot wall you need to move your chest away from
Imagine your whole spine to be like a flag pole that can not bend

Tactile : Teacher use fingers to trace / follow the proposed movement of the scapula

Compare the movement by using inhalation and exhalation for the different scapula movements
Focus on breathing into the upper back on the scapula forward movement (chest away from the wall)
Practice with the hands in differing positions and the arms at various heights.

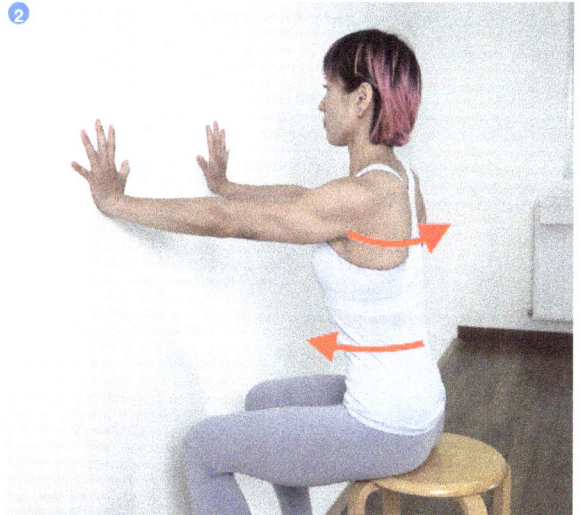

Shoulder blades move towards the wall
Ribcage moves backwards

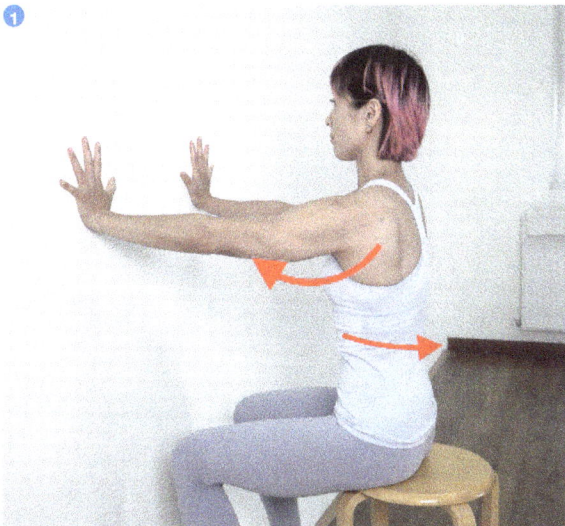

Shoulder blades move towards each other
Ribcage moves forwards

PM8 - Supine Arms

Benefit

Helps to improve proprioception and mobility of the shoulder girdle.
Increases range of movement of the shoulder joint.
Helps to balance tension between the opposing muscles of the shoulder joint.
Helps to integrate the shoulder girdle into the rib cage thus allowing for the

Setup

Lie in a supine position with legs in the 'triple flexed position'. Arms are extended out in front at ninety degrees with the fingers pointing to the ceiling and back of the hands placed against each other.

Movement

Bring the arms out to the sides at ninety degrees to

the body, without rotating the arms or wrists, until the palms of the hands touch the floor. Sweep the arms towards the hips and then lift the arms to the start position. However now the hands have 'rotated outwards ninety degrees' so that the thumbs are now pointing towards each other and the palms are facing the feet.

Bring the arms down to the floor again at ninety degrees so that the edge of the hand is now touching the floor. Sweep the arms down towards the hips as before and the palms of the hands will now touch your hips.

Lift the arms back to the start position and you will find the palms of the hands now face each other.

Repeat the movement of the arms to the floor and you will find the back of the hands touches the floor. Sweep the arms down to the hips and the little finger will touch the hips.

Bring the arms to the start position and you will find the palms are now facing your head. Bring the arms down to the floor as in the previous moves however you will probably find this starting to get difficult now as the shoulder joint has to rotate outwards in order to allow the thumbs to touch the floor.

Now sweep the arms towards the hips again and you will probably be struggling to get the back of the hands to touch the hips. Your goal would be to now lift the arms to the start position but with the back of the hands touching each other and the thumbs pointing to the feet !

You have now completed one set of four repetitions where the set has taken the arms and hands through all the possible positions for the shoulder joint.

Repeat the exercise until you have completed five sets.

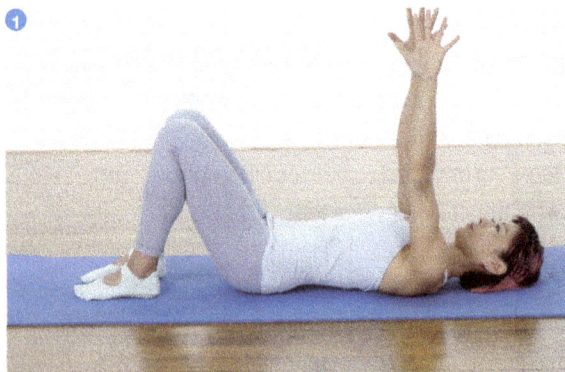

Palms face outwards
Shoulder internally rotated

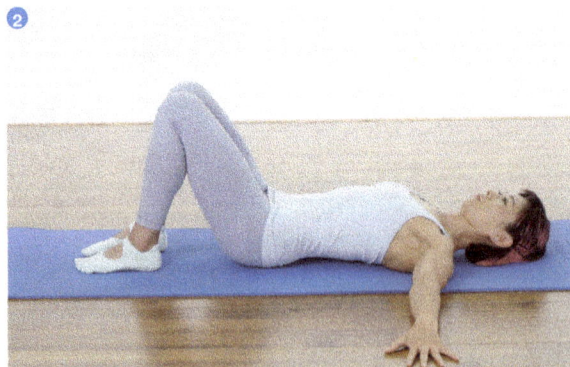

Palms to floor

3

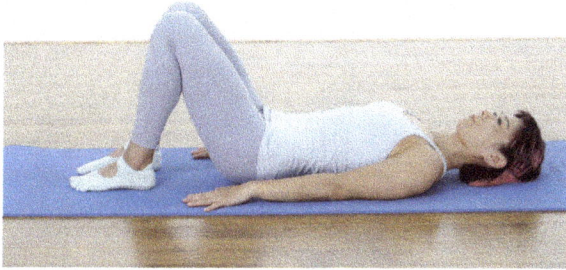

Palms downwards by hips

4

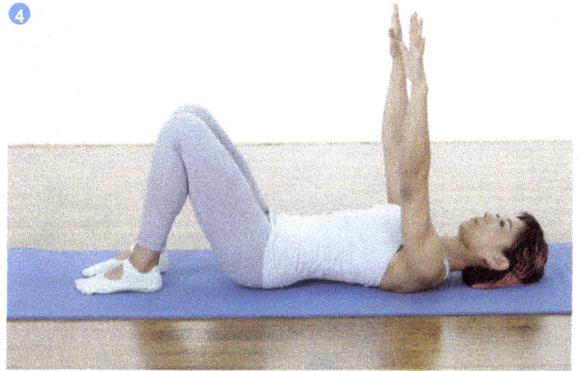

Thumbs point to each other

5

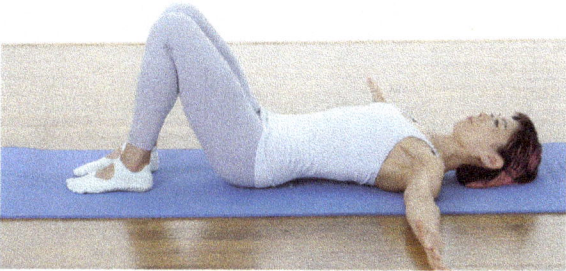

'Knife hand' to floor

6

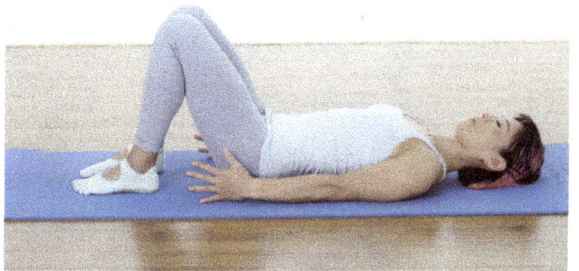

Palms face hips at side

7

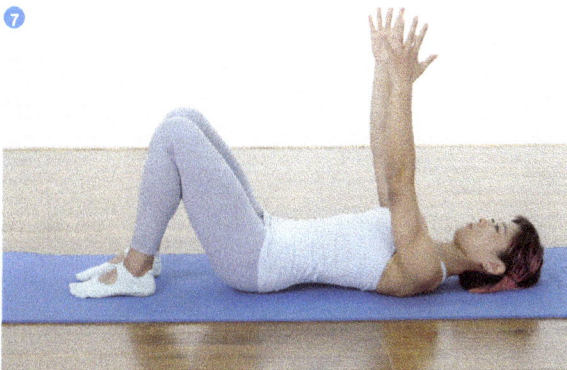

Palms face each other

8

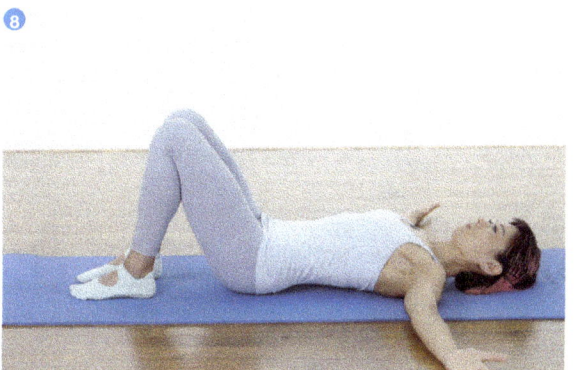

Palms face up

⑨

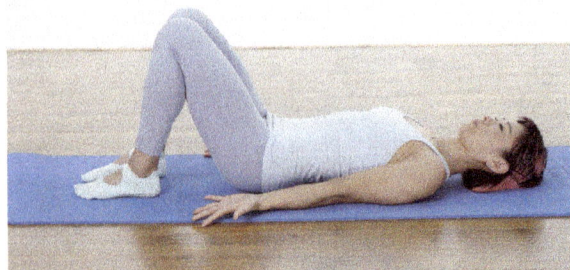

Palms face up at hips

⑩

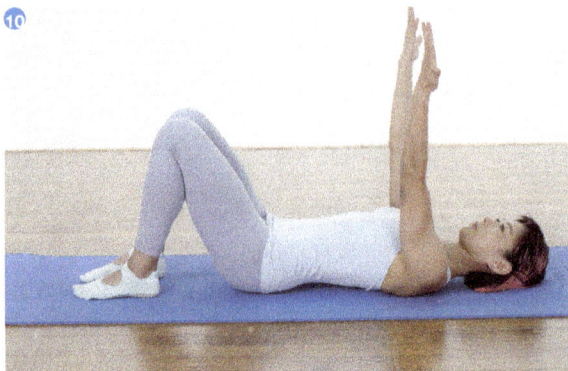

Palms face head

⑪

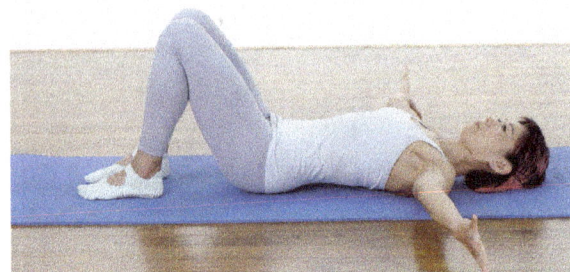

Face face head with thumbs to floor

⑫

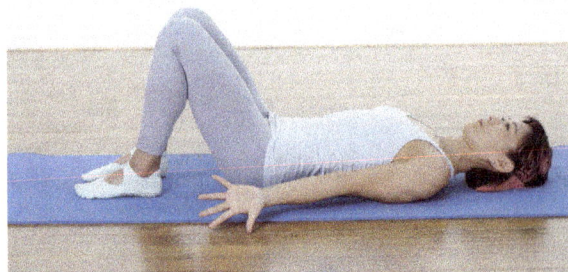

Palms face outwards, thumbs to floor

⑬

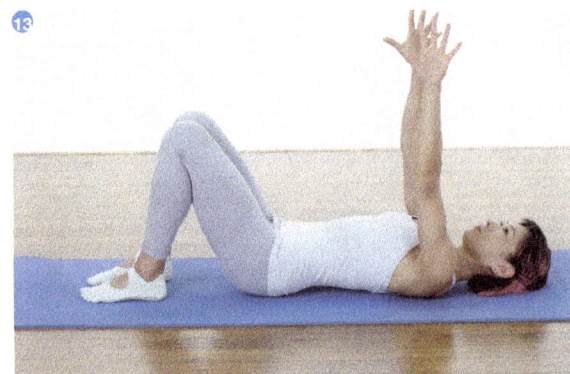

Palms face outwards, thumbs point at knees, shoulder externally
rotated

⑭

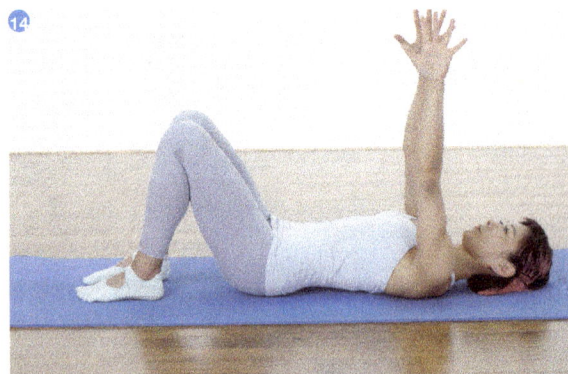

Return to start position.
Palms face outwards, shoulder internally rotated

Scan the QR code to view the exercise - Supine Arms

PM9 - Mermaid 1

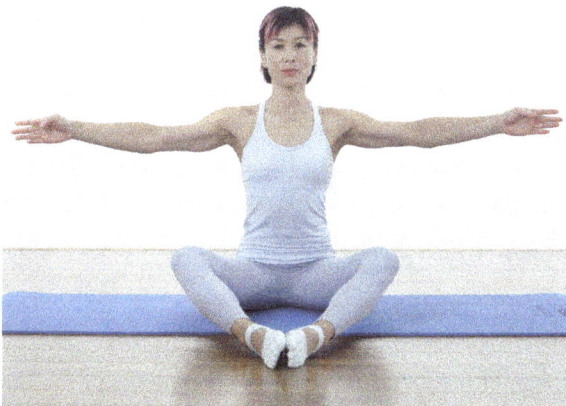

Principles

Organization of the shoulder girdle
Core control
Spinal articulation in side bending

Benefits

Improves forward shift of the ribcage
Helps improve side bending movement of the spine.

Helps improve certain shoulder restrictions
Helps to open up and improve breathing to the side of the ribs
Mobilization of the rib cage may often help with persons suffering from low back pain.

Cues

Verbal : Imagine your ribs as Venetian blinds opening or closing
Inhale to open the ribs
Exhale to close the ribs

Tactile : Teacher use fingers to trace / follow the side bending of each vertebra/

Setup

There is a choice of 3 different starting positions :

a) Seated on a chair with hips and knee flexed. Legs should preferably be hip width apart although a little further is ok.

b) Seated on the floor with the hips and knees flexed and the legs dropped out to the side keeping the feet together in the midline.

c) Similar to option 'b' except that you sit on a small raised platform or box.

The setup principle is the same for all 3 options in that the pelvis must be in an upright neutral position sitting on top of your sit bones. The hands should be resting or hanging comfortably by the hips.
The reason to perform the exercise seated as opposed to standing is to take away the influence of

the ankles, knees and hips in the side bending movement. If a person lacks spinal mobility then he or she will over compensate by increasing inversion or eversion at the ankle joint or pushing the pelvis out to the side. Therefore this exercise helps limit the accessory movements of the pelvis and lower body thereby placing an emphasis on mobilizing the spine to reduce tension in the spinal joints and muscles.

Movement 1

Draw the shoulder blades down the back of the spine as though you can reach the tip of each shoulder blade into the corresponding back pocket. You should feel the chest lift and open as a result.

Float both arms upwards and out to the side so that the arms are held extended just below shoulder height with the palms facing the front and approximately 15 cm in front of the body. Imagine you are about to reach the arms out and forwards to give somebody a big hug !

Bring you right hand across to the lower left rib cage and as in the exercise Thoracic Rotation (PM4) slide the right hand down and across to the right ASIS whilst simultaneously rotating the ribcage to the right bringing the left arm with you.

Notice how the the position of the left shoulder did not change - ie the left humerus did not horizontally abduct or adduct in the joint. The center of your ribcage should be now facing diagonally across to your right side.

Raise your right arm so that the shoulder bade is in a similar position to the start position and then rotate the ribcage with the arms held out to the side back to the start position.

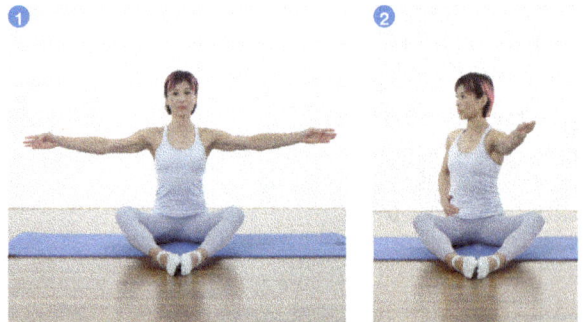

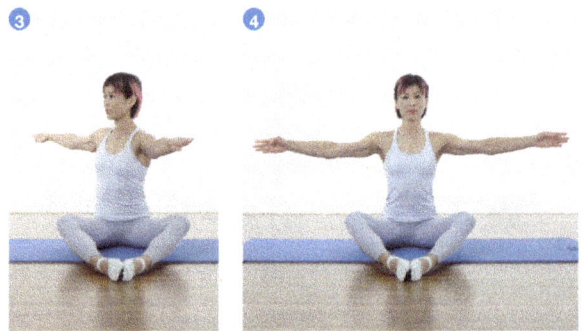

Movement 2

Begin in the same position as movement 1 with the arms held outwards to the side but with the hands slightly in front of the body so that the arms ar in line with the 'scapular plane'.

Raise the left arm directly overhead with the palm of the hand facing to the right.

Pay particular attention to the space between the left ear and the shoulder. There should be as much space as possible

Begin a right side bend by bringing the right ear towards the right shoulder, however as you do so relax through the right side of the ribs to allow the whole spine to side bend to the right. Maintain a long C shaped curve in the spine when viewed from behind without the middle vertebrae excessively being pushed out to the side.

Also bring your awareness to maintaining a good space between each ear and shoulder so that the head is positioned optimally over the spine.

As you bend to the side try to visualize the ribs on the right side moving towards each other and the ribs on the left side being opened. You may think of the movement of a Venetian blind as it opens one side and closes the other.

Take a deep breath into the left side of the rib cage and see if you can feel the ribs expanding further.

To return to the start position bring each vertebrae on top of the one below stacking them on top of each other from the side.

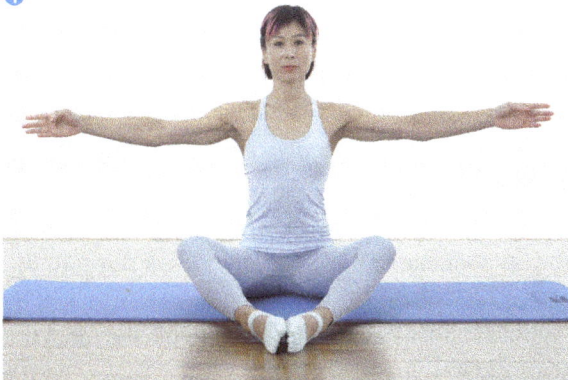

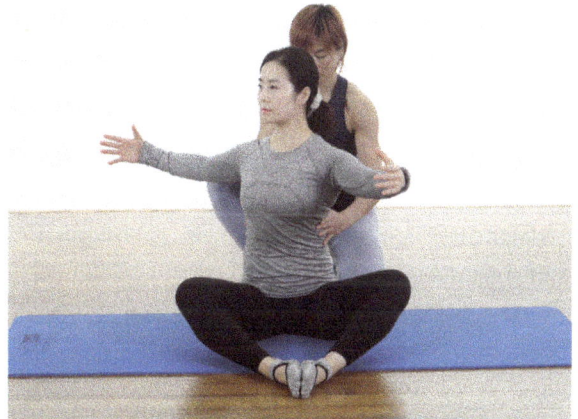

Compare the movement by using inhalation and exhalation for the different scapula movements

Focus on breathing into the upper back on the scapula forward movement (chest away from the wall)

Practice with the hands in differing positions and the arms at various heights.

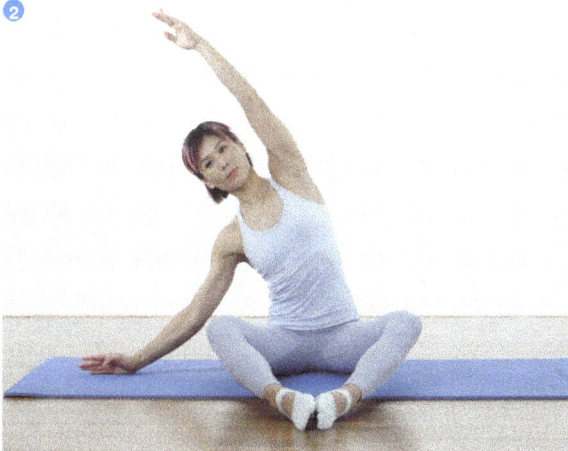

Teacher guided or assisted cue for Mermaid exercise

PM10 - Assisted Roll Down

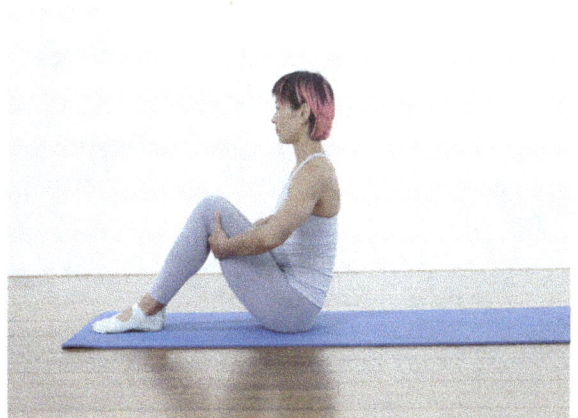

Contraindications & Precautions

Flexion exercises are considered
contraindicated for persons with steoporosis.

Principles

Core control
Articulation of the spine in flexion

Benefits

Helps improve ribcage positioning over pelvis
Helps to 'engage the core'
Releases lower and upper back tension

Cues

Verbal : Curl your tail towards you pubic bone
Hollow your abdominals
Peel your spine on and off the floor like a piece of
sticky tape

Tactile : Teacher use fingers to trace / follow the
placement of each individual vertebra on and off
the floor.
Teacher may use very light touch of thumb and
forefinger to cue the abdominal hollowing.

Set Up

Begin in a sitting position with your feet placed in
front of you on the mat, both hands hold behind the
back of the thighs close to the back of the knees and
your weight very slightly behind your sit bones.

The arms should be in a 'rounded position' with
shoulders relaxed and your spine will be slightly
flexed due to the upright position of the head over a
slightly posterior pelvis.

Take a moment to practice breathing into the sides and
back of the ribs whilst hollowing your abdominals.

Curl you tail towards your pubic bone to initiate a
scoop of the sit bones towards the back of the knees
and feel how your pelvis begins to 'roll backwards,.

Continue the posterior movement of the pelvis and
see if you can feel each of your lumbar vertebra
being placed down on the mat one bone at a time. A
restraint in this exercise is that you are not allowed to
either straighten nor bend you arms any more than in
the start position.

You should feel the feet slowly get lifted into the air
as you continue to curl your spine back down to the
mat.

Continue curling your spine down to the mat until the
head rests on the floor.

To return to the start position begin by lifting the
head and looking towards your knees as you roll the
spine back up to the start position.

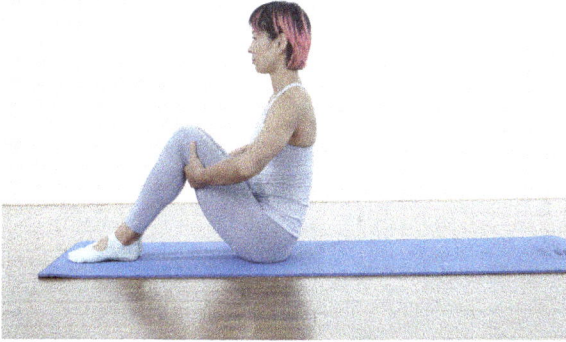

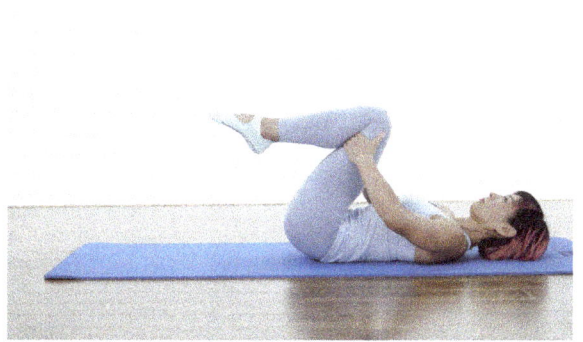

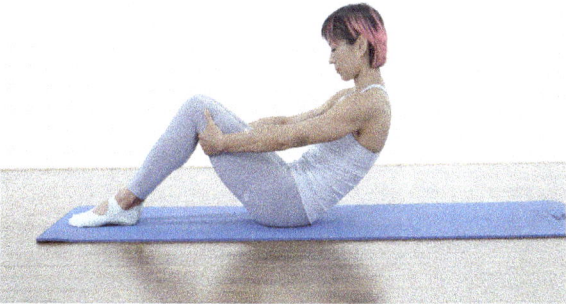

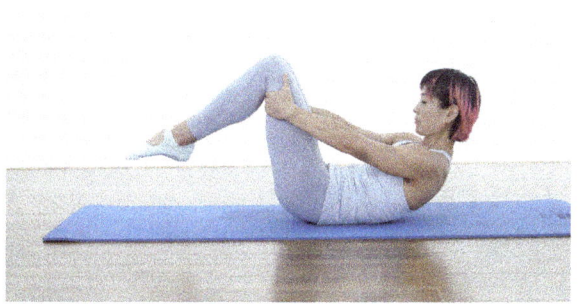

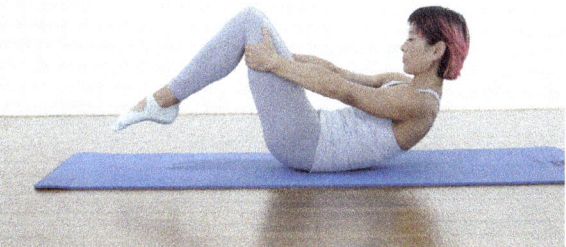

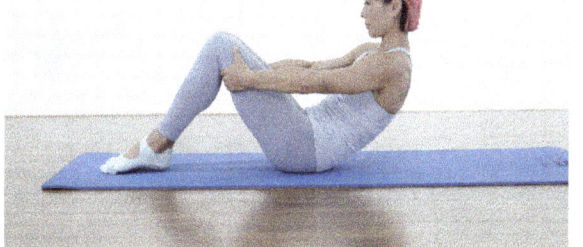

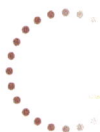

⑦

This is a great exercise to help learn to use the correct abdominal muscles for a flexion movement. In everyday life we would naturally move the pelvis backwards as bend over however this movement is quite often accompanied with overusing the rectus abdominus muscle which in turn is associated with compression of the spine and disc injuries. Learning to use a competent strategy for spinal flexion may go a long way to helping support the spine when having to use spinal flexion in daily life.

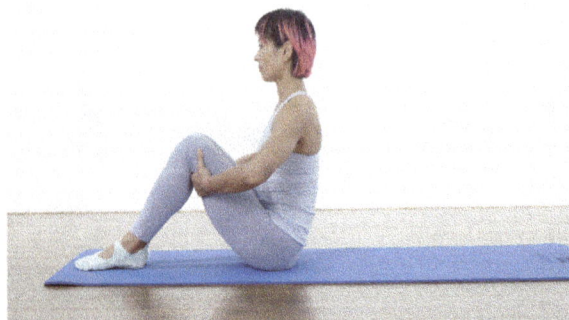

How slow can you succeed whilst maintaining a speed that is fluid and smooth but allows you to stop at any position at any time...

Scan the QR code to view the exercise Assisted Roll Down

Contraindications & Precautions

Flexion exercises are considered contraindicated for persons suffering with osteoporosis.
Persons with acute disc problems should not attempt this exercise.
This is more of a 'preventative" as opposed to a 'treatment exercise' therefore any persons with acute or existing back pain should avoid this exercise.

PM11 - Standing Roll Down

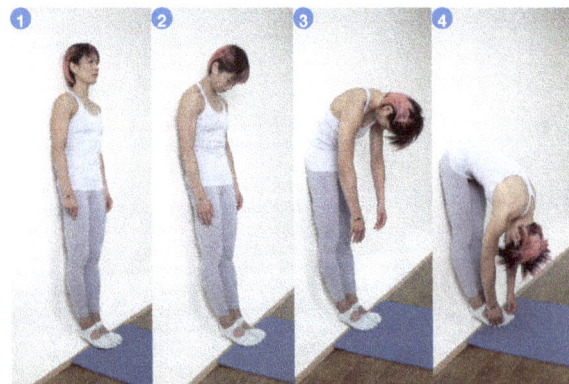

Set Up

Stand against a wall with your sacrum and upper back touching the wall. Your lumbar spine and head should be approx 1- 2 cm away from the wall (1-2 finger widths) and your feet should be at a position away from the wall appropriate for your level as follows :

15 cm - beginner
10cm - intermediate
5 cm - advanced

Your arms can be held by your sides or with the hands gently placed across your pelvis / lower abdomen.

Movement

Draw the abdominals deeply inwards and upwards. Relax the chin to your chest by imagining you can slide and lift your ears up and over the top of your head. As the head moves towards the chest allow the collar bones to soften and move downwards. See if you can feel a reciprical movement in your upper back of the ribs and vertebrae moving apart as the ribs in the front 'move together'. There should be a 'lifting feel' from the back as the front flexes and moves towards the floor. Continue to flex the spine one vertebra at a time and imagine a piece of sticky tape that gets peeled from the wall.

See how long you can keep your lower spine against the wall as you flex forwards.

Take as many breaths as you need as you move towards the floor.

Allow yourself to stay for 3- 5 breaths in the end position before reversing the movement and stacking the spine one vertebra at a time all the way back up. You will find that the difficulty for this exercise is to perform the movement without falling over ! The close to the wall your feet are - the more difficult the exercise.

Principles

Core control
Articulation of the spine in flexion

Benefits

Improves abdominal muscle strategy for con-traction.
Helps improve ribcage positioning over pelvis
Helps to 'engage the core'
Releases lower and upper back tension

Cues

Verbal : Hollow your abdominals
Peel your spine off the wall like a piece of sticky tape
Imagine a wire just above your hip joints - as you bend over don't touch the wire with your belly.
Imagine the ribs closing at the front and opening at the back
Imagine an invisible hand lifting and holding the abdominals as you bend forwards.

Tactile : Teacher use fingers to trace / follow the placement of each individual vertebra on / off the wall.
Teacher may use very light touch of thumb and forefinger to cue the abdominal hollowing.

How far can you flex without falling over ?
How does changing the distance of the feet from the wall change the exercise ?

PM12 - Prone Extension 1

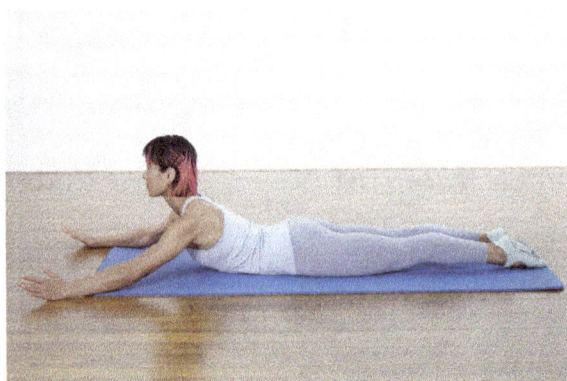

Many people suffer from low back because their upper back and ribcage is unable to extend meaning that the movement comes from the lower back which is compensating for the lack of movement further up the spine. The ability to extend through the thoracic spine is an essential skill for all persons wishing to perform sport, improve posture or treat any form of low back pain.

Set Up

Lie face down on the mat the arms overhead with the hands placed the width of the mat apart. Before beginning the exercise perform a mental check list as follows :

1) Feet are pointed and on the mat
2) Knees are lifted from the mat
3) Legs are placed as close together as is comfrotable
4) ASIS's are 1 or 2 finger widths from the mat
5) Abdominals are drawn in (imagine an ice cube under your belly)
6) Head is lifted from the floor 1 - 2 cm

7) Arms are held mat width apart with the 'knife edge' part of the hand towards the floor.

Movement

Slowly lift the eyes and imagine you can slide your ears downwards to the bottom back of the head. At the same time imagine your collar bones are butterflies floating, lifting and pulling the breast bone in a scooping movement forwards and upwards from the mat.

As the breast bone scoops and lifts the edge of the hands press into the floor 'stiffening' the underneath of the arms so that they can help 'pull' the ribcage further forwards and upwards from the mat.

Only go as far in this extension movement as your last ribs. The end of the movement is just before the bottom ribs are about to be lifted from the mat.

Remain in this 'thoracic extended' position and observe :

1) *What happened to the pelvis ? If the pelvis tilted forwards excessively the ASIS' will both be on the mat. Bring them back from the mat in a manner similar to the pelvic clock exercise from before.*

2) *What would happen if you placed a ball at the base of the head and let go ? Would it roll down immediately to the lower back or can you imagine that it would roll down to the mid part of the upper back as it relaxes and sinks to the floor.*

3) *Inhale-exhale : on the exhalation relax the back of the ribs and scoop and lift the front ......*

4) *Imagine a ball placed between the shoulder blades. See if you can relax the ribs enough to allow the ball to sink and drop into the front of the ribcage.*

Stay in this position for 5 breaths and then allow yourself to relax back down to the mat

①

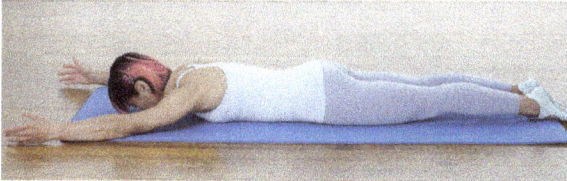

②

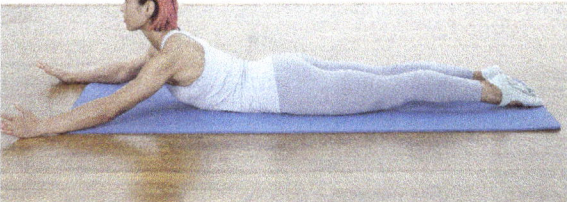

③

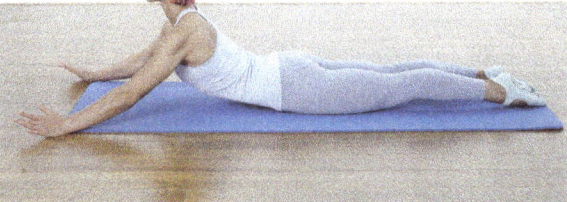

Benefits

Releases lower and upper back tension
Improves thoracic extension
Relieves neck and shoulder tension
Improves upper body posture

Cues

Verbal : Start by looking upwards
Imagine you can slide your ears to the base of your head
Imagine your collar bones like 2 butterflies floating and flying upwards
Imagine your breast bone like a feather floating away
Imagine a ball between the shoulder blades that you can let 'sink' to the front
Use your underarms to pull yourself forwards and upwards

Tactile : Teacher can use fingers to trace / articulate the spinal segment movement
Teacher can gently help scoop the ribcage forwards and upwards
Teacher can place fingers gently onto the sternum and manubrium to cue the extension

Principles

Thoracic extension (articulation in extension)

Pay particular attention to the lower back. As soon as you feel the movement reach the lower back vertebra - back off and breathe for a few moments to see if you can relax the upper body and ribcage into more extension.

Scan the QR code to view the exercise - Prone Extension I

Scan the QR code to view the exercise - Prone Extension II

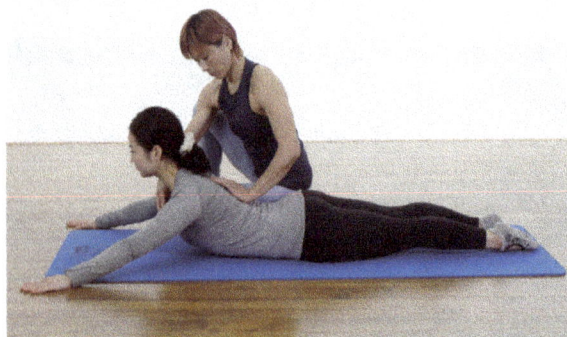

Teacher guided cue for Prone Extension exercise

PM13 - Thoracic Figure of Eights

Setup

Sit on a stall with hips and knee flexed. Legs should preferably be hip width apart although a little further is ok.

Sit on top of your sit bones with the pelvis in an upright position and the spine stacked over the pelvis in a neutral position. Place the palms of each hand against your breast bone.

Movement

Begin by performing a side bend to the right and then the left side. Note that the fixed or stable pelvis results in the 'top down' movement as each vertebra moves or bends on top of the one below. Pay attention to how the ribs 'close' on the side you are bending towards and 'open' on the other side.

Now perform the rotation exercise as before (PM6), but without the hand slide by rotating the ribcage to the right and pause in that position. Your left elbow will now be pointing diagonally out to the left side in front of the body and the right elbow will be pointing in the opposite direction behind you.

Now perform a 'left side bend' maintaining the 'right rotation' position of the body. The right elbow now points diagonally to the right behind you and the left elbow is directly opposite pointing in front. From this position rotate to the left maintaining the left side bend position of the body.

Now make a right side bend maintaining the left rotation position followed by a right rotation - you should now be back in 'position 3' of right side bend with right rotation.

Make 'half a side bend to your left to come to an upright position and finally half rotate to the left to return to the start position facing the front.

Now combine all these movements into a smooth fluid motion for approximately 1 minute before changing the direction for another minute.

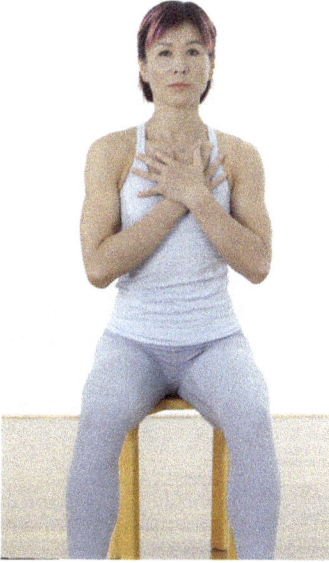

Start position

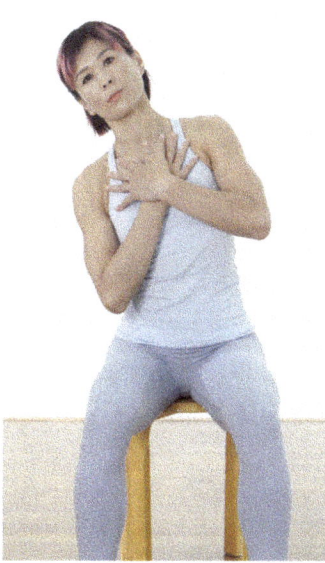

Side bend right

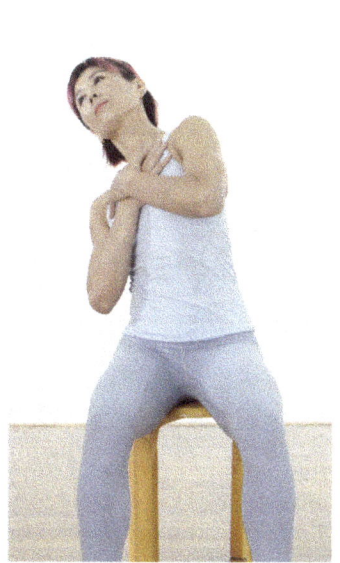

Rotate right

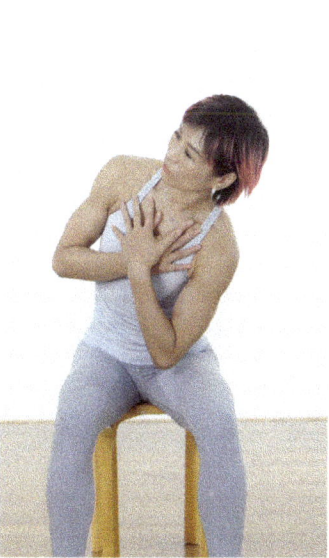

Side bend left

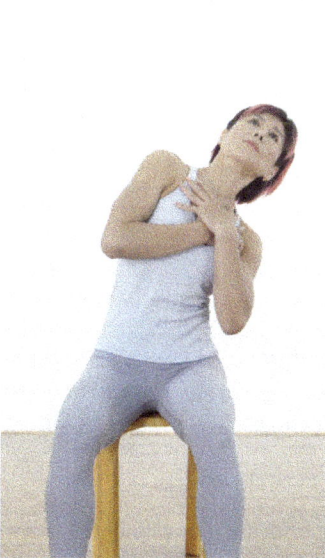

Rotate left

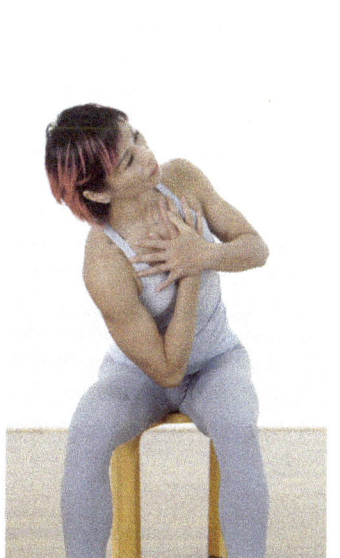

Side bend right

⑦

⑧

⑨

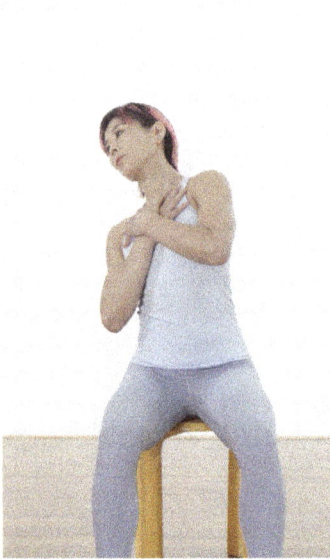

Rotate right

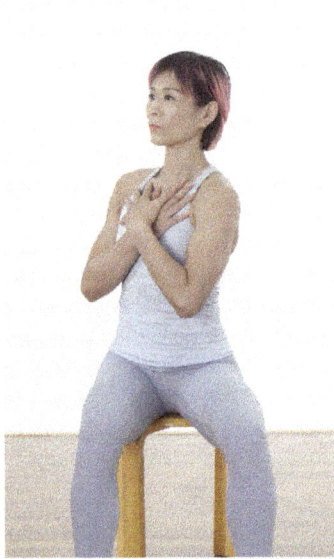

Half side bend left

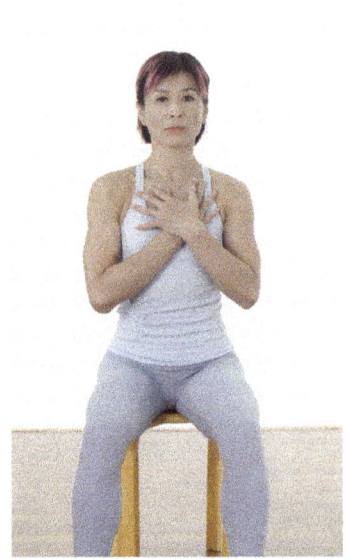

Half rotate left

Principles

Articulation of the spine in all 3 planes of movement

Benefits

Improve spinal mobility
Improve mobility of the whole ribcage
Helps improve breathing
Helps release neck and shoulder tension
Helps release lower back tension
Helps relieve low, middle and upper back pain

Cues

Verbal : Imagine your ribcage like a Venetian blind opening on one side and closing on the other.
Imagine each vertebra side bending or rotating on the one below it.
Keep the tips of the shoulder blades pointing towards you back pockets

Tactile : Teacher uses very light touch with the hands to guide the rib cage in the appropriate direction

Perform the side bending and rotation movements with both inhalation and exhalation and observe how this changes the movement.
Pause in between positions to observe how the breathing affects the position and ribcage

Scan the QR code to view the exercise - Seated Figure Eight

PM14 - Book Openings (Top Down)

Setup

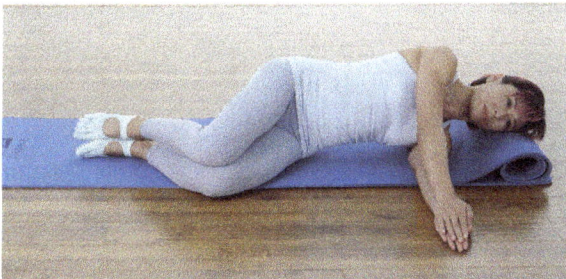

Begin in a sidelying position with the shoulders stacked upon each other and one palm resting on the one below with arms outstretched.

The pelvis and spine should be held in a neutral position and the spine should be in a straight line viewed from behind . Hips, knees and ankles flexed.

The head can rest on a long pillow or cushion no more than 8cm thick

Movement 1

Begin by sliding the right hand forwards and backwards on the left arm 3- 5 times and observe the small rotations being made in the upper ribcage.

Benefits

Improve rotation of thoracic spine (the mid to upper spine where all the ribs attach) - improve breathing and takes tension away from the lower back.

Helps mobility of the ribcage - improve breathing and takes tension away from the lower back.

Helps release tightness and shortness in front of shoulder and upper chest - helps to bring the head back to a better position over the ribcage thus being very beneficial for the neck and shoulders.

Now slide the right hand along the left arm drawing a line along the middle of the arm until the fingers touch the right shoulder joint.

In this position extend the the left elbow so that the left hand points to the ceiling.

From this position continue the movement as before looking at the thumb the whole time until the limit of the rotation is reached. Return the left arm to the vertical position and sweep the extended arm back to the start position.

It is important to maintain the integrity of the shoulder joint and rotate from the ribcage without overextending the shoulder joint throughout the whole exercise.

The return to the start position is initiated from the ribcage with the right lower ribs moving towards the left ASIS (remember Thoracic Rotation - PM4 ?)

Movement 2

Whilst lying on your right side begin to lift and sweep

your left arm up in the air and across over to the other side as though painting a brush stroke up the wall, across the ceiling and down the opposite wall. You should be looking at the thumb and index finger of the left hand throughout the movement so that your head will turn and face the left side at the end of the movement.

The restraint to the exercise is to keep your hips, pelvis, knees and ankles stacked on top of each other with no movement throughout the exercise. You should thus feel a comfortable stretch across the waist and your left upper chest area.

Return the left arm and hand to the start position maintaining focus on the ability of the ribcage and thoracic spine to move freely with each individual vertebra 'rotating' on the vertebra below it. If you don't know how many vertebra you have in your thoracic spine see if you can count them !

Movement 1

1

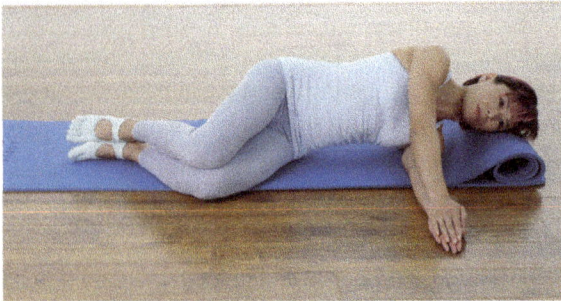

2

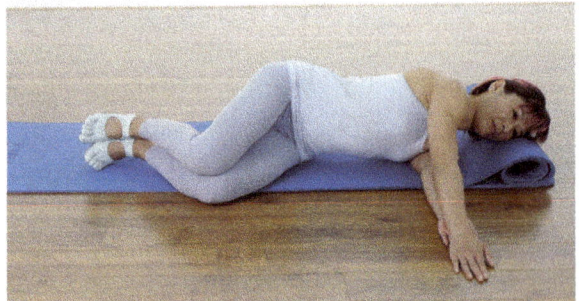

Hand slides forwards and backwards along lower arm

3

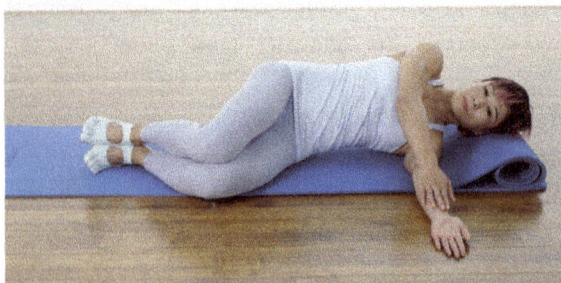

4

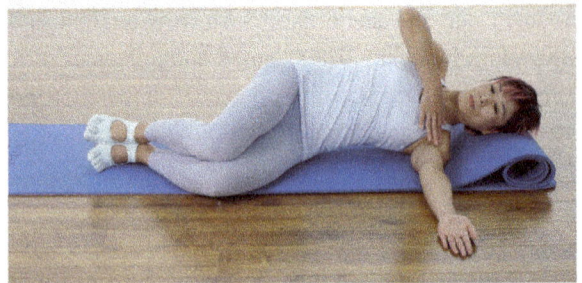

Hand slides back towards the elbowt

Hand stops at shoulder joint

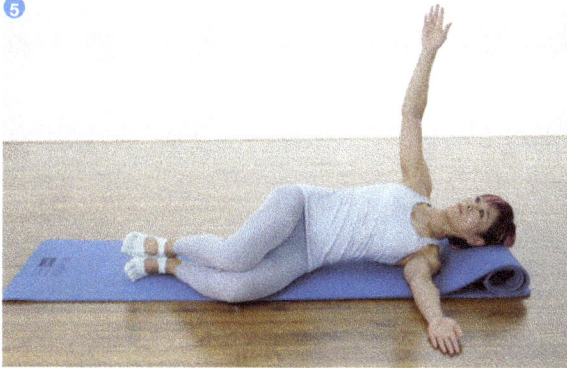

Arm extends towards ceiling

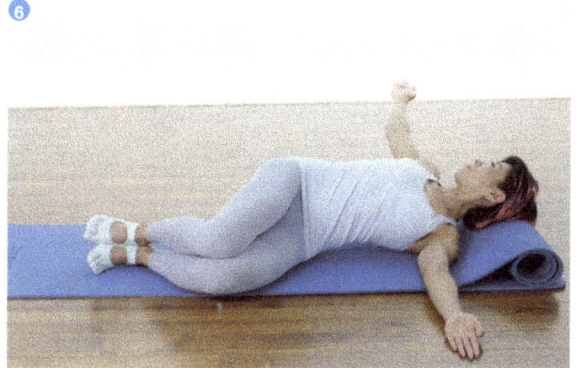

Ribcage rotates to allow arm to lower towards the floor

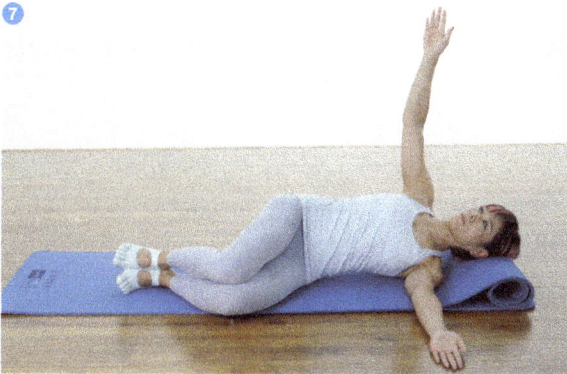

Movement to start position begins in ribcage

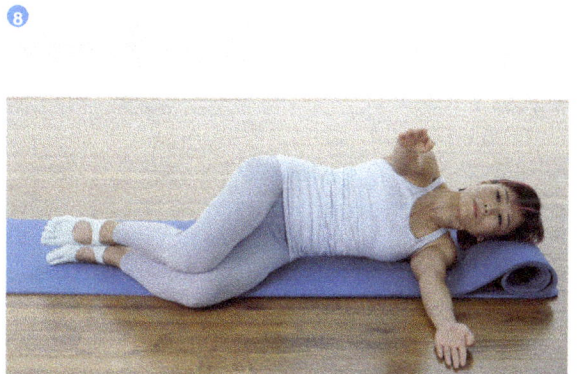

Arm remains extended on return movement

Movement 2

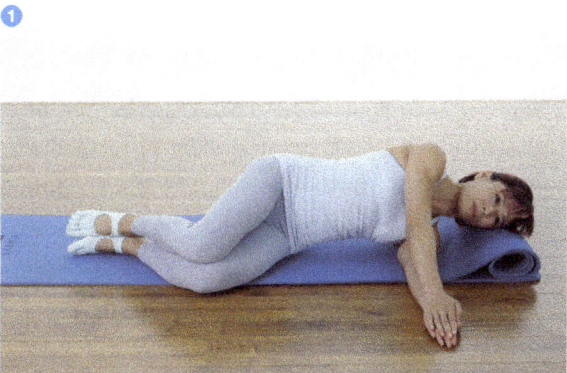

Start position

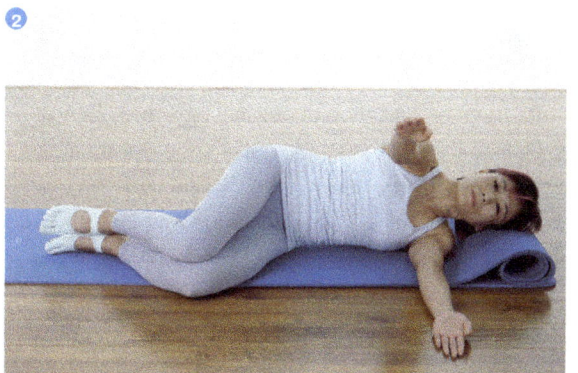

Hand and arm lift away from bottom arm

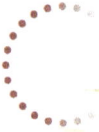

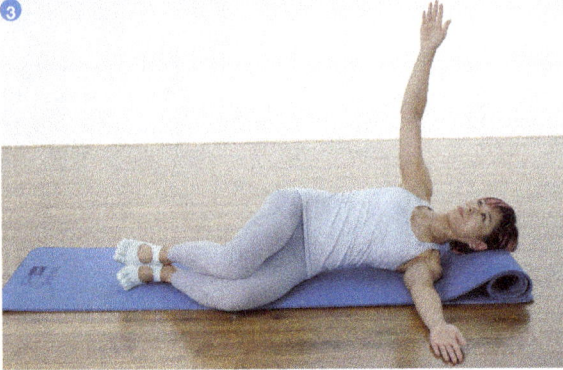

Arm rotates to 90 degrees

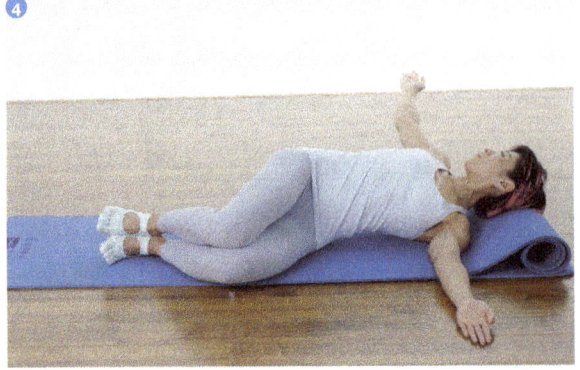

Ribcage rotates to allow arm to lower towards the floor

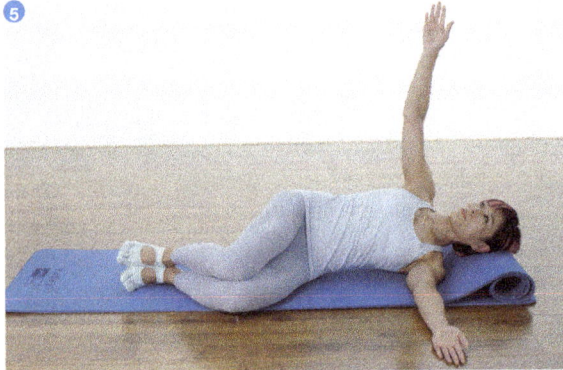

Movement to start position begins in ribcage

Principles

Articulation in rotation for thoracic spine
Organization of spine and ribcage

Scan the QR code to view the exercise - Book Openings

Benefits

Improve organisation of pelvis, spine and ribcage
Release lower back, neck and shoulder tension
Improve rotation of thoracic spine (the mid to upper spine where all the ribs attach) - improve breathing and takes tension away from the lower back.
Helps mobility of the ribcage - improve breathing and takes tension away from the lower back.

Helps release tightness and shortness in front of shoulder and upper chest - helps to bring the head back to a better position over the ribcage thus being very beneficial for the neck and shoulders.

Cues

Verbal : Imagine a paint brush in your right hand and draw a big circle up the wall, across the ceiling and down the opposite wall.

Tactile : Teacher sites on the right side of client facing the head and uses gentle touch to bring proprioceptive feedback to the client for the rotation.

Use an inhalation for the rotation out and exhalation to return to start position.
Use exhalation for the rotation out and inhalation to return to start position.
Make multiple inhalations and exhalations in the end position.
How dod all these variations on the movement feel.
What is the difference between Movement 1 and Movement 2

PM15 - Head lift

Contraindications & Precautions

Neck pathologies such as spondylosis or disc problems may be exacerbated by this exercise.

Benefits

Strengthens the deep muscles of the neck that help stabilize the head and neck.
Helps alleviate neck pain
Helps alleviate headaches
Improves the position of the head over the ribcage which will help improve neck and shoulder issues.
Is an important basic component of many Pilates Mat exercises.
Helps activate the gluteal muscles (your butt) - good for posture and taking tension away from the lower back.

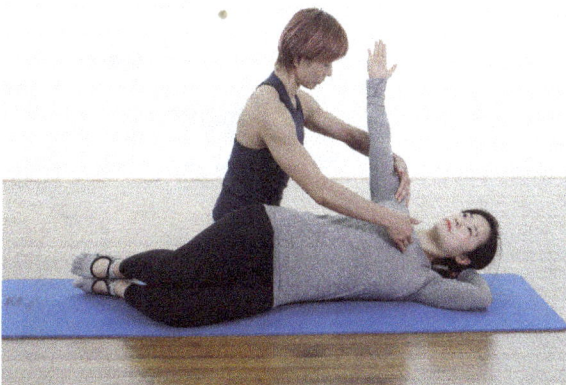

Teacher guided cue for Book Openings exercise

Setup

Lie on the mat in a supine position with the legs in a triple flexed position with your hands placed by your sides. If you feel uncomfortable in your neck in this position you can place one hand under the back of the head.

Movement

Begin by tilting the head backwards and forwards by lifting the chin to the ceiling and then dipping towards the chest. Find the 'halfway position' to bring the head to rest in a 'neutral position'.

Imagine a ball placed at the top of your head on the floor. Lengthen through the spine to try and push the ball away from you so that your head floats away from the mat (or your hand).

The head should lift no more than 1.5 - 2 cm from the floor (the width of your mobile phone !)

You should feel the deep flexor muscles in the front of your neck engage to support the weight of the head from the floor.

The chin will be very slightly tilted towards the chest as though you are holding an oversized tennis ball between the chin and the chest.

Hold this position for 5 slow counts and then slowly lower the head to the floor.

Before performing the next repetition allow 30 - 60 seconds rest with some gentle rotations of the head to relax the neck muscles.

Perform 3 to 5 repetitions of holding the head in this position for a count of 5 each time.

Important note :

The muscles we are targeting are the deep neck muscles. If performed incorrectly you will over engage a muscle called the sternocleidomastoid (SCM) which will make you will feel very uncomfortable. This is an easy muscle to find on the left and right side of the neck as it 'pops out' when the deep muscles are not being used properly. You can observe this muscle in action by tuning your head to one side and then lifting the head against some resistance VERY GENTLY.

WARNING : This exercise is designed to help recruit the deep muscles at the front of the neck. No matter what is your perceived level of fitness you should perform no more than 3 repetitions for the first time. Many persons have extremely weak muscles here and it is very common to acquire some discomfort or pain in these muscles when practicing this exercise the first time. Although you will not be damaging or

hurting yourself it is quite possible to feel a degree of soreness and/or pain in the neck area the next day if your muscles have not been trained properly to perform this exercise.

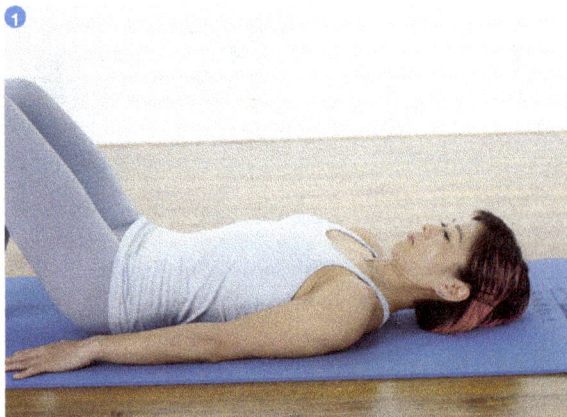

Relaxed head on the mat

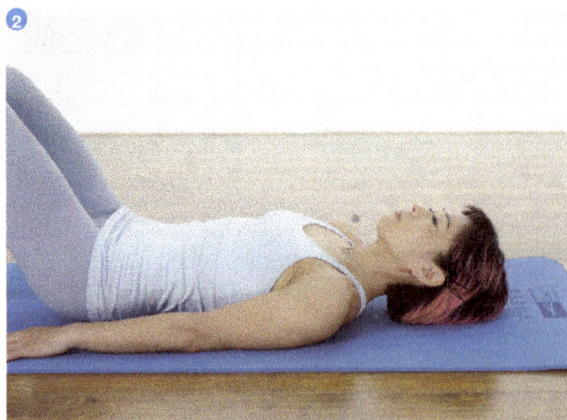

Use the deep muscles of the neck to lift the head

Principles

Functional unit alignment
Stabilization of the shoulder girdle
Articulation of the spine (cervical spine in flexion)

Cues

Verbal : Imagine a ball placed at the top of the head - try to move the ball.
Imagine you can slide your ears up towards the top and front of the head.
Feel the neck and upper ribcage lengthen and the ribs sink to the mat.
Imagine you are holding an oversized tennis ball between your jaw and the chest.

Tactile : Teacher can stabilize / cue the jaw with one hand whilst cueing the head into 'the lifted position' with the other hand

Use an inhalation to lift the head and then use an exhalation to lift the head. What difference does the breathing make ?
Can you identify between when the superficial muscles work to do the exercise and when the deeper muscles are activated ?
What happens if you lift the head without the 'pre contraction' of the lower abdominal muscles ?

PM16 - Chest Lift

Contraindications & Precautions

Neck pathologies such as spondylosis or disc problems may be exacerbated by this exercise.

Setup

Lie in a supine position with the legs in a triple flexed position.
Begin with fingers interlocked and the hands behind the back of the neck at the base of the skull. Use the 'knife edge' of the hands to help 'lift the head' from the bottom and give a slight stretch to the neck
The elbows should be lifted from the floor far enough that you can see them from the corner of each eye so that the arms are helping support the head and lengthen the neck.

Movement

Imagine you have a hose pipe inserted through the mouth and down the throat. Begin the exercise with the Head Lift and the hands behind the back of your neck at the base of the skull supporting the head.
Make sure your elbows are held in a position to the side but slightly in front of the head so that you can see them out of the corner of your eyes. Begin to curl the head followed by the chest from the floor paying attention to a number of things :

  • *See if you can visualize the articulation / movement of each vertebra as it 'peels way' from the one below*
  • *Feel the length being created in the back of the neck and upper back.*

• Pay attention to the imaginary hose pipe and make sure it does not kink or reduce the flow of air (or imaginary water) travelling through the pipe.

• As the head and upper chest lifts from the floor feel the narrowing of the waist and hollowing of the abdominal muscles whilst the pelvis and lower back remain stable. Imagine a glass of water on the lower belly that does not spill as the head is lifted.

• You may 'allow' a slight tilting back of the pelvis as the chest lifts however be sure to check that the lower back does not flatten into the floor.

Continue lifting the head and chest curling your way through the spine one vertebra at a time until you can not lift anymore or you feel your belly begin to 'pop out' as the abdominal muscles lose the ability to hollow out. The ideal position to stop will be when you feel the back of the last 2 or 3 ribs still in contact with the floor.

In this 'chest lifted position' take 3 deep inhalations into the back of the ribs to maximise your possible posterior expansion of the ribcage.

Benefits

Helps improve recruitment strategy of the abdominal muscles
Strengthens the deep muscles of the neck that help stabilize the head and neck.
Helps alleviate neck pain
Helps alleviate headaches
Improves the position of the head over the ribcage which will help improve neck and shoulder issues.
Is an important basic component of many Pilates Mat exercises.

Principles

Functional unit alignment
Stabilization of the shoulder girdle
Articulation of the spine (flexion)

Cues

Verbal : Imagine a tube/hose pipe in your mouth and down the throat. Don't kink the pipe as you flex through the spine.
Inhale- exhale - relax the eyes, nose, jaw, throat, collar bones and ribs.
Feel the ribs at the back open and the ribs at the front close as you flex.
Imagine holding a tennis ball between your jaw and the chest as you flex through the rib cage

①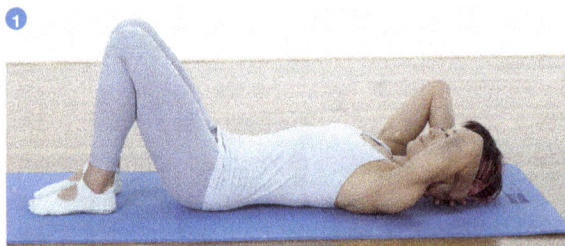

②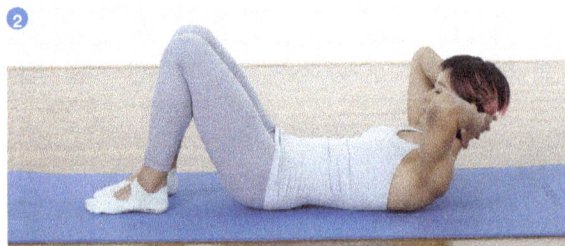

Look past your knees as you flex and curl the rib cage upwards.

Tactile : Teacher can use fingers of one hand to cue the sternum and fingers of the other hand to cue the upper spine.

Use an inhalation to lift the head and then use an exhalation to lift the head. What difference does the breathing make ?
Can you maintain distance between the pubic bone and the bottom of your ribs ?

Scan the QR code to view the exercise - Chest Lift

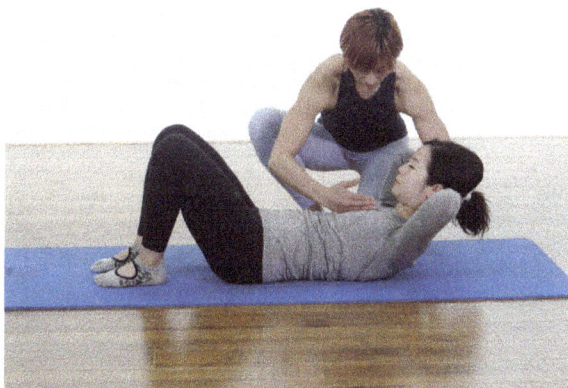

Teacher guided / assisted cue for Book Openings exercise

PM17 - Hip Flexor Stretch

This is just one of those exercises that 'everybody does' Or maybe 'should do'. The act of sitting for such long periods every day plays havoc with our hips, lower back and spine by shortening the muscles that pull our pelvis forwards away from an optimum position and placing huge amounts of tension on the spine all the way up to the neck and head.
This is one of those exercises we should devote at least 10 minutes to practicing everyday !

Contraindications & Precautions

Persons with knee pain may find this difficult however a thicker mat or rolled up towel may help take the pain or tension away from the knee.

Benefits

Improves overall posture
Helps improve position of head, ribcage and pelvis alignment
Helps take tension away from lower back
Helps improve mobility for hip extension movements

Set Up

Kneeling lunge position standing on the left leg flexed at the hip and knee 90 degrees in the front and kneeling on the right knee also flexed at the hip and knee 90 degrees.

The left knee is directly over the left ankle.

The right knee is directly under the right hip.

The spine is upright.

The right hand is placed over the right buttock and the left hand over the lower right pelvic area.

Note: You may hold on to a chair or other support if the balance is too challenged for this exercise.

Movement

Part 1

Pivot backwards to stick your butt out the back and then smoothly return to the start position by contracting the right butt muscle as hard as you can. You can use your right hand to feel if the muscle is contracting properly. In this position you should have a 'rock hard butt'.

Hold this 'butt squeeze' for 3 seconds. The pelvis and spine should be upright with the spine as straight as possible.

Depending on your flexibility you will feel a stretch:

Across the front of the right thigh
Across the front of the right hip
Across the front of the right thigh and the right hip.

Move backwards and forwards in a fluid smooth manner for 8 - 10 repetitions holding the butt squeeze for a 3 count each time.

Part 2

Now move the left foot 25 cm further in front.

Pivot the pelvis and spine together towards the left knee. Ensure the spine stays in a line with the right thigh.

Repeat this movement 8 - 10 times.

Hold the forward position and hollow the abdominals as much as possible to pull upwards into a thoracic extension position with the head looking upwards.

Hold this position for 5 breaths.

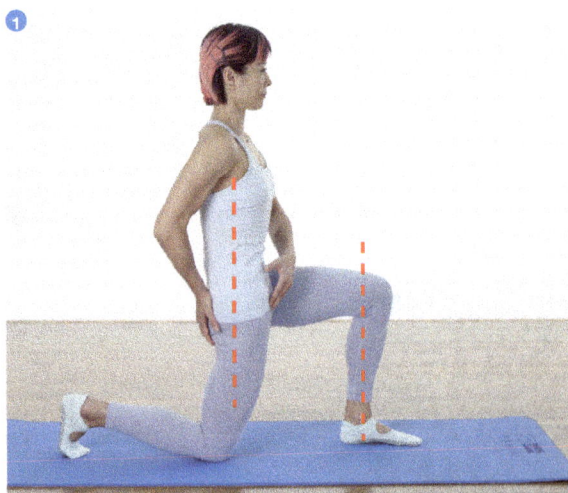

Start position

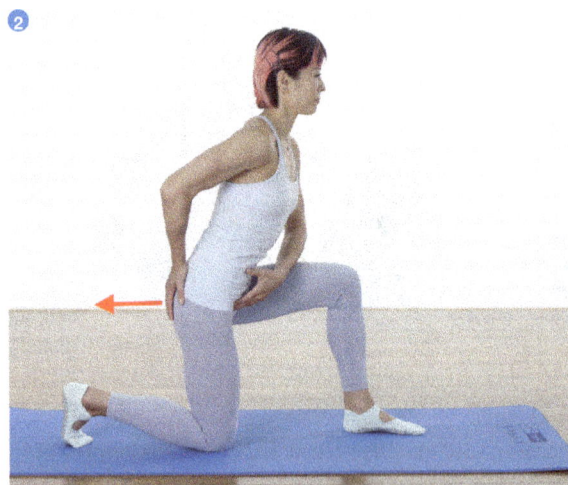

Butt goes back

3

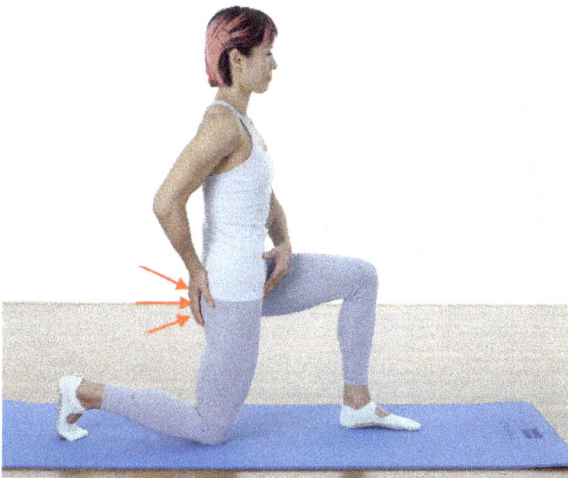

Butt goes forwards and squeezes

4

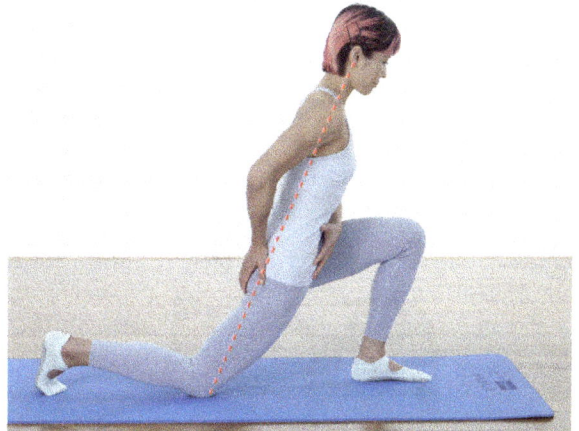

Pelvis moves forwards

5

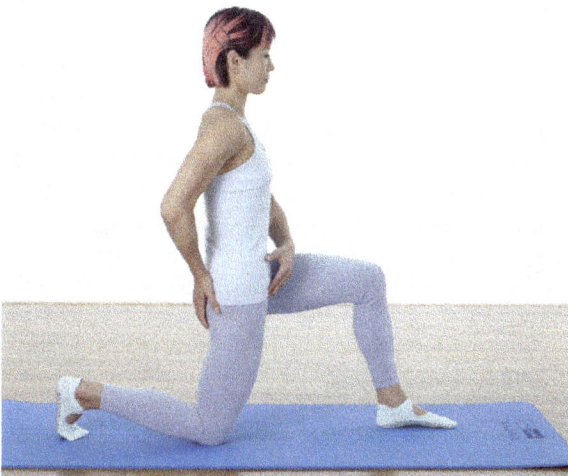

Foot moves forwards

6

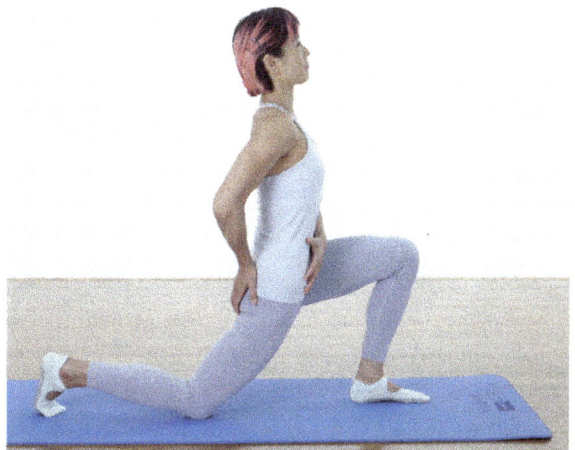

Extend the spine

Where do you feel the most stretch ?

Scan the QR code to view the exercise - Kneeling Hip Flexor Stretch

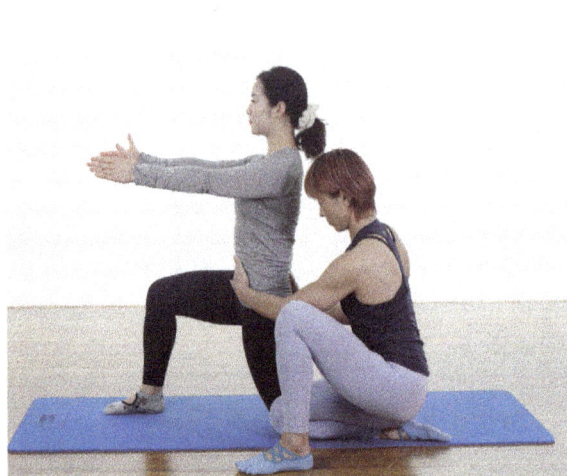

Teacher guided cue for Kneeling Hip Flexor Stretch exercise

Principles

Functional unit alignment
Core Control
Lumbo Pelvic Hip Complex mobility and stability

Cues

Verbal : Squeeze your butt as much as possible
Imagine a ruler from your lumbar spine the sacrum. Keep it straight and don't bend
For the last movement pull the collar bones as far away from your tail bone as possible

Tactile : Instructor places one hand over the 'butt hand' and one hand over the 'abdominal hand' of the client to monitor unwanted movement of instability of the LPHC

PM18 - Pelvic Lift

"The Mother of All Butt Exercises"
Not so much 'the mother' because it is so difficult but moreover because it is the exercise that allows you to really find the Gluteus Maximus muscle and has many variations.

Benefits

This is a wonderful exercise to help release lower back tension, relieve low back pain and strengthen your gluteal muscles or 'butt'.
If you perform this exercise with your arms away from the floor it will also considerably help stabilise the spine.

Setup

Supine position with legs triple flexed and hip width apart. The pelvis and spine are in neutral position and the arms are placed on the floor slightly away from the body.
This is one of those exercises that is helped by performing certain movements with a particular breath.

Movement

Begin with an inhalation followed by a strong exhalation. On the exhalation initiate a 'pull' on the pelvic floor muscles as the waist narrows and you have a feeling of the pelvic floor being pulled up towards your belly button.

On the next inhalation maintain the stability of the pelvis and waist and simultaneously lift the pelvis towards the ceiling whilst pressing the feet firmly 'through' the floor. The pelvis and spine should lift as a single unit with no bending or arching. In the end position the thighs of the legs and the spine should make one continuous line to the shoulders. However the common mistake in the movement is to try and lift using the back muscles which forces the back to arch pressing the ribs forwards and towards the ceiling.

In the top position pause for a moment and re-arrange the ribcage if needed so that it does not protrude or stick out to the ceiling.

Hold this position for 5 exhalations and inhalations focusing on :

• Stability of the pelvis and spine
• Contraction of the butt muscles to press the feet into the floor
• Position or alignment of the ribcage in relation to the pelvis.
• Inhalation to the back and sides of the ribcage.

Use the final exhalation to return to the start position by softening the collarbones and sternum at the top of the ribcage and allowing the back of the ribs to sink into the floor bringing the vertebra of the spine with them. The 2 common analogies used are :

Imagine the spine is like a string of pearls being held taut in this position. Now allow each pearl one at a time to be released into the floor until the pelvis is back to the start position.

Imagine the spine is like a bicycle chain held taut. Allow each vertebra (link in the chain) to relax and be lowered to the floor one by one until the pelvis returns to the start position.

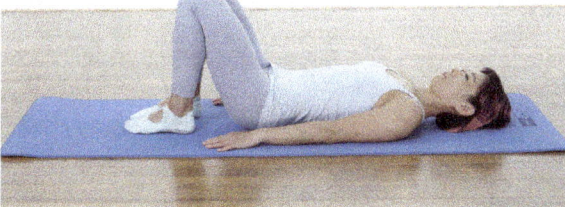

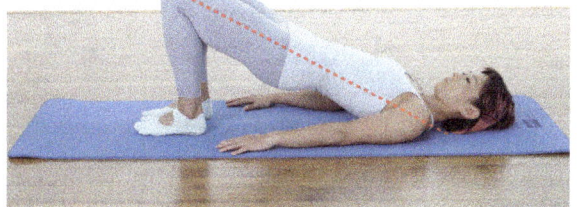

③

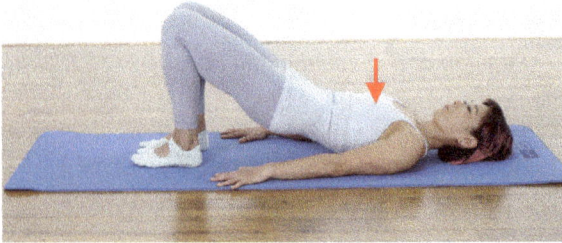

④

⑤

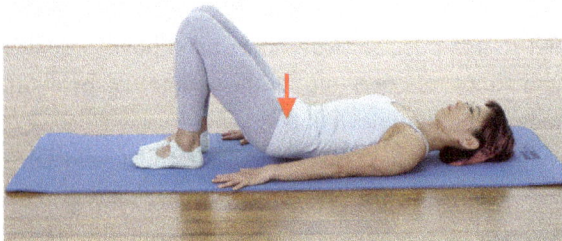

⑥

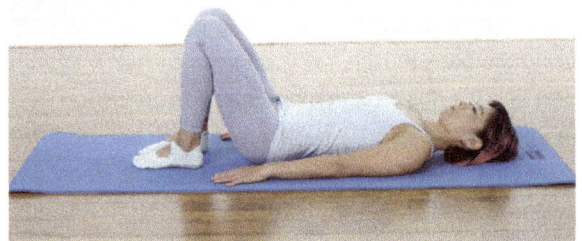

Principles

Functional unit alignment
Core Control
Lumbo Pelvic Hip Complex mobility and stability
Spinal Articulation

Cues

Verbal : Press your feet into the floor
Maintain the connection between the ribs and pelvis
Imagine the spine is like a string of pearls. Allow each pearl one at a time to be released into the floor until the pelvis is back to the start position.

Imagine the spine is like a bicycle chain held taut. Allow each vertebra (link in the chain) to relax and be lowered to the floor one by one until the pelvis returns to the start position.

Tactile : Use one hand under the pelvis and spine and the other over the abdomen and ribs to cue the pelvis and spine throughout the movement

Use different breathing strategies for the up and down movement - what changes ?
Practice with hands and arms in different positions - hands on pelvis / hands by your sides. What is the difference between the 2 positions ?

Scan the QR code to view the exercise - Pelvic Lift

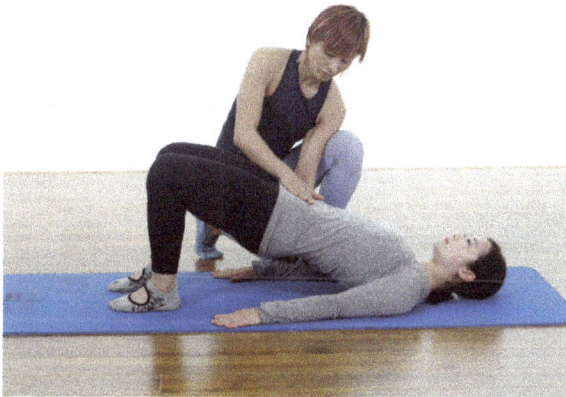

Teacher guided cue for Pelvic Lift exercise

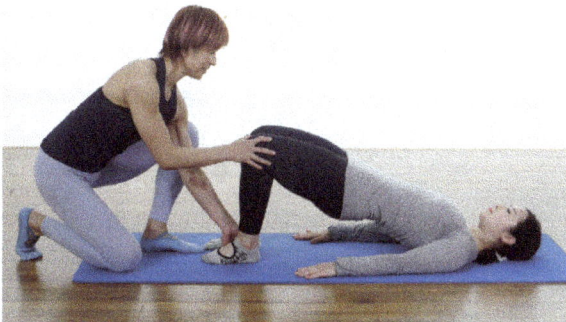

Teacher resisted cue test for Glute Max activation

Ensure the pelvis returns to the neutral position.

PM19 - Pelvic Curl

The pelvic curl may be considered a variation of the Pelvic Lift. The difference between the 2 exercises is that whilst the Pelvic Lift emphasizes the stability of the pelvis and spine in the lifting phase of the movement the Pelvic Curl has an emphasis on the mobility of the pelvis and spine.

Set Up

Supine position with legs triple flexed and hip width apart. The pelvis and spine are in neutral position and the arms are placed on the floor slightly away from the body.

Movement

Exhale to curl your tail bone towards your pubic bone (pelvic floor activation).

Curl the tail followed by the pelvis upwards and forwards towards the back of the knees so that the spine is pulled taut in a straight line. At the end of the movement.

Ensure the feet are pressing strongly into the mat and the butt muscles are squeezing tight.

In this top position pause for a moment and re-arrange the ribcage if needed so that it does not protrude or stick out to the ceiling.

Hold this position for 5 exhalations and inhalations focusing on :

  • *Stability of the pelvis and spine*
  • *Contraction of the butt muscles to press the feet into the floor*
  • *Position or alignment of the ribcage in relation to the pelvis.*

• Inhalation to the back and sides of the ribcage.

On an exhalation - soften the collarbones and sternum at the top of the ribcage and allowing the back of the ribs to sink into the floor bringing the vertebra of the spine with them.

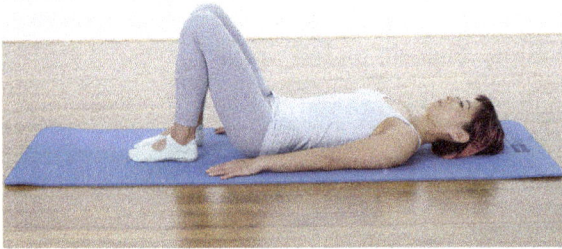

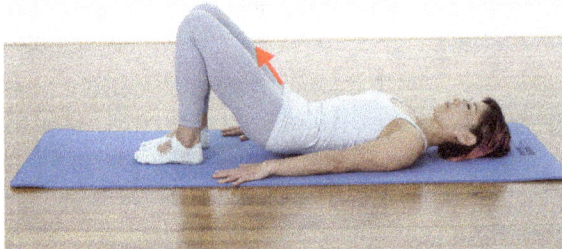

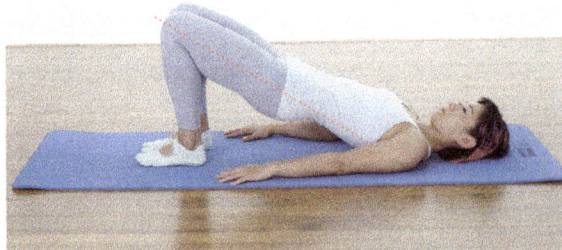

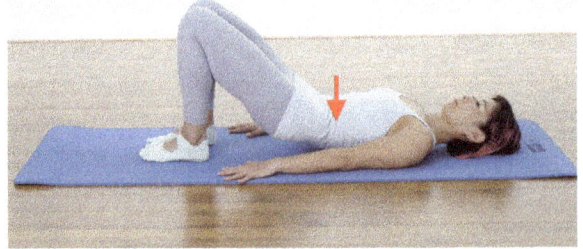

Principles

Functional unit alignment
Core Control
Lumbo Pelvic Hip Complex mobility and stability
Spinal Articulation

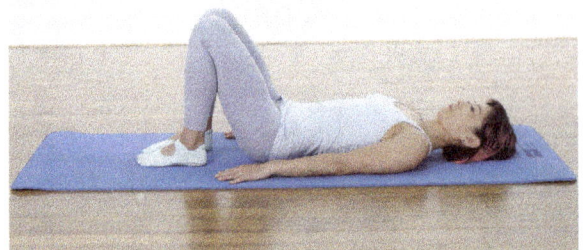

Cues

Verbal : Press your feet into the floor
Scoop your tail towards the pubic bone
Scoop the pelvis upwards and towards the back of the knees

Tactile : Use one hand under the pelvis and spine and the other over the abdomen and ribs to cue the pelvis and spine throughout the movement

Scan the QR code to view the exercise - Pelvic Curl

Benefits

Helps balance out the spinal and abdominal muscles

Helps relieve low or upper back pain

Improves activation of the abdominal muscles

Improves activation of the gluteal (Butt) muscles

Movement

Press your feet firmly into the floor whilst performing a 'scoop' of the tail bone towards the back of the knees. Continue to scoop the pelvis up and forwards whilst articulating through the vertebrae of the spine until you reach the bridge position.

Maintain this position and with an exhalation begin to lift the head and chest from the floor. Use your butt muscles to resist the movement of the upper body lifting from the floor by reluctantly lowering the spine and pelvis to the floor. Now repeat the lifting of the pelvis to the bridge position but resist the movement by reluctantly lowering the upper body to the floor.

In other words you continue to make a 'see saw' type movement by lifting the head, chest and upper spine as you lower the pelvis and lumbar spine and then conversely lift the pelvis and lumbar spine as you lower the upper spine, chest and head.

The common mistake that people make is that they lower one end in order to raise the other end. The correct form is to ensure you lift one end first and the other end lowers towards the floor because it is forced to due to the raising of the other end.

Ensure the pelvis returns to the neutral position.

PM20 - Chest lift & Pelvic Curl

Setup

Lie on your back with your legs in the triple flexed position. Hands are interlocked behind the neck at the base of the head and elbows slightly in front of the head.

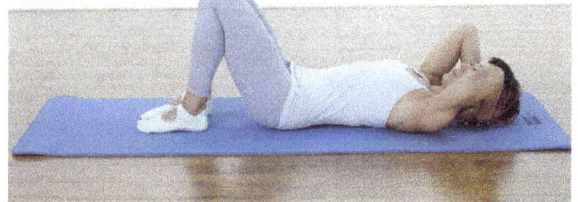

Start position

2

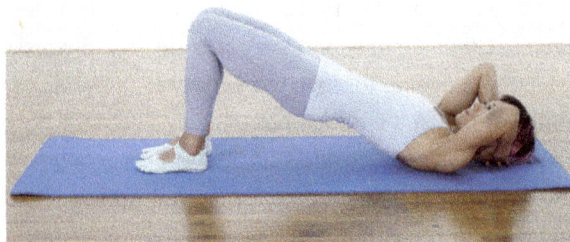

Lift to bridge position

3

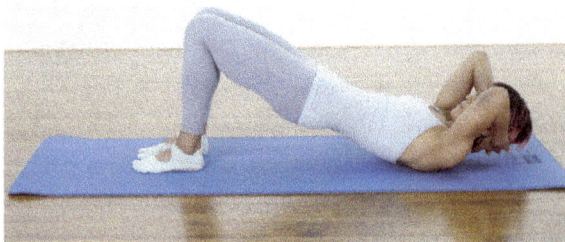

Begin to lift head and chest

4

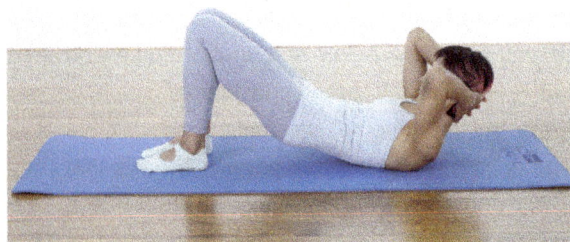

Resist upper body movement using the lower body

5

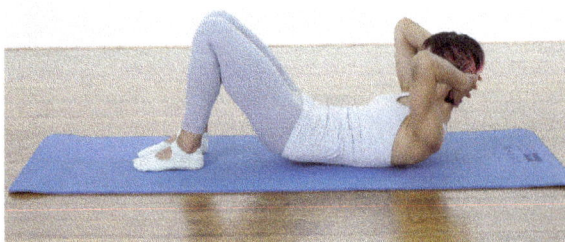

Reluctantly allow the pelvis to lower

6

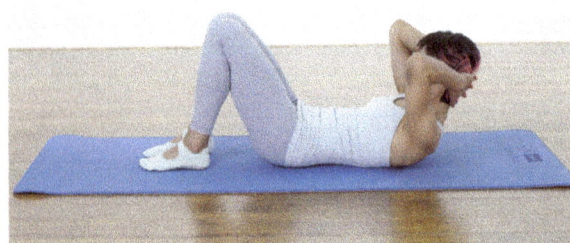

Pelvis on the mat

7

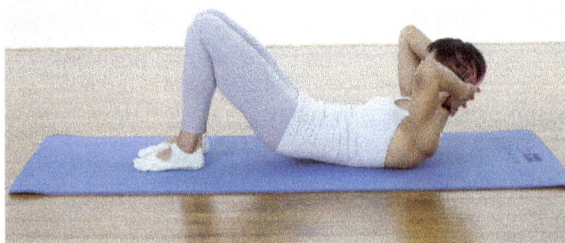

Scoop and lift the pelvis whilst resisting with the upper body

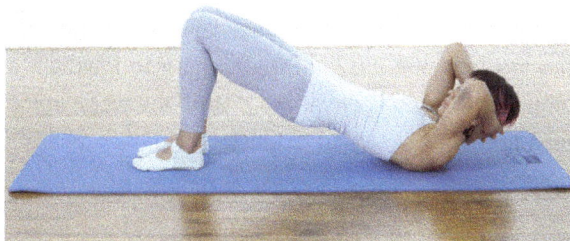

Lift to bridge position

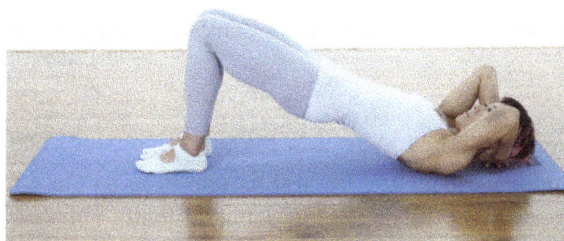

Reluctantly allow upper body to the mat

Principles

Functional unit alignment
Core Control
Lumbo Pelvic Hip Complex mobility and stability
Spinal Articulation

Which movement feels easier to resist : upper or lower body ?
Can you feel the spine is like the rocker on a rocking chair

Scan the QR code to view the exercise - Pelvic Curl Chest Lift

PM21 - Quadruped

Cues

Verbal : Press your feet into the floor
Scoop your tail towards the pubic bone
Scoop the pelvis upwards and towards the back of the knees
Resist the chest coming up by using your glutes and lower body
Resist the pelvis coming up by using the upper body

Tactile : Use one hand under the pelvis and spine and the other over the abdomen and ribs to cue the pelvis and spine throughout the movement

Benefits

Helps balance
Helps teach stabilization of the LPHC
Helps organization of contralateral (left / right) movement

The Quadruped exercise has a number of variations however we will focus on the basic movement here that places an emphasis on the stability between contralateral sides against a rotational component.

Set Up

Kneeling on all fours with the knees perpendicular under the hips and hip width apart. The hands are placed directly under the shoulder joints shoulder width apart.

Pelvis and spine are held in a neutral position with the head, ribcage and pelvis held in alignment.

Movement

Part 1

Imagine a glass of water on top of the pelvis and another glass between the shoulder blades. Flex the right shoulder and slide the fingers of the right hand along the mat in front of you until just the tips of the fingers are touching the floor. Observe what happened to the (imaginary) 2 glasses of water - If you think some of the water has spilled you will need to adjust your position slightly to bring the glasses level again.

Now float the right arm up from the floor as high as you can go whilst maintaining good organization of the shoulder girdle, rib cage and spine. Some persons may only be able to lift a few centimeters whilst others may be able to bring the arm level with the shoulder joint. The focus is on the quality of the movement whilst maintaining stability of pelvis, spine, ribcage and shoulder girdle.

Bring the right arm and hand back to the start position and then repeat the movement again however this time make 5 short pulsing movements up and down when the arm is held out.

Part 2

Gently lift the left knee a couple of centimeters from the mat without disturbing the imaginary glass of water. Now slide the foot backwards by extending the leg from the hip joint taking care to maintain a stable pelvis and again not to disturb the water in the (imaginary) glass. Upon extension of the leg make a number of check points :

The ball of the foot should be on the mat
The back of the knee should have no creases
The left butt muscles and hamstring muscles should be activated.
The pelvis should be level and not slanted
The pelvis should not be side lifted / hoiked towards the shoulder
The pelvis should not be rotated
There should be no side shift of the ribcage
There should be no rotation of the ribcage

Now plantar flex the ankle (point the foot) so that the toes are resting gently on the paint of the mat.

Reach through the leg to initiate an extension movement to float the leg from the floor. Similarly to the arm you should only lift the leg as high as you are able to maintain the checklist above regarding the pelvis and ribcage. Again this may be only a few centimeters or it may even mean being able to pass the 'horizontal point'.

Return the leg to the start position.

Repeat the movement again but this time perform 5 up and down pulses with the leg from the hip joint.

Part 3

Now combine parts 1 and 2 into one movement.

A reminder that focus if on the quality of the movement in regards to the stability of the pelvis, spine, ribcage and shoulder girdle whilst the arm and leg move in their respective joints along with appropriate movement of the scapula on the side that the arm is lifting.

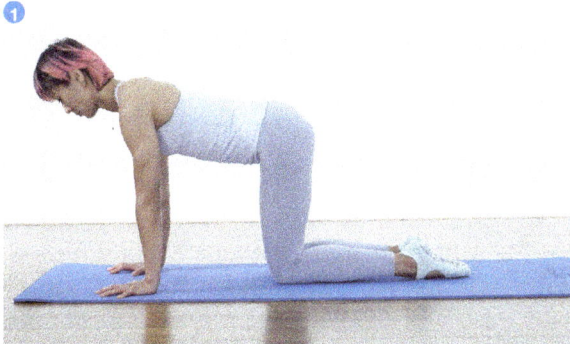

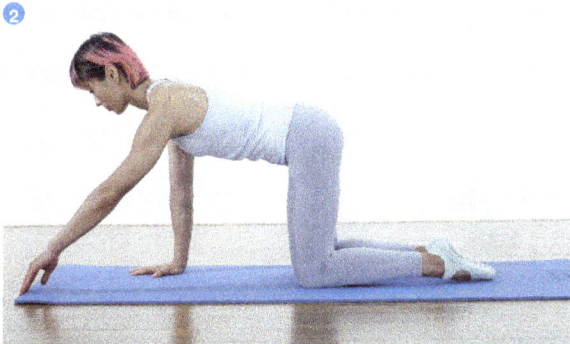

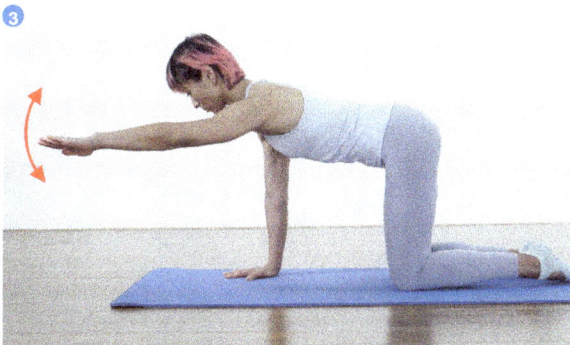

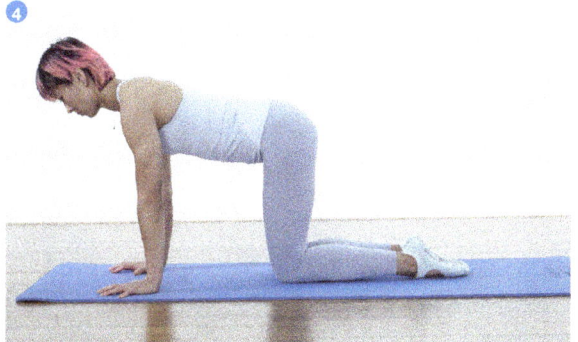

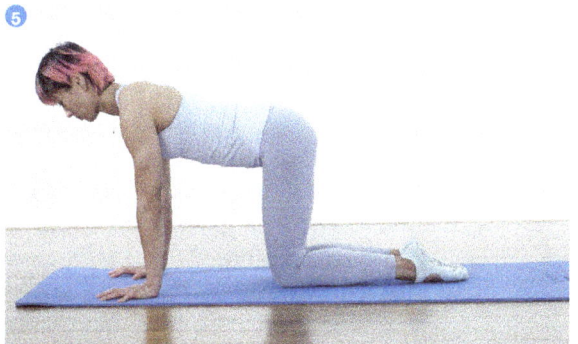

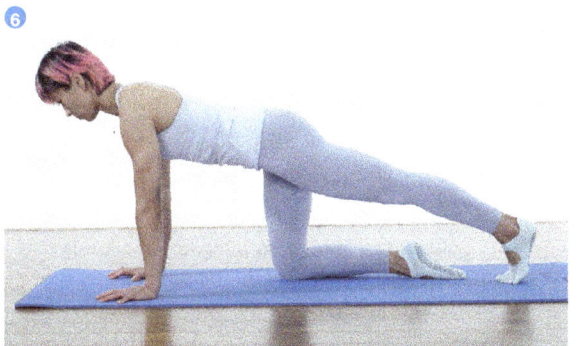

⑦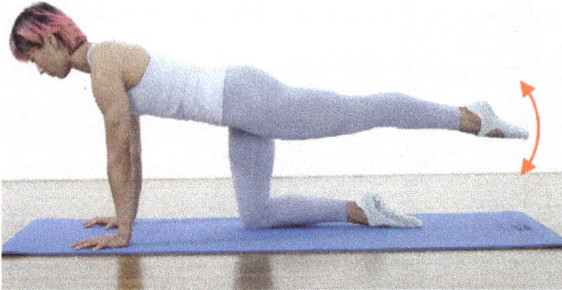

⑧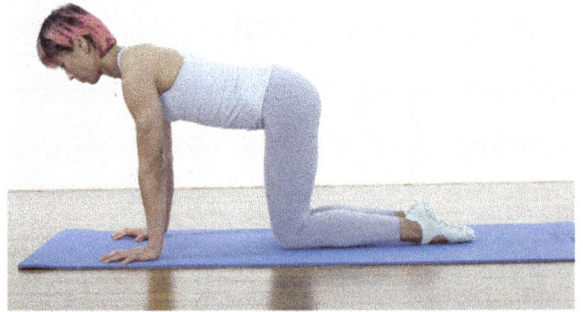

⑨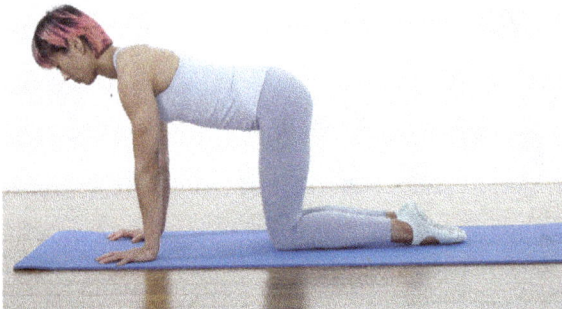

⑩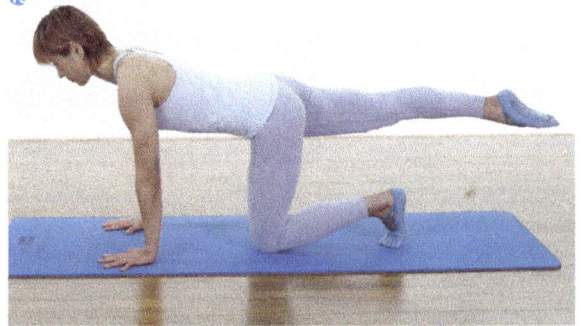

⑪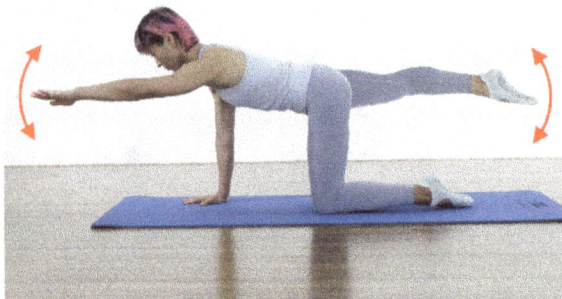

Principles

Functional unit alignment
Core Control
Lumbo Pelvic Hip Complex stability

Cues

Verbal : Imagine a rod through your head to your tail
Lengthen the leg to lift it.
Avoid shifting the pelvis
Tactile : Use one hand under the lower abdominals and the other over the lumbar to give proprioceptive feedback of the position.

Scan the QR code to view the exercise - Quadruped

Can you feel the abdominals engage to avoid a pelvic shift ?
Compare the movement to allowing a side shift of the pelvis and ribcage.

PM22 - Side to Side

This is one of those exercises that really exemplifies what Pilates is well known for when you hear somebody say " Oh yeah, Pilates thats the thing where you use all your little muscles". From the outside it appears that very little is happening but on the inside there is a lot of work going on.

This would be one of those movements where master teacher Michael King would say "Show me your Pilates face" meaning that the practitioner is showing no signs of effort from the outside despite the hidden amount of work on the inside.

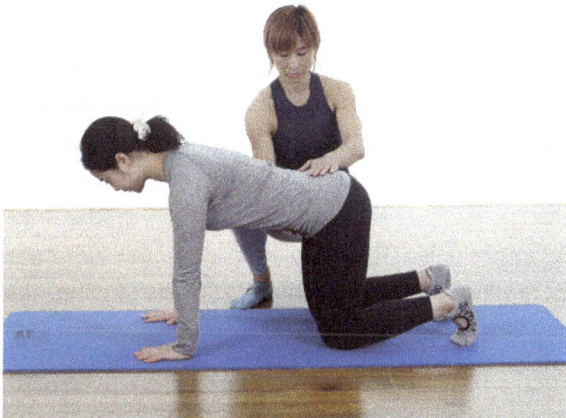

Teacher gives Guided cue for Quadruped exercise

Contraindications & Precautions

This is actually a great exercise for Post Natal recovery however care must be taken to begin with, and become proficient with the basic version before progressing.

Post natal women having had a cesarean should not attempt this exercise without guidance from a qualified medical or exercise professional due to the pressure it can exert on the lower abdominal musculature and tissue.

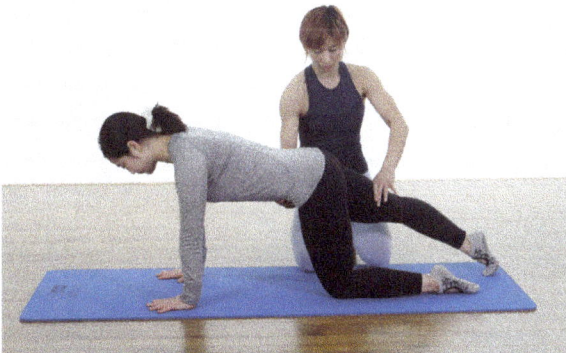

Teacher gives resisted cue test for Glute Max activation in Quadruped exercise

Set Up

Lie on your back in the triple flexed position with your hands either resting by your sides or over the lower abdomen.

Your knees and ankles are touching each other as though held together with glue. Pelvis is in a neutral position.

Benefits

Helps address left / right lower abdominal imbalances

May help in rebalancing the pelvis for a transverse plane rotation

Strengthens the lower abdominal muscles

Helps strengthen the pelvic floor

Helps post natal recovery

Helps stabilize the SI joint

Helps take tension away from the lower back

Movement

Exhale to engage the lower abdominal muscles and float your feet from the mat far enough to slide a piece of paper under them.

Your feet are now 'floating' on the mat just touching the 'paint on the mat'.

Ensure your lower back has not arched from the floor and the belly did not 'pop out'. One thing you can try is to place a paper cup over the lower abdomen. Your goal is to stop the cup from lifting / popping up in the air as you float your feet from the floor.

From this position you will slowly lower the left and right legs to the left side :

• *Imagine (or use) a small ball between the knees. The ball will need to roll in a counterclockwise direction when the legs go left and a clockwise direction when the legs go right.*

• *The leg is not the driver ! So in fact you don't lower the legs to the side - in fact you need to 'lift' the right leg from below by lifting the right pelvic half. Try to touch the left knee with the right ASIS. This is achieved by 'shortening' a diagonal line from the left*

lower ribs to the right ASIS.

• *The right side of the pelvis lifts from the mat and the pelvis and torso rotate to the left approximately 30 degrees.*

You may press into the floor using the right arm to engage the right latissimus dorsi muscle to help the movement. Remember the latissimus dorsi muscle inserts into the thoracolumbar fascia so the contractions of the right lats helps engage the core muscles through its' attachment.

Return to the start position and repeat to the other side.

A progression of the exercise can be made by simply increasing the lever length and performing the movement with the legs at a 90 - 90 (table top) position.

Scan the QR code to view the exercise Side to Side

❶

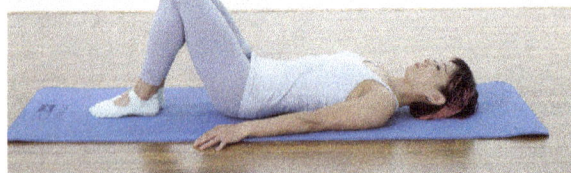

Start position

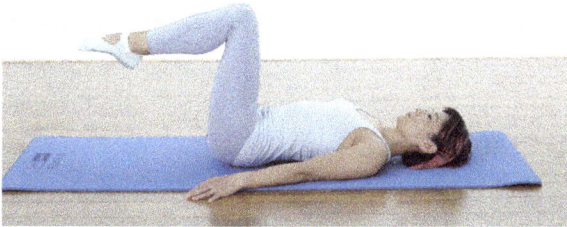

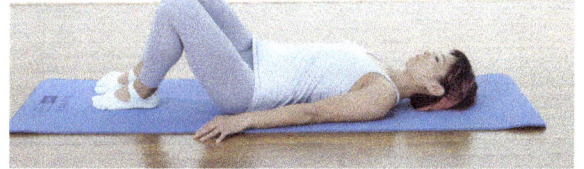

Legs move left

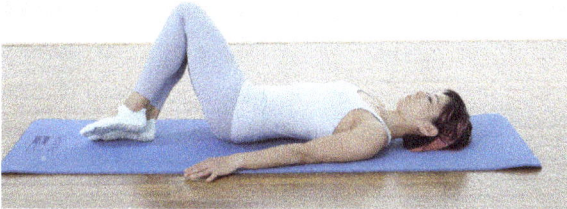

Legs move right

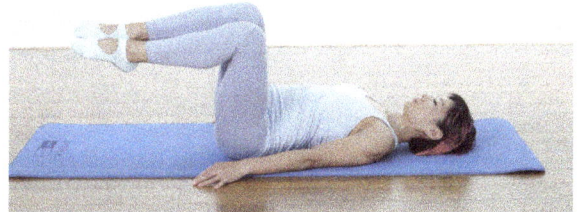

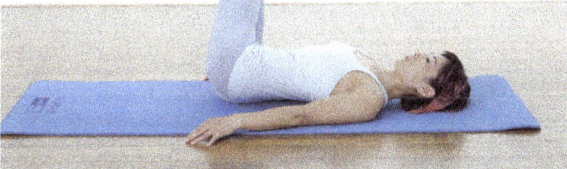

Progression

Cues

Verbal : Bring your right ASIS towards your left knee
Bring the bottom of your left ribcage towards your right ASIS
Do not disturb a paper cup on your lower abdomen

Tactile : Use a small ball between the knees to guide the legs

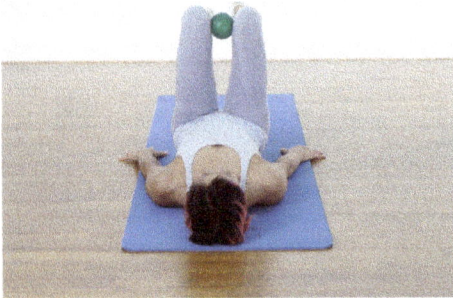

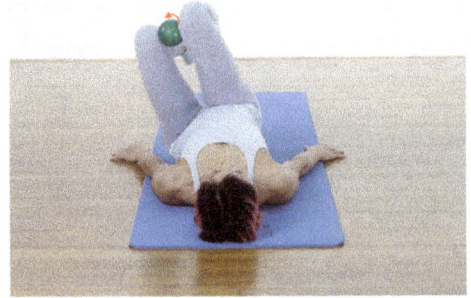

Right leg moves 'up and across' - ball rotates counter clockwise

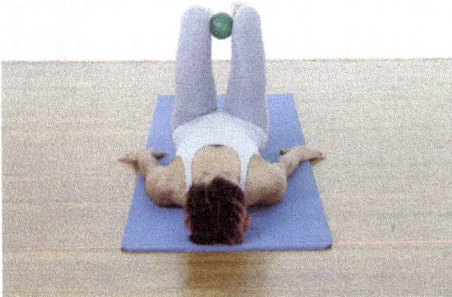

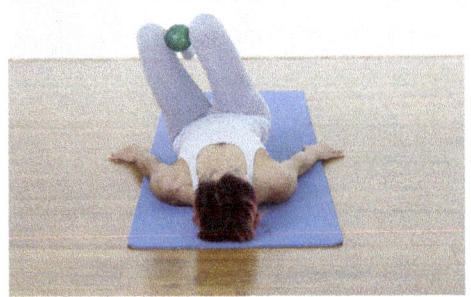

Right leg 'drops' - ball does not rotate

What is the difference between using the arms as support and not using the arms ?

Experiment with using various degrees of rotation / ranges of movement. What differences are there when you move a small, medium and large range of motion ?

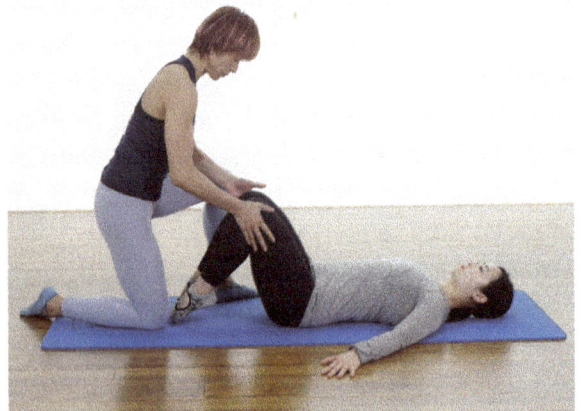

Teacher guided cue for Side to Side exercise

CHAPTER

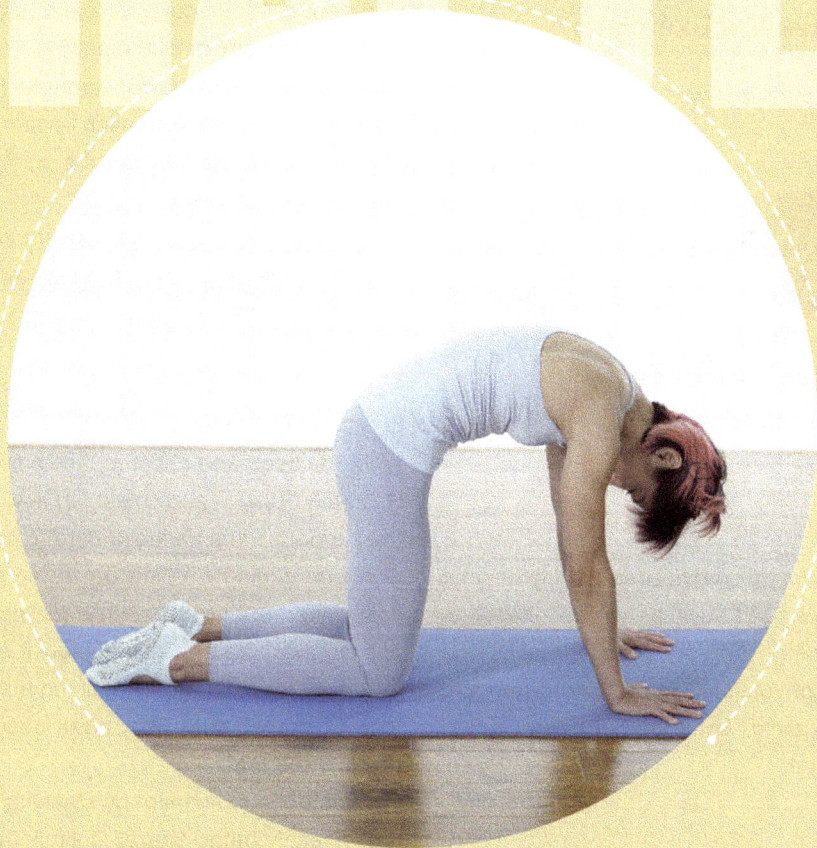

Eight

The Pilates Mat Exercises (M)

8.1 ▶ The Pilates Mat Exercises

M1 - Roll Up

Contraindications & Precautions

Pregnancy
Flexion movements are contraindicated for persons suffering from Osteoporosis

Set Up

The classical position to start is already lying on your back with arms averhead however we will choose to begin in the sitting position position with legs extended in front of you, ankles are dorsi flexed and legs adducted together. Arms are held extended in front at chest height.

Movement

Curl your tail towards your pubic bone to initiate a posterior movement of the pelvis.

Continue to curl down through the spine one vertebra at a time feeling each vertebra resting on the mat as it 'pulls away' from the vertebra above it in one continuous chain.

Finish with the arms held overhead and a long straight spine on the mat feeling how the abdominal muscles can squeeze from the sides to stabilize and lengthen the spine.

Reach the extended arms to the ceiling and when they are approximately 90 degrees to the chest begin to lift the head and chest in the same manner as the Head Lift (PM-15) and Chest Lift (PM-16) but without the support of the hands under the head.

Continue curling / rolling up to the sitting position, again one vertebra at a time feeling each vertebra peeling away from the one below it as you come up to the sitting position maintaining a flexed spine in a 'big C curve' with the arms reaching forwards towards the feet.

Complete the movement by stacking the vertebra on top of each other one at a time from the bottom

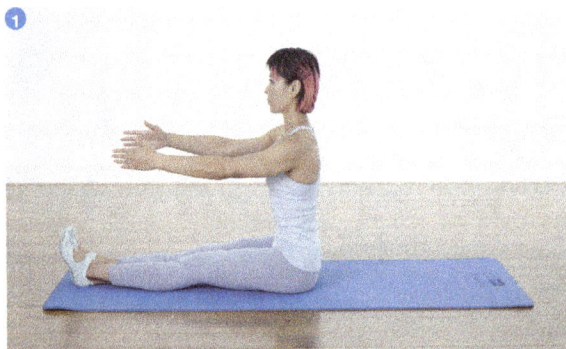

Start position

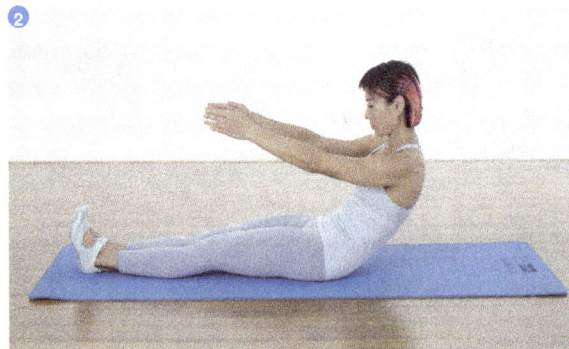

Curl the tail and begin rolling backwards

③
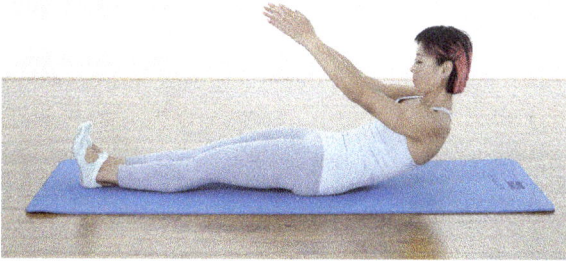
Curl the spine to the mat

④
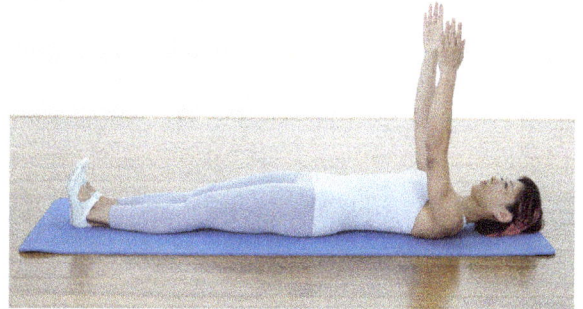
Arms to the ceiling

⑤
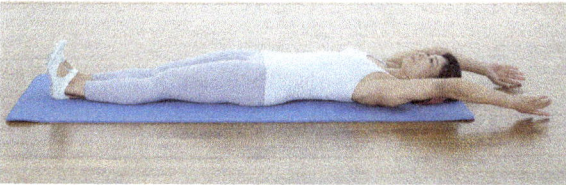
Arms overhead

⑥
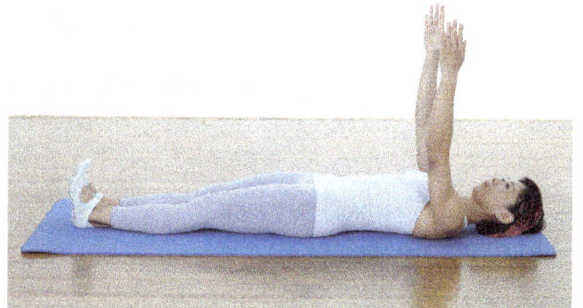
Bring arms back to 90 degrees again

⑦
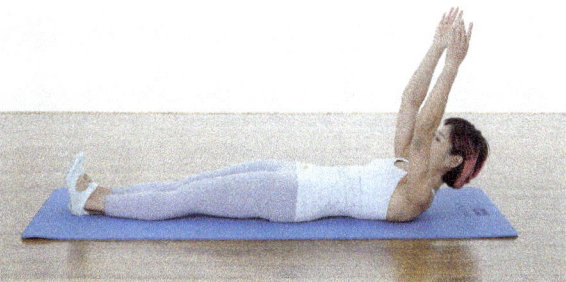
Begin to curl away from the mat

⑧
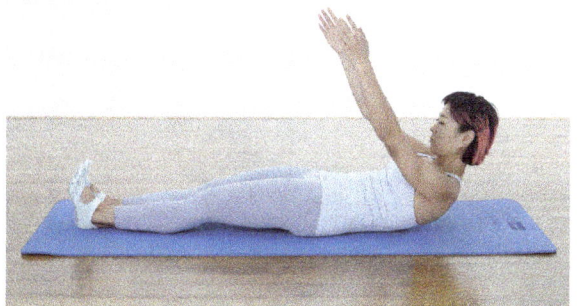
Continue peeling the vertebrae from the floor

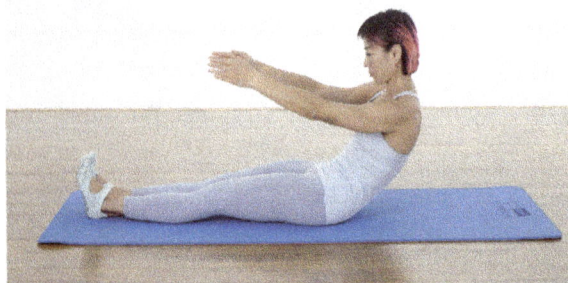

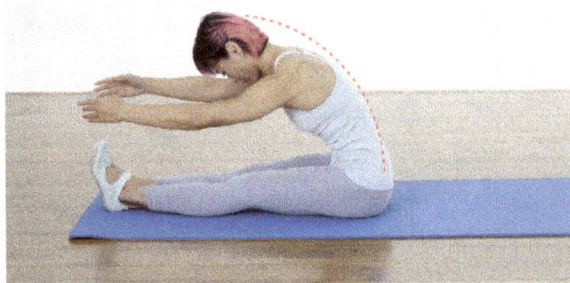

Finish in a C' curve

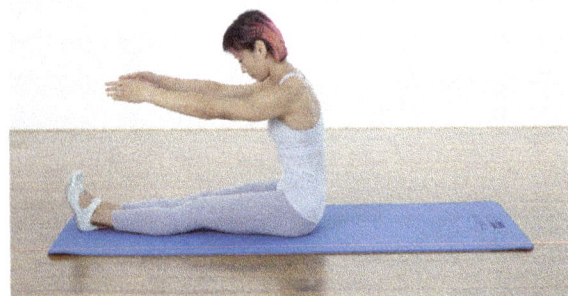

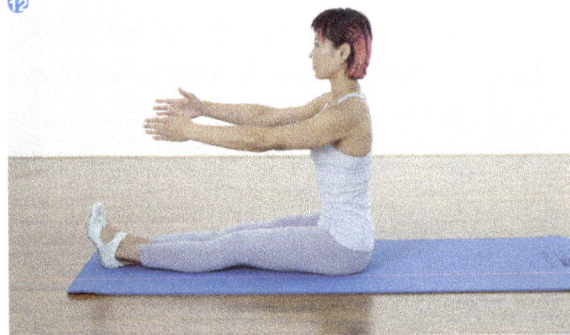

Stack the spine

Benefits

Helps improve spinal flexion
Helps abdominal muscle activation strategy
Builds spinal and pelvic awareness

Principles

Core Control
Spinal articulation into flexion

Cues

Verbal : Scoop your tail towards your pubic bone
Count the vertebra on your spine as you place
them one at a time on to the mat
Peel your spine from the floor

Tactile : Teacher can use gentle guided touch at
abdominals and vertebra levels

Scan the QR code to view the exercise - Roll Up

Teacher resisted cue for Roll Up exercise

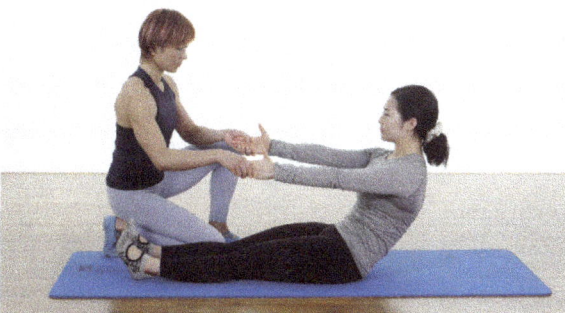

Teacher assisted cue for Roll Up exercise

upwards to finish with the spine in a vertical position.

Contraindications & Precautions

This exercise may be contraindicated for persons with some hip pathologies

M2 - Single Leg Circle 1

Set Up

Supine position with the legs extended and arms by your sides or resting gently on your pelvis.

Movement

Slide the sole of your left foot towards your left sit bone until the left knee is perpendicular to the left hip.

Extend the left leg without moving the left hip - the thigh remains perpendicular to the mat and plantar flex the foot.

This is now your 'center point' from which you will draw a circle with your left leg.

Imagine your left foot is a brush that paints a circle on the ceiling in a counter clockwise direction. As the leg moves right and downwards internally rotate the thigh in the hip joint. As the leg moves outwards and back up externally rotate the hip and also bring the leg past the vertical position.

Perform 5 - 8 repetitions and then change direction.

An alternative imagery is to imagine your femur head is like a pencil drawing a small circle in the hollow of your acetabulum.

The circle made by the leg can maintain the same size or you can increase the size as you continue moving. Either way the focus of the movement is

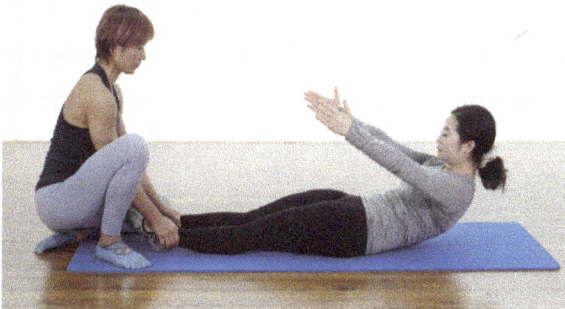

1

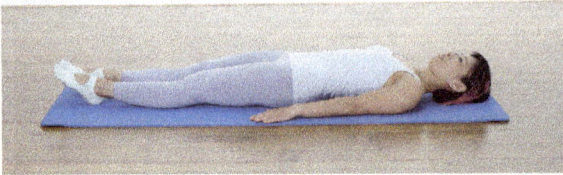

Start position

2

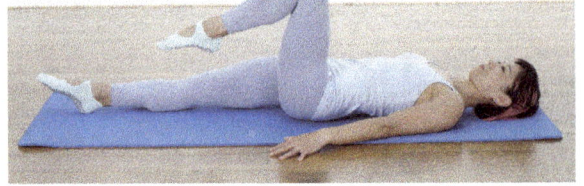

Flex knee and hip

3

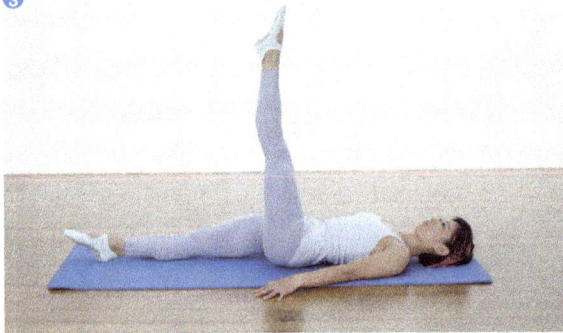

Extend the leg

4

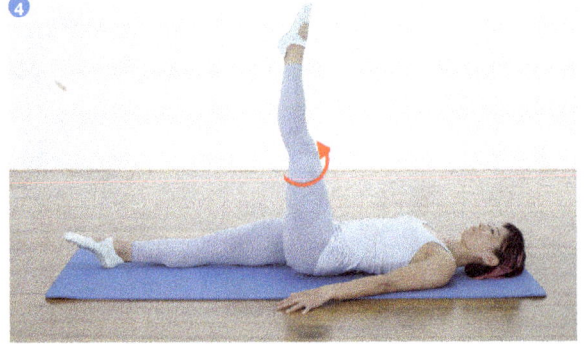

Move right and internally rotate

5

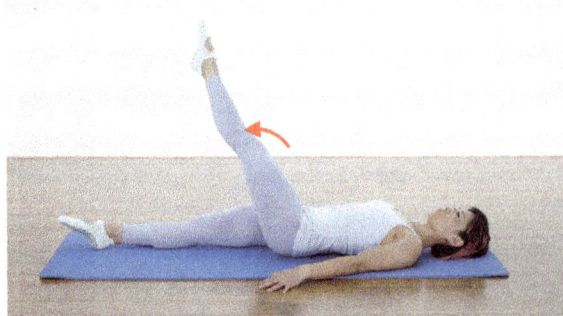

Lower right and internally rotate

6

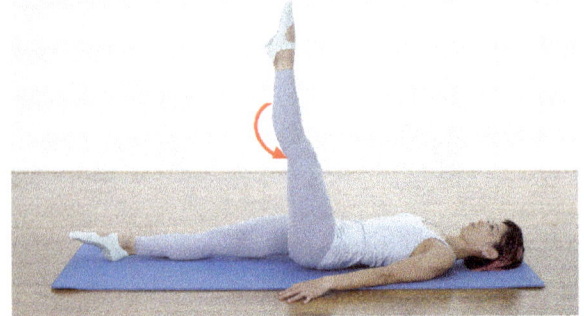

Move to left and externally rotate

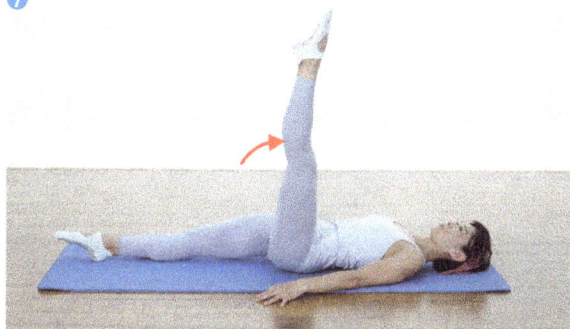

Move up and left and externally rotate

on mobility of the hip joint including the internal and external rotation components whilst keeping a stable pelvis throughout the movement.
For added stability press both arms into the floor.

Note

The Single Leg Circle exercises has a pre requisite of hamstring flexibility. If the muscles in the back of the leg are not flexible enough the leg will not be able to go to vertical position resulting in excessive tension in the synergistic hip flexors and reducing pelvis stability.
Therefore it is a good idea to 'test' the appropriate position of the leg before before commencing the exercise. If the leg can not be extended in the vertical position then the exercise should be regressed so that the thigh is vertical to the hip joint and the knee is flexed to the appropriate point.

Benefits

Builds core stability
Helps build awareness of the lumbar pelvic hip complex
Improves hip mobility

Cues

Verbal : Imagine your foot is a paint brush drawing a circle on the ceiling
Imagine your femur is a pencil drawing a small circle in your acetabulum

Tactile : Teacher can place one hand under the lower back and the other over the lower abdomen to help cue the pelvic stabiity
Teacher can help guide the internal and external rotation of the femur in the hip joint

Principles

Core Control
Lumbo Pelvic Hip Complex stabiity
Ability for the hip joint to 'disassociate' / be independent from the pelvis

What is the difference between performing the exercise with the arms pressed into the floor by your sides and resting gently over your lower abdomen.

Scan the QR code to view the exercise - Single Leg Circles 1

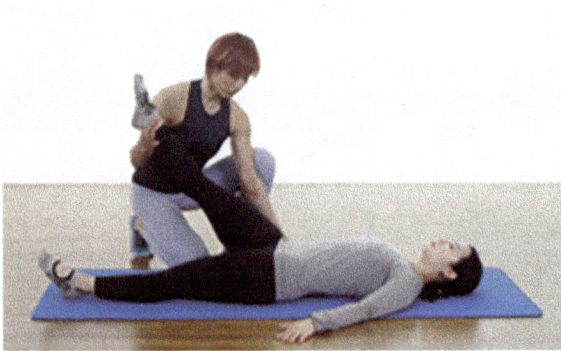

Teacher tests the hamstring flexibility with a stable pelvis for the Single Leg exercise. If the leg is unable to go vertical then the exercise should be performed with a slightly flexed knee but maintaining a vertical thigh over the hip joint.

M3 - Single Leg Circle 2

Contraindications & Precautions

This exercise may be contraindicated for persons with some hip pathologies

This movement differs from the Leg Circle 1 in that the previous exercise has an emphasis on the mobility of the hip joint whilst stabilizing the pelvis. This version however allows the movement of the pelvic halves to mobilize / stretch the tight areas of the 'outer butt' and lower back all the way up to the neck and shoulders.

Set Up

Supine position with the legs extended and arms extended approximately 45 degrees out by your sides.

Movement

Slide the right leg to the upright position as in Leg Circle 1.

Bring the leg over to the left side of the body with the aim to get the foot to the floor without lifting the right shoulder from the mat. If you are unable to do then placing the foot on the floor is the priority so do this with as little movement of the shoulder as possible.

Internally rotate the femur in the hip socket as you bring the leg over.

Maintain contact between the right foot and the floor and sweep the foot towards and over the left leg to continue to the right side using the ribcage as the driver.

Bring the right leg out to the right side of the body as far as is comfortable whilst externally rotating the femur in the hip socket and 'lift' the leg from the floor maintaining a stable pelvis to repeat the movement again.

Perform 5 - 8 repetitions before changing direction.

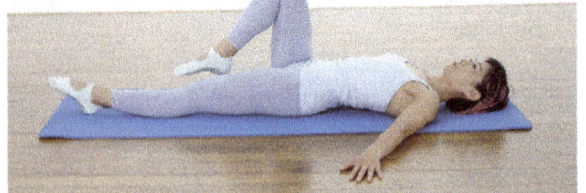

Start position

2

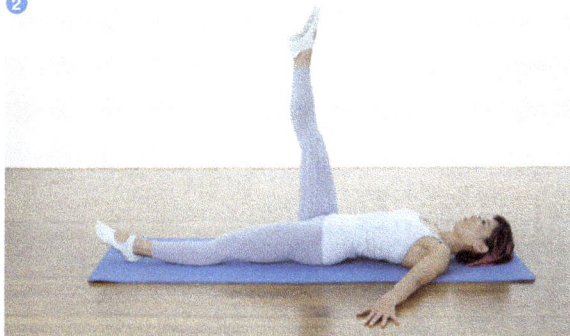

Straighten leg

3

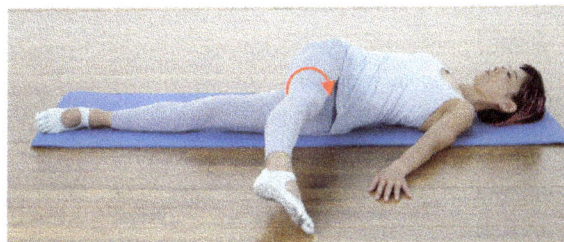

Lower leg to the left

4

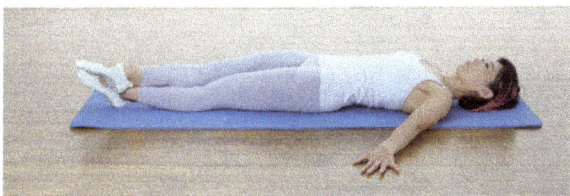

Sweep across the floor and over the other leg

5

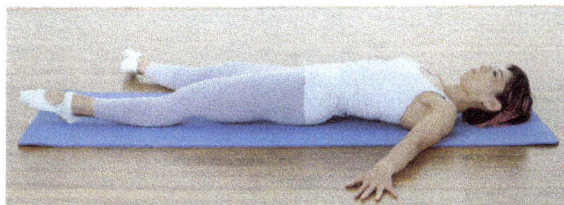

Sweep to the right side

6

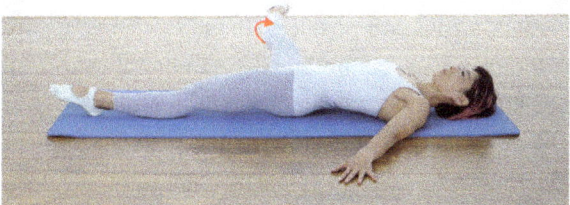

Lift from right side using inner thigh muscles

7

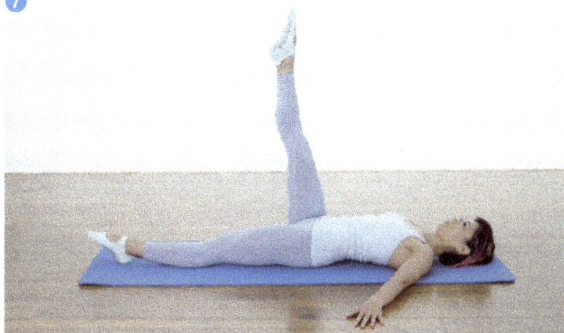

Return to start position

Benefits

Releases the lower back

Helps improves hip mobility

Improves spinal mobility

Releases the back of the leg

Helps build hip muscle strength

Integrates the oblique and latissimus dorsi muscles

Cues

Verbal : Imagine your foot is like a magnet sweeping across the floor

Keep the shoulder on the mat

Press the arm into the mat

Move from the ribcage

Move from the leg !

Feel how the ribcage can pull the leg over the other leg

Tactile : Teacher can gently lead the leg as it sweeps around

Teacher guides the ribs to lead the leg

Principles

Core Control

Lumbo Pelvic Hip Complex organization and mobility

Spinal articulation

Ability for the hip joint to 'disassociate' / be independent from the pelvis

What is the difference between performing the exercise with the arms pressed into the floor by your sides or holding out at 45 degrees ?

Scan the QR code to view the exercise Single Leg Circles 2

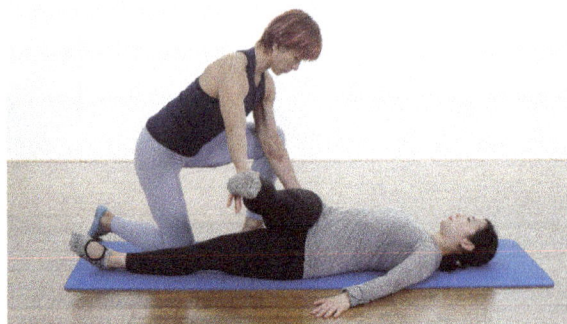

Teacher guided cue for Single Leg Circle 2 exercise

M4 - Roll Like a Ball

The Pilates mat repertoire contains a number of movements that involve some form of rolling on the back in a rounded position. These movements vary in the degree of control needed to control the spinal position throughout the movement.

The Roll Like a Ball exercise is the basic movement that maintains a flexed spinal position without having to transition into other positions. It is usually considered to be a good spinal massage but moreover it is a good preparation for the next exercise in the sequence - Single Leg Stretch.

Set Up

Sit on the mat with your weight slightly behind your sit bones. Exhale to help curl your tail towards your pubic bone and initiate a long deep 'C' curve with a hollowing of the abdominal muscles.

The hips and knees are flexed with the knees close to the chest and the hands either interlocked or placed over each other at the front of the shins.

The arms should be wrapped around the bent legs with the elbows pointed slightly outwards to keep the elbows flexed as though hugging a ball.

The head is held close to the knees but not touching as though you are holding a small ball between the forehead and knees.

Movement

Press the legs into the arms whilst simultaneously resisting with the arms. You should feel an immediate connection into your core muscles as your abdominals hollow and your spine. The arms expand sideways as though holding a beach ball that is being inflated whilst the hands stay in contact with each other to resist the ball inflation.

Curl your tail towards your pubic bone to deepen the curve and feel the weight shift further back behind the pelvis. As the weight shifts back the body should begin to roll backwards.

Allow the body to 'roll like a ball' until you reach the area between the shoulder blades. Pause for just a moment in this position and then return to the start position by rolling back up.

Practice this rolling motion at the 'slowest speed possible'.

The legs, spine, arms and head should stay in the same position throughout the movement with the feeling that you can stop at any position at any time. The slower the speed the more advanced the movement.

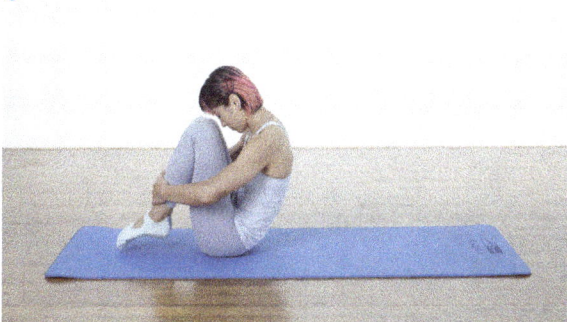

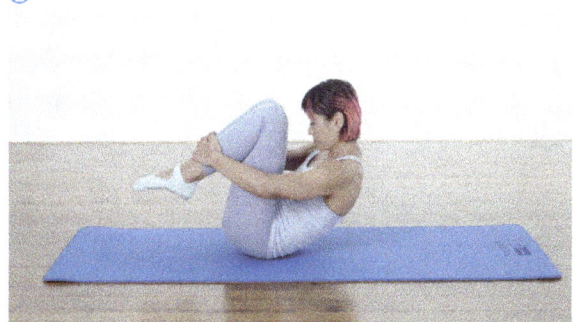

❸

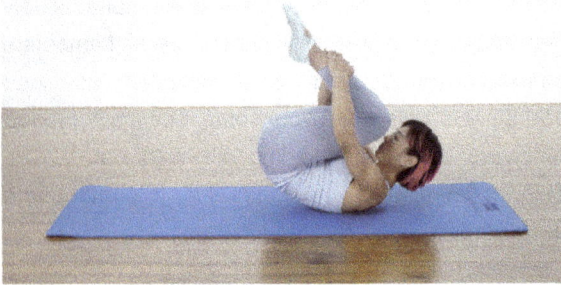

❹

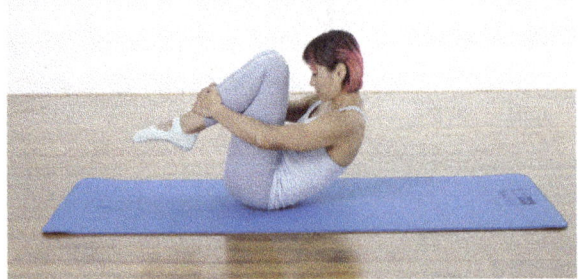

❺

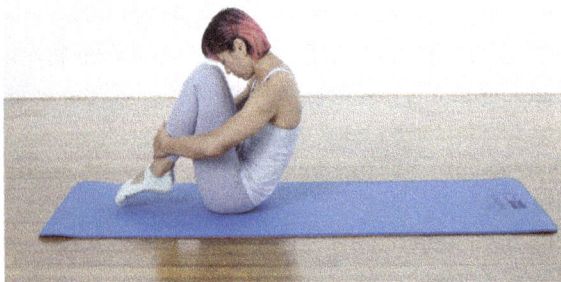

Benefits

Helps release the back muscles
Improves spinal mobility
Increases abdominal control

Principles

Core Control
Spinal articulation

Cues

Verbal : Imagine you are a ball rolling
Imagine the ball can stop at any time
Keep the legs pressed into the arms & the arms
pressed into the legs
Feel the abdominal connection when you tense
the arms and legs
Keep the head still

Tactile : Teacher can gently lead and help with the
rolling motion
Teacher should check the abdominal hollowing

What is the difference between practicing at
different speeds ?
What happens if you release the tension between
arms and legs ?

Scan the QR code to view the
exercise - Roll Like a Ball

M5 - Single Leg Stretch

Considered to be the first exercise of the 'Big Five' in the abdominal series.
We will look at 2 versions.

Version 1

Set Up

Begin in a sitting position with the right leg extended on the mat in front of you and the left leg in the triple flexed position. Your left hand holds the bottom of the left shin and the right hand clasps the top of the shin and knee area.

Movement

Curl your tail to wards the pubic bone to initiate a rolling down to the mat. Finish with the right leg extended the appropriate distance from the floor* (see below). The left leg is pulled firmly towards the chest with both arms however the leg also pushes away from the body against the resistance of the arms to produce an abdominal connection similar to Roll Like a Ball.

The chest and head is lifted with the gaze looking beyond the knees.

Inhale to the back and sides of the ribs and feel the expansion of the ribcage along with the stabilization of the abdominals. Exhale to feel the contraction and 'squeezing' of the abdominal muscles.

In one swift and smooth motion switch positions of the legs so that the left leg is now extended and the right leg pulled towards the chest.

Make another inhale and exhalation to bring the attention to the ribcage and abdominals again.

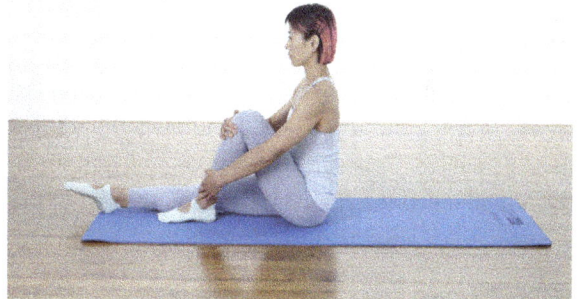

Start position

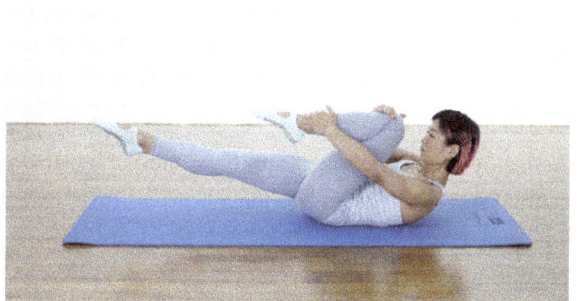

Arms and leg resist each other to connect into the abdominals.

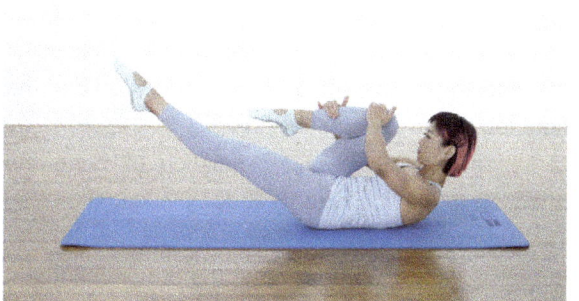

Arms and leg resist each other to connect into the abdominals.

Version 2

Set Up

Begin in a sitting position with the right leg extended on the mat in front of you and the left leg in the triple flexed position. Your left hand holds the bottom of the left shin and the right hand clasps the top of the shin and knee area.

Movement

Curl your tail to wards the pubic bone to initiate a rolling down to the mat. Finish with the right leg extended and suspended the appropriate distance from the floor* (see below). The left hip is flexed past 90 degrees so that the shin is parallel to the floor in a 'table top' position. The left hand is placed against the bottom side of the left shin and the right hand press gently into the inside of the left knee. Both hands ae now placing counter rotational forces into the left leg.

The chest and head is lifted with the gaze looking beyond the knees.

Inhale to the back and sides of the ribs and feel the expansion of the ribcage along with the stabilization of the abdominals. Exhale to feel the contraction and 'squeezing' of the abdominal muscles. Compare these feelings with version 1.

In one swift and smooth motion switch positions of the legs so that the left leg is now extended and the right leg pulled towards the chest.

Make another inhale and exhalation to bring the attention to the ribcage and abdominals again.

The Appropriate Distance from the floor.

In both versions the position of the outstretched leg is very important. The leg should be low enough to place a challenge on the abdominal muscles but high enough that it does not cause stress and strain through the spine due to either short tight hip flexor

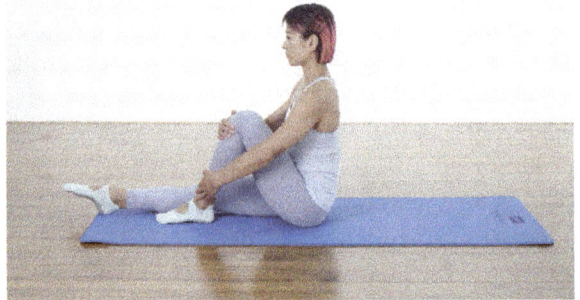

Start position

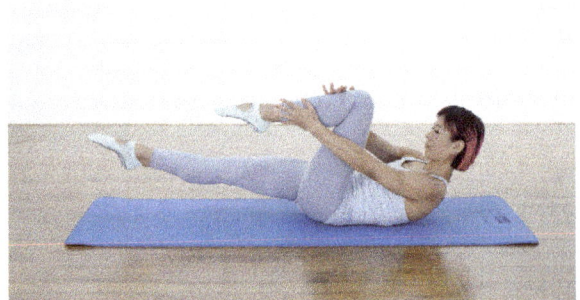

Left hand presses inwards, right hand presses outwards.

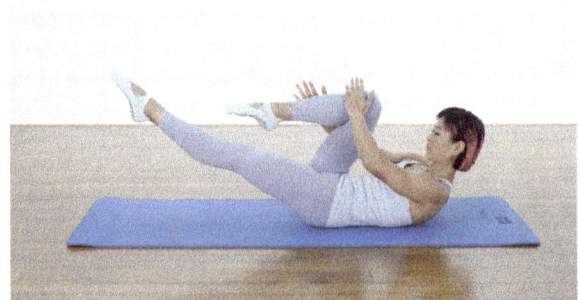

Left hand presses inwards, right hand presses outwards.

muscles and/or lack of support from the core musculature.

A good test to see an optimum height to place the leg is for the teacher to ask the client to lie supine with legs outstretched and the lower spine in contact with the floor or mat.

The tester then holds outstretched leg in a high position whilst placing one hand under the lower back. The tester then slowly lowers the outstretched leg towards the floor feeling for the moment that :

1) *The pelvis begins to rotate anteriorly*
2) *The lumbar spine begins to lift from the floor*

The teacher then informs the client that this is the best position for the outstretched leg for this exercise as any lower down and there will be a loss of lumbo pelvic hip stability placing unwanted tension into the lower back.

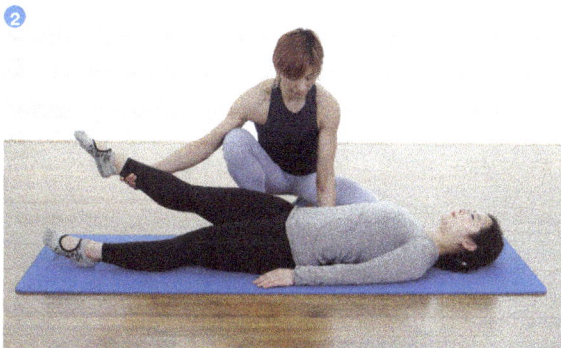

Tester lowers the leg towards the floor looking for the first point at which either the pelvis rotates forwards or the lumbar spine lifts from the floor.

Benefits

Strengthens abdominal muscles
Improves lumbo pelvic hip complex stability
Helps release tension in the lower back
Helps integrate the upper extremity to the core

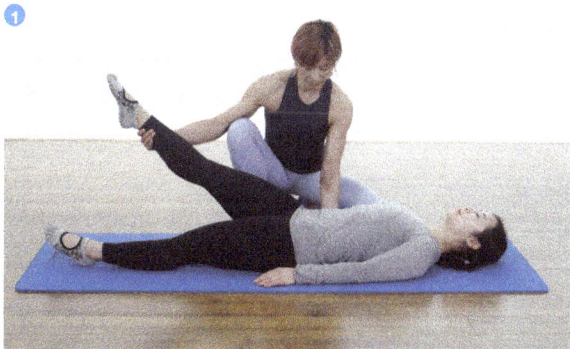

Client is supine with lower back in contact with the floor

Tester places one hand under the lower back and lifts / supports the outstretched leg.

Cues

Verbal : Any 'core' verbal cues may be used.
Any pelvic floor verbal cues may be used

Tactile : Teacher places one hand under the lower back and one hand on lower belly feeling for stability of the LPHC

Principles

Core Control
Spinal articulation
LumboPelvic Hip Complex stability

How do the 2 versions compare with each other ?

How does the degree of hip flexion for the bent leg affect the exercise ?

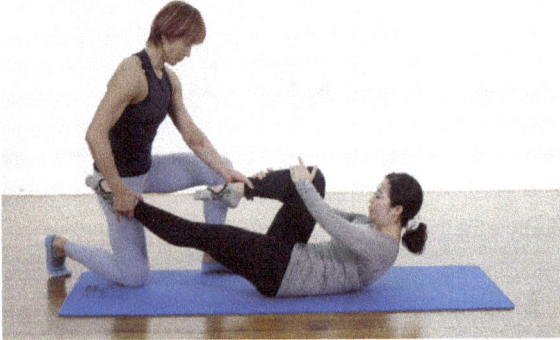

Teacher resisted / assisted cue for Single Leg Stretch exercise

Scan the QR code to view the exercise Single Leg Stretch

M6 - Double Leg Stretch

This is considered to be No.2 in the 'Big Five' sequence of abdominal exercises.

Set Up

Lie on your back with with legs in the triple flexed position and hands placed at the base of the head.
Perform a chest lift
Lift both legs at the same time to pull the knees towards the chest.

Bring your hands so that they now wrap around the front to hold the front of the shins.
You are now in the start position.

Movement

Pull both legs firmly towards the chest with both arms however at the same time push the legs away from the body against the resistance of the arms to produce an abdominal connection similar to Roll Like a Ball.
The chest and head is lifted with the gaze looking beyond the knees.
Inhale to the back and sides of the ribs and feel the expansion of the ribcage along with the stabilization of the abdominals. Exhale to feel the contraction and 'squeezing' of the abdominal muscles.
In one swift and smooth motion :

Extend both legs out in front of you at the appropriate height

Sweep and reach the arms overhead in a manner that enables you to maintain the same position of the head and chest without dropping or lowering the upper body.

Pause for a moment in this position
Smoothly bring the legs back to the start position whilst sweeping the arms to the start position holding on to the front of the shins.
Make another inhale and exhalation to bring the attention to the ribcage and abdominals again before repeating the movement.

①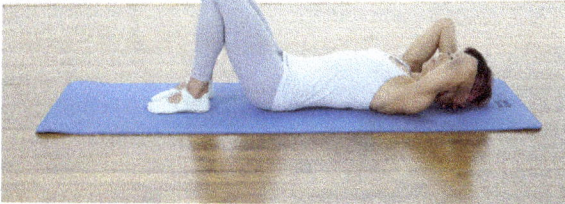

Preparation_01

②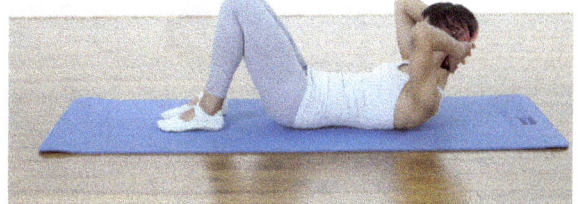

Preparation_02

③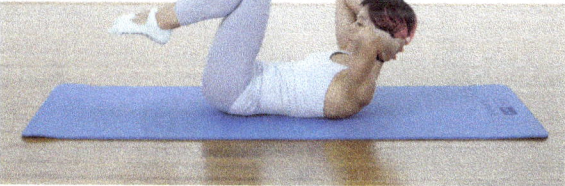

Preparation_03

④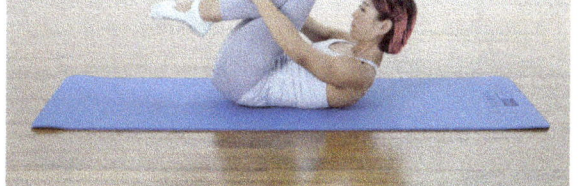

Start position

⑤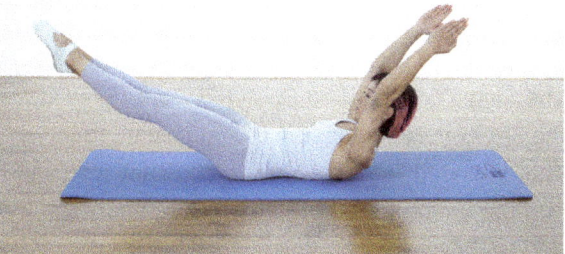

Extend legs and arms

⑥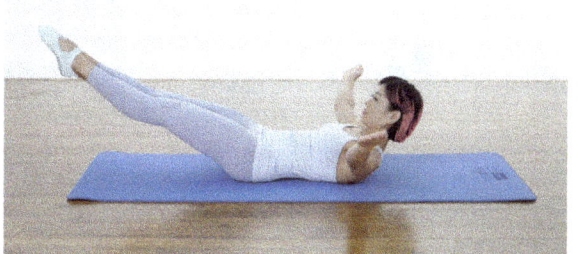

Sweep the arms back towards the legs

7

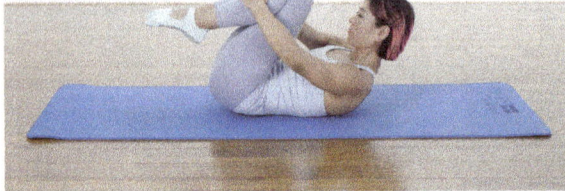

Return to start position

How do the 2 versions compare with each other ?
How does the degree of hip flexion for the bent leg affect the exercise ?

Scan the QR code to view the exercise Double Leg Stretch

Benefits

Strengthens abdominal muscles
Improves lumbo pelvic hip complex stability
Helps release tension in the lower back
Helps integrate the upper extremity to the core

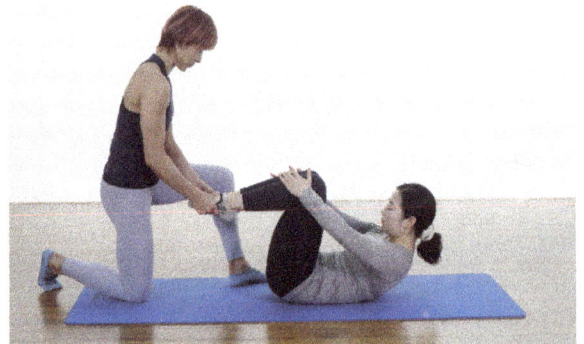

Teacher resisted / guided cue for Double Leg Stretch exercise

Cues

Verbal : Any 'core' verbal cues may be used.
Any pelvic floor verbal cues may be used

Tactile : Teacher places one hand under the lower back and one hand on lower belly feeling for stability of the LPHC

M7 - Single Straight Leg Stretch

The Single Straight Leg Stretch is considered to be the 3rd exercise in the 'Big 5' abdominal sequence. The extended legs maintain a constant long lever into the lumbo pelvic hip complex to challenge the core stability meaning that this would be considered a progression from the Single and Double Leg Stretches.

Principles

Core Control
Spinal articulation
LumboPelvic Hip Complex stability

Benefits

Strengthens abdominal muscles
Improves lumbo pelvic hip complex stability

Set Up

Supine position with the hands supporting the neck and head and legs in triple flexed position.

Movement

Lift the head and chest until you are gazing past your knees.
Float both legs in the air so the knees are over the hip joints with the thighs perpendicular to the floor.
Extend the legs and wrap both hands around the left lower leg close to the knee joint.
Pull the left leg firmly towards the chest with both arms however resist the movement with the muscles at the back of the leg and feel the connection to the abdominals as they hollow and contract to stabilize the spine.
Extend the right hip so that the leg moves to the appropriate distance from the floor.
Inhale to the back and sides of the ribs and feel the expansion of the ribcage along with the stabilization of the abdominals. Exhale to feel the contraction and 'squeezing' of the abdominal muscles.
In one swift and smooth motion :

Switch the position of both legs so that you are now holding th eright leg with the left leg extended away from you whilst maintaining the same position of the head and chest without dropping or lowering the upper body.

Pause for a moment in this position and then repeat the same 'scissor' type movement as many times as necessary.

①

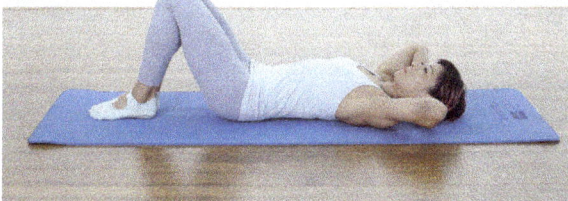

Start position

②

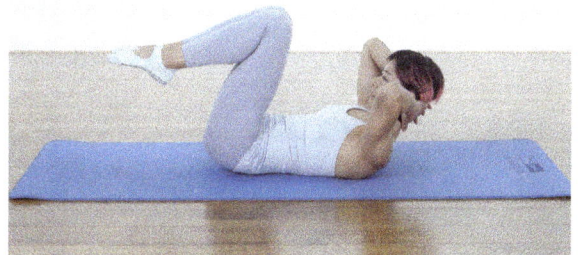

Feet together, knees apart

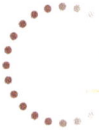

③
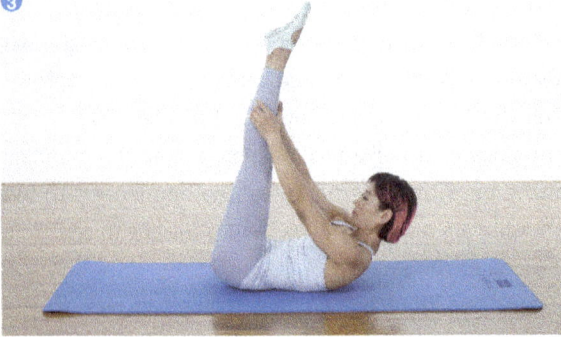

Extend the legs - hold the left leg

④
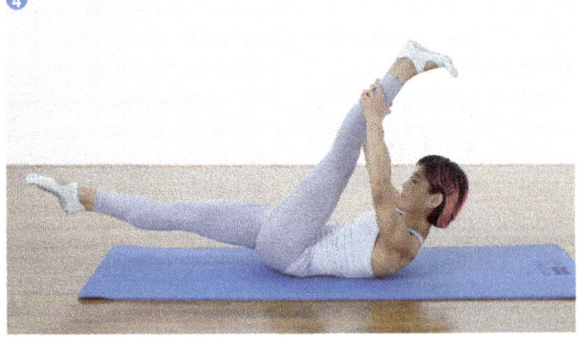

Pull the left - extend the right

⑤
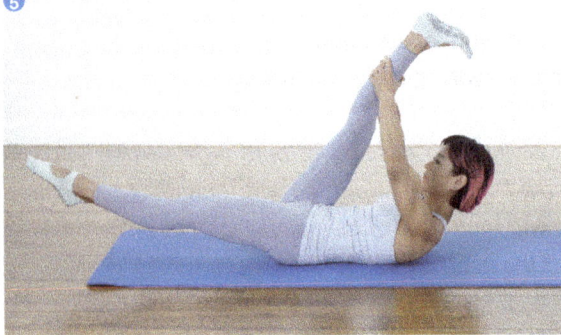

'Switch

Principles

Core Control
Spinal articulation
LumboPelvic Hip Complex stability

Practice comparing the height of the extended leg and the flexion of the opposite leg. How do these compare ?

Cues

Verbal : Any 'core' verbal cues may be used.
Any pelvic floor verbal cues may be used
Feel the connection into the abdominals as you resist with the leg

Tactile : Teacher places one hand under the lower back and one hand on lower belly feeling for stability of the LPHC

Scan the QR code to view the exercise - Single Straight Leg Stretch

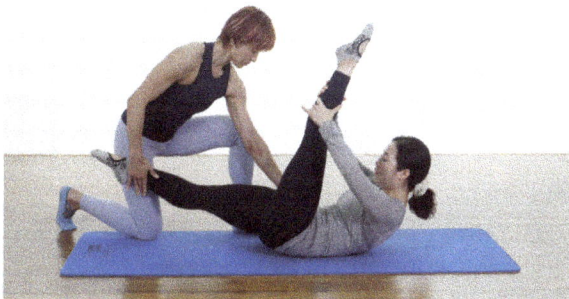

Teacher resisted / assisted / guided cue for Single Straight Leg Stretch exercise

M8 - Double Straight Leg Stretch

The Double Straight Leg Stretch is considered to be the 4th of the 'Big Five' abdominal sequence.

The lowering of both legs produces a considerable long lever load into the lumbo pelvic hip complex to challenge the stability of the pelvis and lower spine.

Contraindications & Precautions

The consistent long lever into the LPHC means that this exercise may not be suitable for persons with lower back pain and / or hip or low back pathologies

Benefits

Strengthens abdominal muscles
Improves lumbo pelvic hip complex stability

Set Up

Supine position with the hands supporting the neck and head and legs in triple flexed position.

Movement

Lift the head and chest until you are gazing past your knees.

Float both legs in the air so the knees are over the hip joints with the thighs perpendicular to the floor.

Extend the legs towards the ceiling with the ankles plantar flexed whilst firmly squeezing the legs together using the inner thigh muscles.

Slowly lower both legs together towards the floor until you feel the point at which either the pelvis begins to 'tip/rotate' forwards or your lower spine begins to arch or lift away from the floor.

Pause in this position and take a strong inhalation to feel the expansion of the ribcage to the back and sides, followed by an exhalation to feel the contraction / squeezing of the abdominal muscles to support the spine.

Dorsi flex the ankles and return the legs to the vertical straight leg position and as you do so see if you can bring your chest towards the knees just a little bit further.

Repeat as necessary.

Remember if the belly bulges during the exercise that you have probably 'lost your core stability'. If this happens then do not go down so far with the legs.

"Move to where your body tells you you can move - not to where you it think it should go"

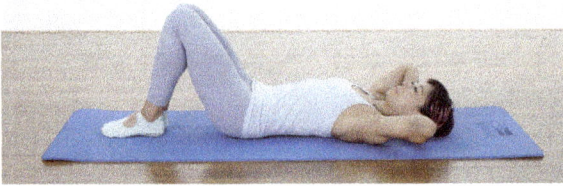

Start position

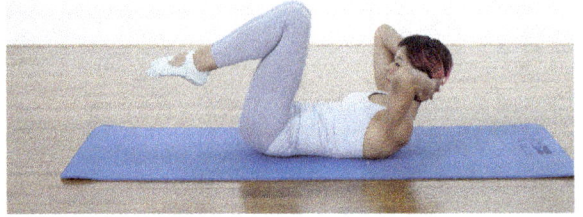

Feet together, knees apart

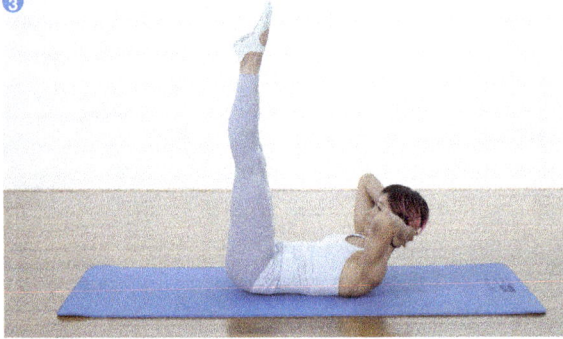

Straighten legs

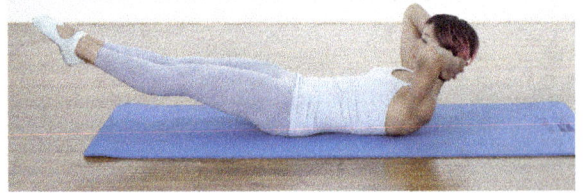

Lower legs

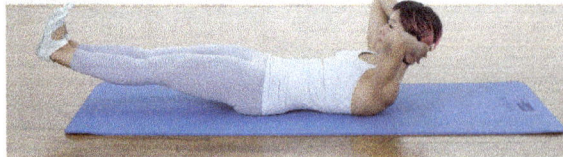

Dorsi flex ankles

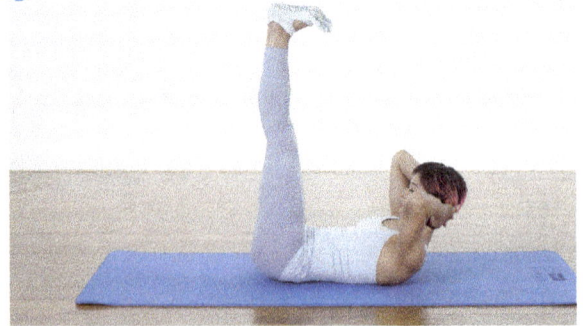

Lift the legs legs

Verbal : Any 'core' verbal cues may be used.
Any pelvic floor verbal cues may be used Hollow the abdominals

Tactile : Teacher places one hand under the lower back and one hand on lower belly feeling for stability of the LPHC

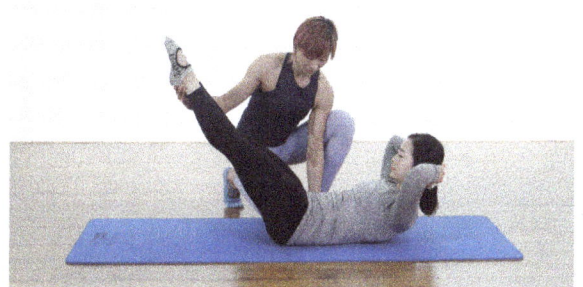

Teacher resisted / assisted cue for Double Straight Leg Stretch exercise

Principles

Core Control
Spinal articulation
LumboPelvic Hip Complex stability

M9 - Criss Cross

The Criss Cross is considered to be the 5th of the 'Big Five' abdominal sequence.

What difference does the dorsi flexion and plantar flexion make in the exercise ?

Contraindications & Precautions

The consistent lever into the LPHC means that this exercise may not be suitable for persons with lower back pain and / or hip or low back pathologies

This exercise contains rotation whilst under load which is not suitable for persons with disc pathlogies

Scan the QR code to view the exercise - Double Straight Leg Stretch

Benefits

Strengthens abdominal muscles
Improves lumbo pelvic hip complex stability

Set Up

Supine position with the hands supporting the neck and head and legs in triple flexed position.

Movement

Lift the head and chest until you are gazing past your knees.

Float both legs in the air so the knees are over the hip joints with the thighs perpendicular to the floor.

Version 1

Extend the right leg to the appropriate distance from the floor whilst rotating the upper body to the left and pulling the flexed left knee towards the chest.

For the rotation of the upper body imagine a line going through the center of the body and the left shoulder and elbow rotating towards the floor.

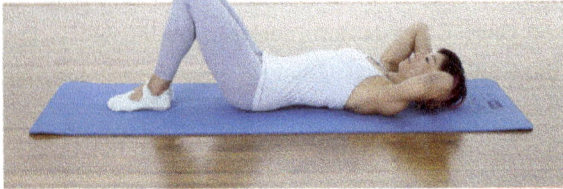

Start position

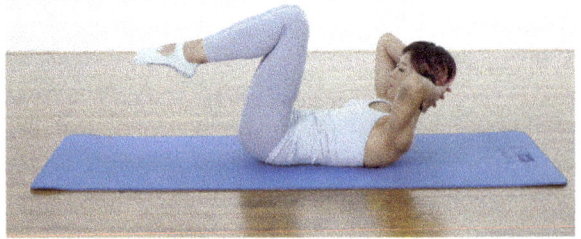

Feet together, knees apart

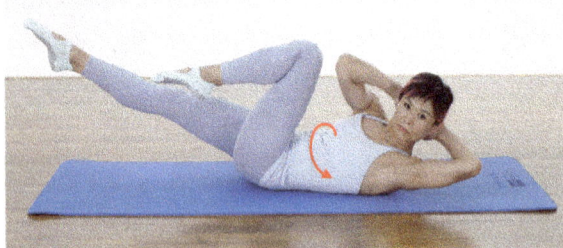

Upper body rotates to the floor

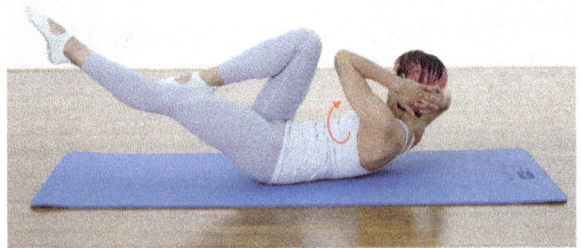

Upper body rotates to the floor

Version 2

Extend the right leg to the appropriate distance from the floor. Place the ankle of the left leg against the inside of the right knee and press to the legs together. The left ankle is now 'glued' to the right knee.

Rotate the upper body to the left by turning the head to look up and over the left elbow. As you turn to look past the left elbow the ribcage will follow.

Pause for a moment in this position and make a one second isometric contraction with the ribcage and left ankle against the right knee.

Repeat other side.

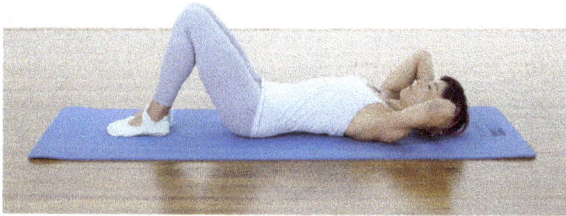

Start position

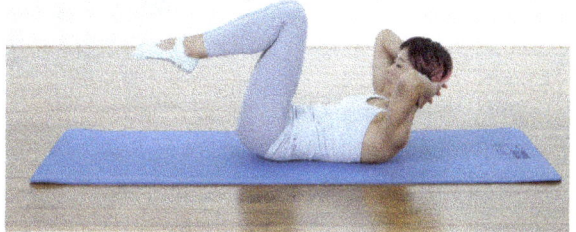

Feet together, knees apart

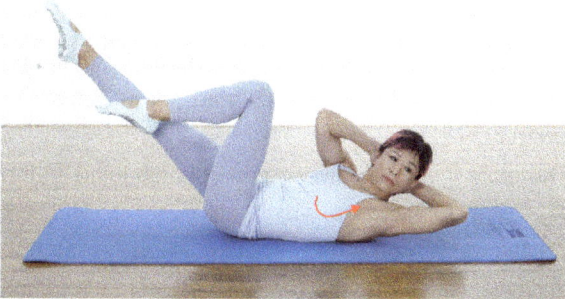

Left ankle presses against right knee
Rotate by looking past left elbow

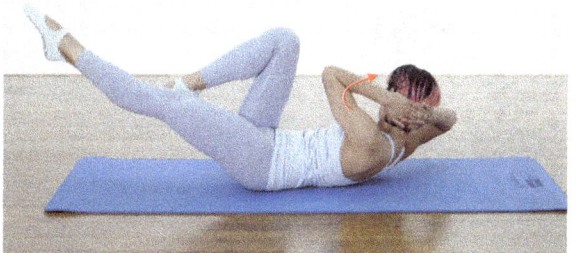

Right ankle presses against left knee
Rotate by looking past right elbow

Principles

Core Control
Spinal articulation
LumboPelvic Hip Complex stability

Cues

Verbal : Any 'core' verbal cues may be used.
Any pelvic floor verbal cues may be used
Hollow the abdominals

Tactile : Teacher places one hand under the lower back and one hand on lower belly feeling for stability of the LPHC

What difference does the dorsi flexion and plantar flexion make in the exercise ?

Scan the QR code to view the exercise - Criss Cross

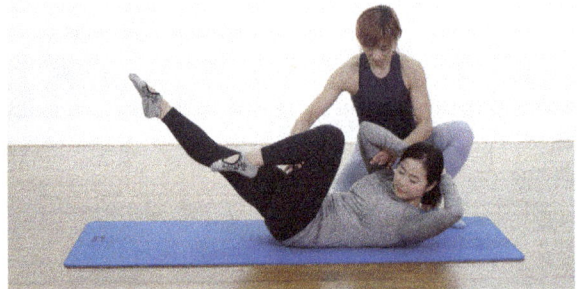

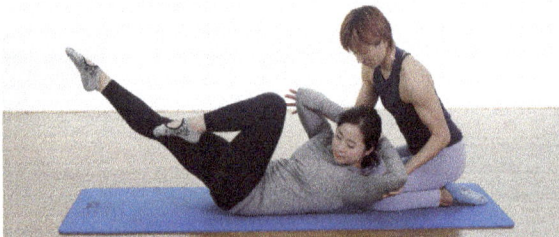

Optional positions for the teacher to give guided / assisted cues for the Criss Cross exercise

M10 - Spine Stretch

Contraindications & Precautions

Flexion exercises may be contraindicated for persons with bulging discs or osteoporosis

The key to this exercise is in the name - make sure you practice a 'Spine Stretch' and not a 'Hamstring Stretch'.
Therefore if you are pivoting on your hip joints trying to reach forward as much as possible you are practicing a hamstring stretch. A spine stretch involves flexion through the spine so there should be a 'rounding / curve' of the back in a 'C shape'.

Set Up

Sitting tall on your sit bones with the legs extended in front of you, dorsi flexed at the ankle and hip width apart. Your arms should be relaxed by your sides. Imagine your spine is resting against a wall behind you.

Movement

Imagine gently squeezing a ball between your legs to switch on your inner thigh muscles.

Raise your arms in front of you with elbows extended just below shoulder height.

Inhale to the side and back of the ribcage and then exhale to squeeze the sides and curl forwards.

First allow the chin to move towards chest. Follow by allowing / relaxing the collar bones and upper ribs downwards whilst 'lifting' the ribs at the back at the same time. The outstretched arms will move towards the feet.

Imagine your spine peeling away from the wall behind you one vertebra at a time. See if you can mentally count all 12 vertebra in thee thoracic spine one by one moving away from the one below.

Stop when you reach the last thoracic vertebra (T12). At this point you ideally want to have the lumbar spine still up against the wall with your abdominals hollowing deeply and your upper back rounded.

Return the spine to the upright position by placing each vertebra back up on the one below.

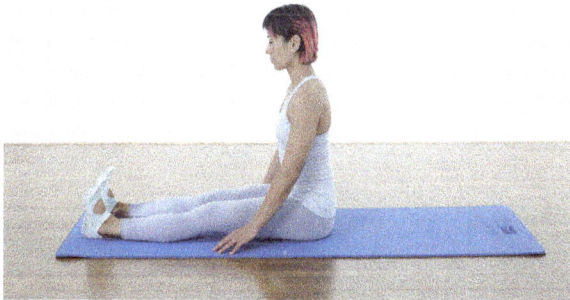

Start position - spine is upright

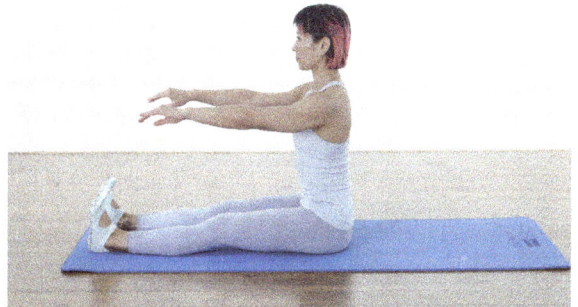

Raise the arms in front

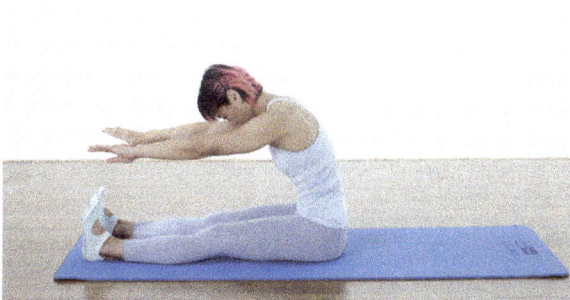

Peel' the spine away from the imaginary wall.

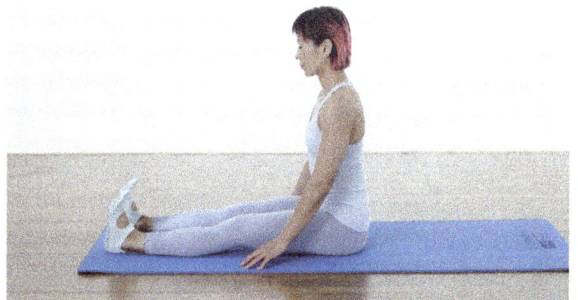

Return to start position

Scan the QR code to view the exercise - Spine Stretch

Practice with and without dorsi flexion - is there a difference ?
Practice with and without the adductors 'switched on' - what is the difference ?
What is the difference if you continue to curl through the lumbar spine ?

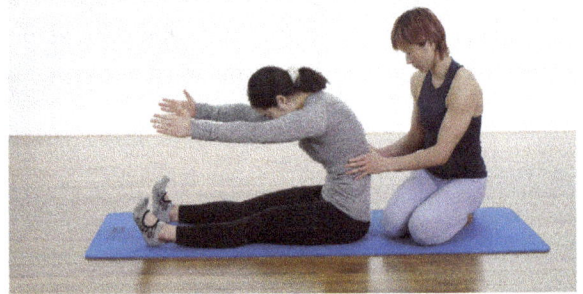

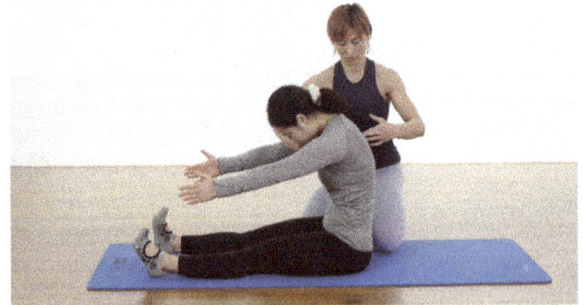

Benefits

Improves mobility of thoracic spine
Takes tension away from neck and shoulders
Takes tension away from low back
Helps improve lateral posterior thoracic breathing

Principles

Core Control
Spinal articulation

Cues

Verbal : Hollow your abdominals
Create a big long C shape in your spine
Peel your spine away from an imaginary wall
Feel each vertebra moving away from the wall one by one
Stack the spine one vertebra at a time to the start position

Tactile : Teacher uses guided touch to help with head and upper chest flexion
Teacher uses assisted touch to help lift the posterior ribs and close the anterior ribs

Assisted and guided cues for the Spine Stretch exercise

M11 - Spine Twist

For the Spine Twist the focus again is on the thoracic ribcage and verterbra. This is very important for persons suffering from low pain as many persons lack the thoracic mobility and try to move from the lower back thus exacerbating the back problem.

Therefore an emphasis in this exercise must be to maintain lumbo pelvic stability and rotate in the upper back and not the lumbar spine.

Set Up

Sitting tall on your sit bones with the legs extended in front of you, dorsi flexed at the ankle and hip width apart. Your arms should be relaxed by your sides. Imagine your spine is resting against a wall behind you.

Movement

Imagine gently squeezing a ball between your legs to switch on your inner thigh muscles.

Raise your arms out to the sides in the scapular plane so that the hands are in your peripheral vision in front of the chest.

Inhale to expand the ribs laterally and posteriorly.

Exhale to close the ribs whilst rotating to the left side.

Alternate between using different drivers for the movement :

- *Left scapula retracts as driver*
- *Ribs as driver*
- *Eyes and head as driver*

Your sternum should now be facing at least 30 degrees to the left side.

Return to the start position.

Contraindications & Precautions

Rotation exercises are usually contraindicated for persons with bulging discs however this is commonly due to the fact that the rotation is coming from the lower spine and not the upper spine. If performed properly under supervision this exercise may be very beneficial for persons with low back pathologies. However if performed incorrectly then the condition may be worsened.

Post Natal women with diastasis recti are usually cautioned against performing rotation exercises however this depends on the direction and location of the diastasis.

1

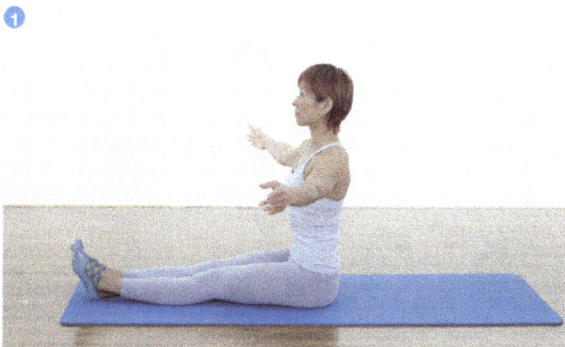

Start position - spine is upright

2

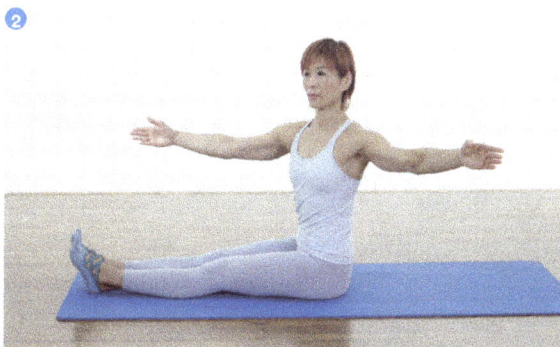

Rotate the ribcage & upper spine

③

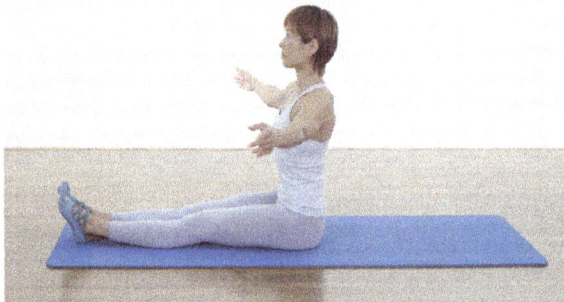

Return to start position

Scan the QR code to view the exercise - Spine Twist

Cues

Verbal : Hollow your abdominals
Feel the ribs open on the front left side and close on the front right side as you turn left
Feel each vertebra rotating away from the wall one by one
Feel the left shoulder blade retract and the right shoulder blade protract as you rotate

Tactile : Teacher uses guided touch to help with head and upper rotation
Teacher uses assisted touch to help rotation

Practice with and without dorsi flexion - is there a difference ?
Practice with and without the adductors 'switched on' - what is the difference ?
What happens if you focus keeping the left shoulder blade still with no retraction ?
What happens if you use the ribcage or shoulder blade as the driver ?

Benefits

Improves mobility of thoracic spine
Takes tension away from neck and shoulders
Takes tension away from low back
Helps improve lateral posterior thoracic breathing

Principles

Core Control
Spinal articulation

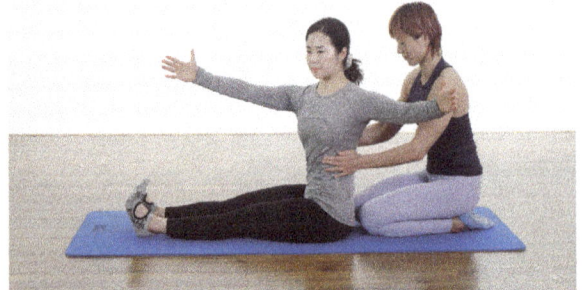

Assisted cue for the Spine Twist exercise

M12 - Saw

The Saw exercise can be seen as being a combination of the Spine Stretch and Spine Twist exercises with one extra 'bit' thrown in. You may observe that the Spine Stretch is very much in the sagittal plane and the Spine Twist in the transverse plane. If we were to combine these 2 planes of movement and now add the frontal plane we get the Saw.

This becomes an excellent movement for stretching muscles in all 3 planes at the same time.

Benefits

Improves mobility of whole spine
Stretches hamstrings and back muscles
Helps 'open up' the upper back
Improves abdominal oblique muscle activation
Stretches QL muscle

Set Up

Sitting position with the legs open to the width of the mat. The ankles are dorsi flexed and the spine is upright.

The arms are held abducted and slightly in front of the body just below shoulder height as in the Spine Twist.

Movement

In one smooth fluid movement and on an exhalation :

- *Rotate the head to the left with the torso*
- *Side bend to the right*
- *Flex the spine forwards so that the little finger on the right hand brushes the outside of the left little toe.*
- *Rotate the left arm inwards so that the thumb points towards the floor - keep looking at the thumb as you move into the position.*

'Micro pause' in this position for a moment and make another exhalation to challenge the body to move further into the position with a strong recruitment of the abdominal muscles.

Return to the start position

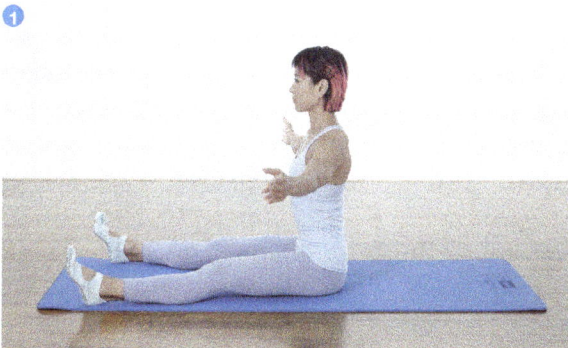

Start position

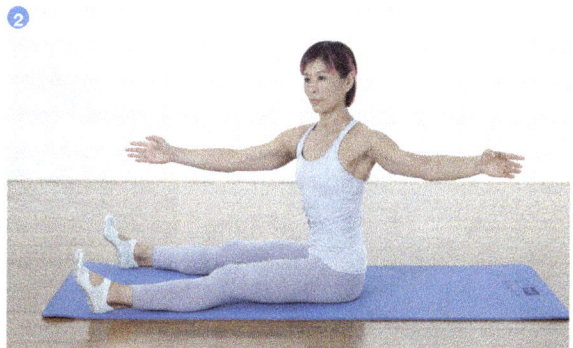

Rotate left

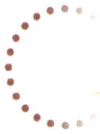
③

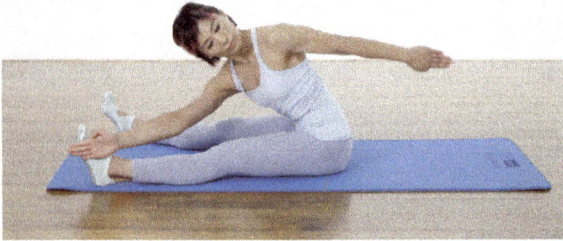

Reach right little finger across left little toe

④

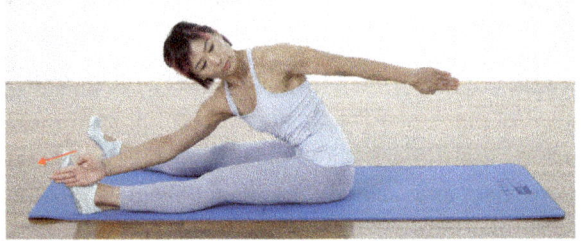

Exhale and quickly pulse further

⑤

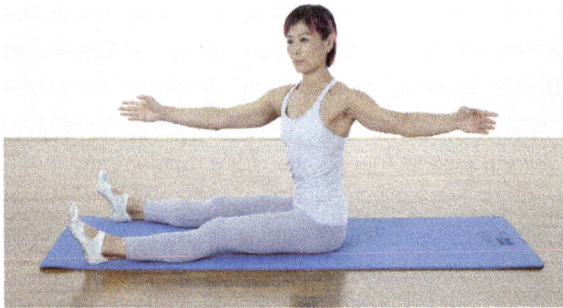

Return upright with rotation

⑥

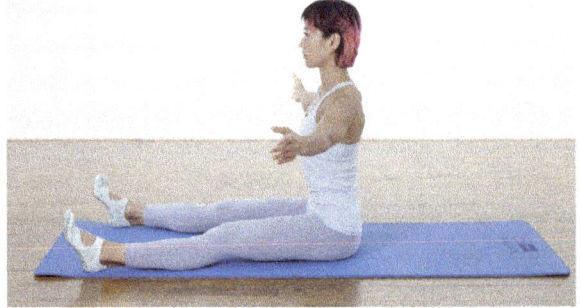

Return to start position

❶

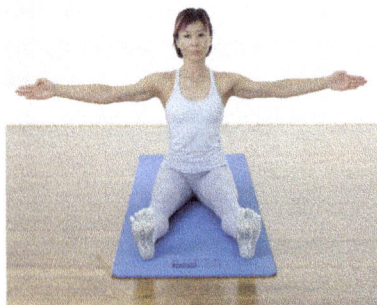

❷

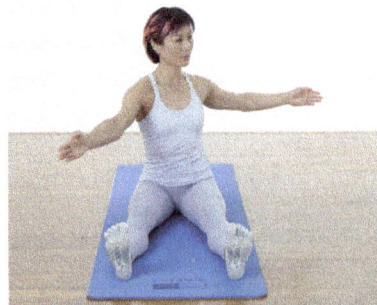

❸

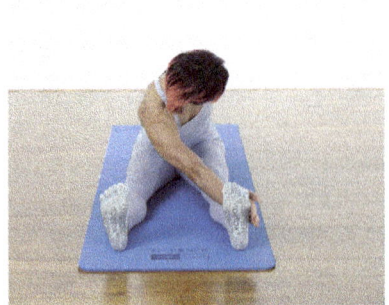

What happens if you focus keeping the left shoulder blade still with no retraction ?
Practice using different drivers of : ribcage / eyes / head / shoulder blade - what difference does it make ?

Scan the QR code to view the exercise - Saw

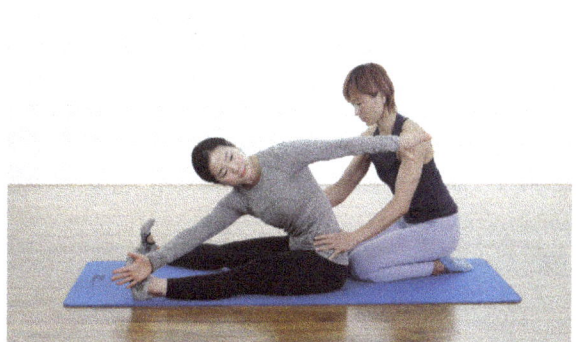

Assisted or guided cue for the Saw exercise

M13 - Open Leg Rocker

The Open Leg Rocker takes the movement principles of the Spine Stretch and Rolling Like a Ball and mixes them together to challenge the core abdominal stability whilst maintaining a stretch / giving a massage to the back tissues with an added challenge to the mobility and stability of the pelvis.

Contraindications & Precautions

Flexion exercises may be contraindicated for persons with bulging discs or osteoporosis

Set Up

Sitting behind the sit bones with the feet lifted from the floor and the hands holding the lower calf of each leg.

Movement

Straighten both the legs whilst keeping hold of the calves so that the body makes a 'V' shape when viewed from the side. The arms pull the legs and the legs push against the arms to create a dynamic

balance into the core muscles with your weight behind the sit bones.

Initiate a curl of the tail bone towards the pubic bone so that the pelvis begins to posteriorly tilt and the spine begins to flex. Continue flexing through the

spine so that it takes the body into a controlled backwards roll whilst still holding the bottom of the legs. Continue rolling until you reach the shoulder blade area before rolling back up to the start position with arms and legs outstretched.

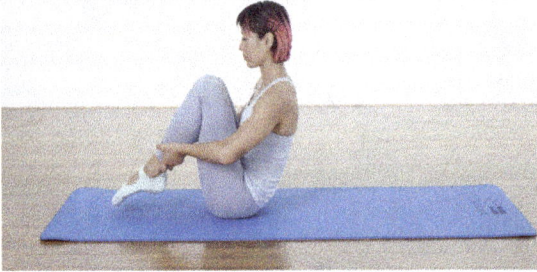

Start position

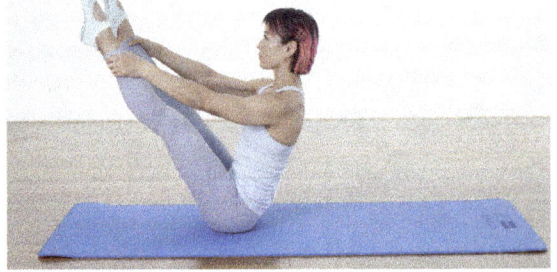

Hold legs in 'V' shape

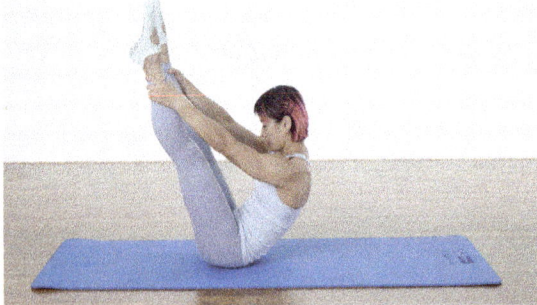

Pelvis rolls backwards

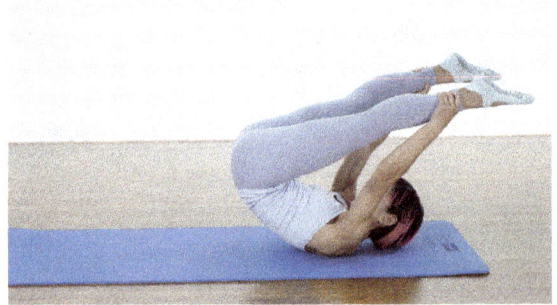

Flex and roll through spine

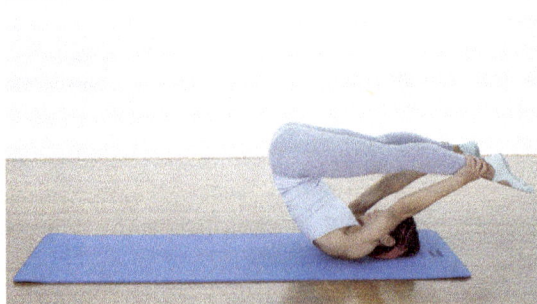

Continue to shoulder blades

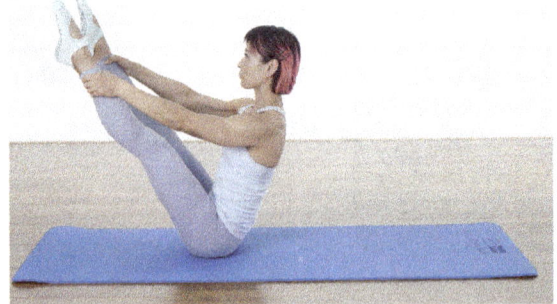

Roll back up keeping legs straight

Benefits

Helps stability of mid back (thoraco-lumbar junction)
Stretches hamstrings and back muscles
Helps 'open up' the upper back
Improves abdominal oblique muscle activation
Stretches QL muscle

Principles

Core Control
Spinal articulation in flexion,
Organization of shoulder girdle
LPHC stability and mobility

Cues

Verbal : Hollow your abdominals
Imagine your spine like a big beach ball that can roll
Pull with the arms - push with the legs

Tactile : Teacher uses guided touch to help stability and abdominal hollowing
Teacher uses assisted touch to help final part of sitting up onto the sit bones

Try practicing with different hand positions on the legs.
Practice exhalation rolling backwards and inhalation to return to start position
Practice inhalation rolling backwards and exhalation to return to start position
Try with legs wide and with legs narrow position.

Scan the QR code to view the exercise - Open Leg Rocker

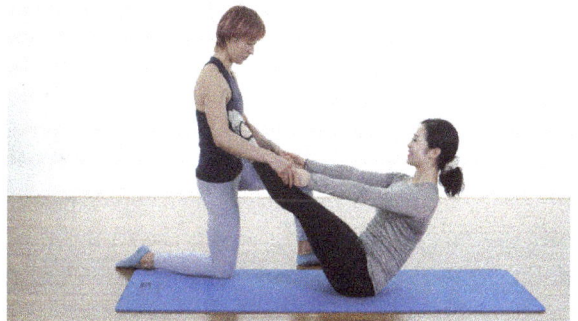

Guided or assisted cue for the Open Leg Rocker exercise

M14 - Single Leg Kick

The Single Leg Kick is a nice practical exercise to help activate the hamstring muscles whilst inhibiting the quadriceps muscles at the front of the leg. This is of importance because many people have weak hamstrings and an over active 'rectus femoris' muscle leading to hip dysfunction and low back pain. Experienced teachers will also observe which direction the calf will face when the client kicks the leg. A short and/or tight lateral hamstring may be identified by observing if the calf 'faces inwards' upon the kick.

Contraindications & Precautions

Extension exercises may be contraindicated for persons with stenosis.

Set Up

Sphinx position with the elbows under the shoulder joint and the forearms parallel in front. Rather than simply resting on your elbows begin with the elbows a fraction in front and have the feeling of trying to pull your self forward along the mat to engage the abdominal muscles and lengthen the spine.

The weight of the body should be on the pelvis either at a level of the hips or slightly higher just below the height of the ASIS's

The legs are parallel close together with the ankles plantar flexed (feet pointed).

The chest is lifted with the head in alignment and the eyes gazing approximately 1 meter in front.

Movement

Flex the left knee to firmly 'kick' the sole of the foot towards the left buttock. At a slower speed return the left foot slightly passed the 90 degree position of the knee and quickly change the ankle position to dorsi flexion and now firmly kick the heel of the foot towards the buttock.

With control extend the leg so that it floats 10 cm above the mat.

You have now completed 1 set on the left leg. Repeat 5 - 8 sets and then perform on the right side. Alternatively you may choose to alternate between one set on the left and then one set on the right. Some notes on the movement :

• When performing the kick pay attention to the feeling in the knee of the kicking leg. Many persons will automatically press the knee into the floor which would in fact engage the hip flexors which is something we do not want to happen. Imagine the knee is floating on a water lily as you kick and do not push the water lily under the water.

• Pay attention to your lower back and maintain the 'lift through your abdominals'. This will help stop the lower back from sagging which will create strain and even pain through the lumbar spine.

• Practice the exercise with a controlled rhythm. Many teachers will accompany the 'kick - kick' with a clicking of the fingers and then a drawn out 'reeeeech' as the leg straightens. The basic rhythm would be " quick - quick - slooooooow / quick - quick - slooooow "

• Make sure the foot of the kicking leg actually is facing and moving towards the buttock of the same side and not going out at an angle whichh would indicate an imbalance of the pelvis and hips.

①

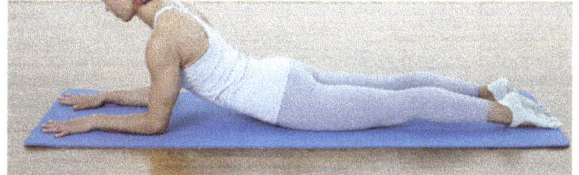

Start position

②

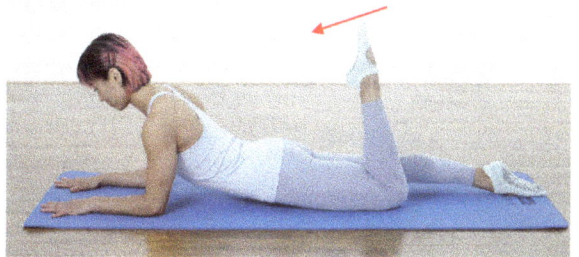

Leg kicks

③

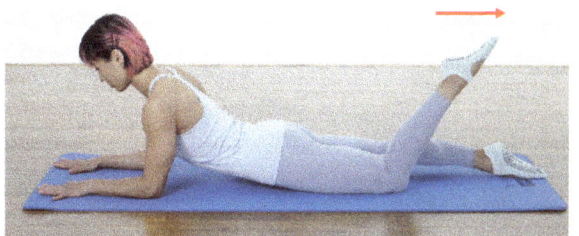

Extend the leg past 90 degrees to knee

④

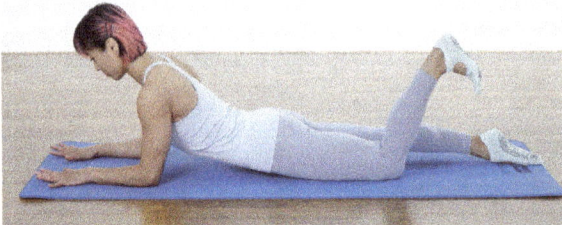

Dorsi flex ankle

⑤

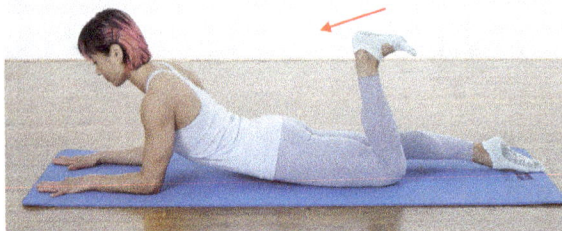

Kick

⑥

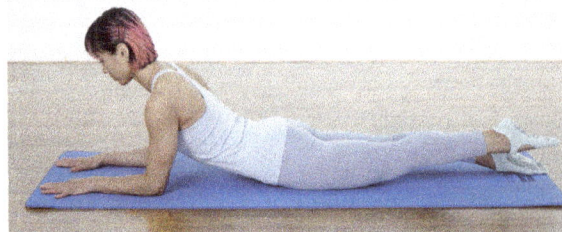

Extend and 'lift' leg

Scan the QR code to view the
exercise - Single Leg Kick

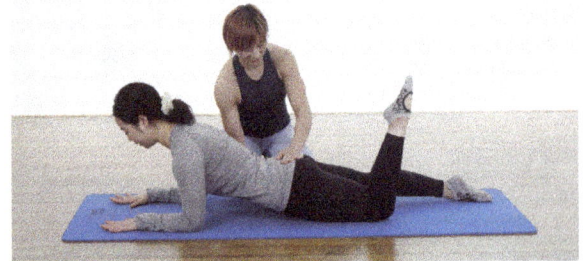

Guided cue for Single Leg Kick exercise

M15 - Double Leg Kick

The Double Leg Kick follows on from the Single Leg
Kick unifying both the left and right posterior
myofascial kinetic chains into one movement.

Contraindications & Precautions

Extension exercises may be contraindicated for
persons with stenosis.

Set Up

Prone position with the hands behind the lower back.
The hands may be placed with fingers interlocked or
one hand holding the 4 fingers of the other hand.
The head is turned in left or right direction with one

cheek on the mat.

Legs are extended and gently pressed together with the knees lifted from the floor to activate the glute and hamstrings muscles. Pubic bone can be gently pressed into the mat and the ASIS on each side is one finger width from the floor.

Movement

Kick both legs towards your buttocks 3 times :

1st kick - plantar flexed ankles
2nd kick - dorsi flexed ankles
3rd kick - plantar flexed ankles

Extend both legs keeping them approximately 10 - 15 cm in the air. As you extend the legs lift the arms away from the spine and extend the spine upwards lifting away from the floor and opening across the chest and front of the shoulders.

Pause for a moment in this position and articulate the spine back down to the mat with the head facing in the opposite direction to before.

Some things to focus on when performing the exercise :

• *Each time you kick pay attention to keeping the pelvis as stable as possible to avoid an anterior tilting movement accompanied with excessive lordosis in the lumbar spine.*

• *Lift the arms away from the body before extending through the spine*

• *When moving into the extension position 'pull your shoulder blades into your back pockets'.*

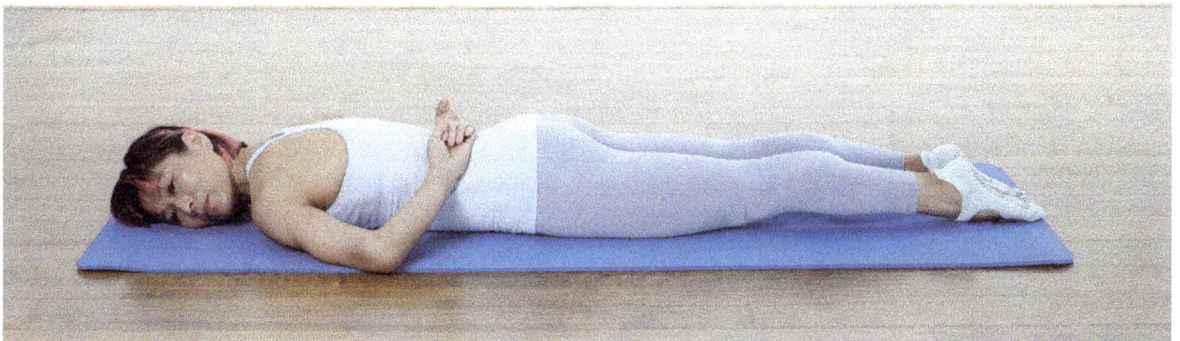

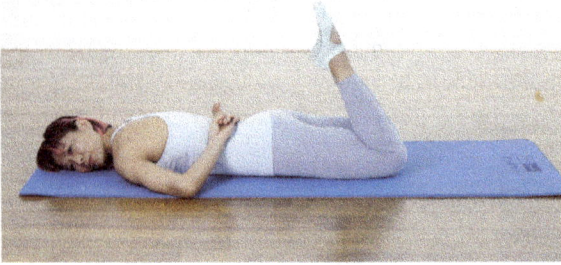

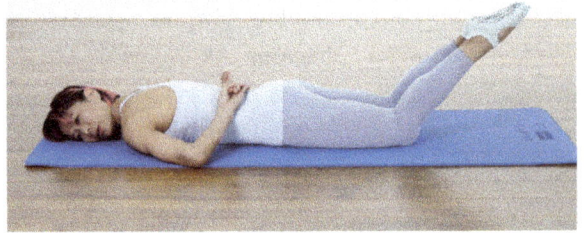

Kick once - planter flex

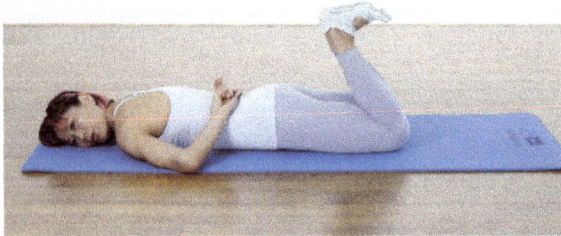

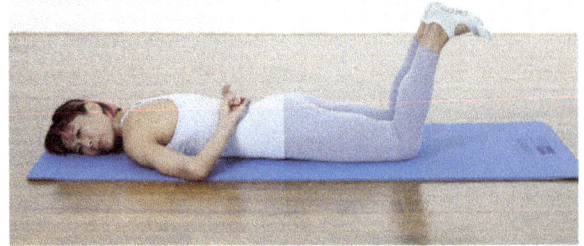

Kick third time - planter flex

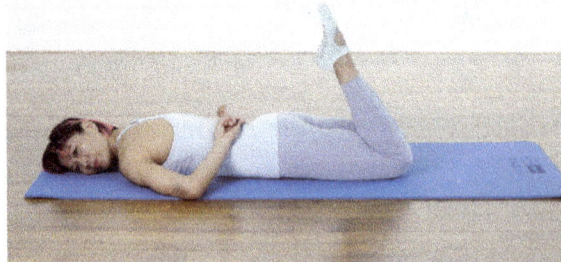

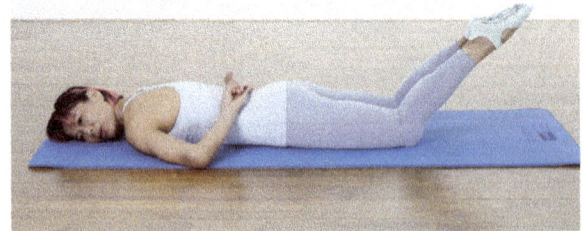

Kick twice - dorsi flex

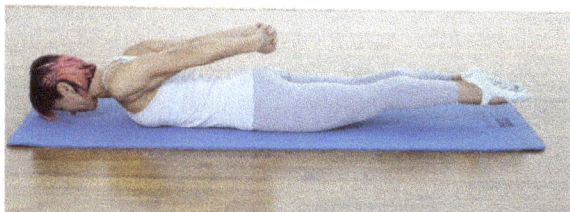

Lift and extend the arms - extend the legs

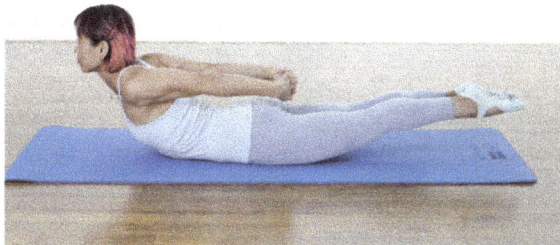

Lift and extend spine

Benefits

Helps with LPHC stability
Improves back strength
Helps improve hamstring muscle imbalances
Releases tension at front of hips

Principles

Core Control
Organization of shoulder girdle
LPHC stability and hip differentiation
Spinal articulation in extension

Cues

Verbal : Pull your abdominals away from the floor
Imagine your knees are resting on water lilies - do
not push them under when you kick
Squeeze your abdominals as you kick
"quick - quick - quick - slooooooow "

Tactile : Teacher uses guided touch for
proprioceptive feedback on LPH stability
Teacher places fingers under the knees to cue
hamstring contraction
Teacher can gently press pelvis into the mat to
cue glute activation

Perform the spinal extension by extending the
arms with the movement - compare to lifting the
arms away from the body first ...... how do the
movements compare ?
Perform 3 kicks with plantar flexed ankles. How
does this compare to the sequence listed above ?

Scan the QR code to view the
exercise - Double Leg Kick

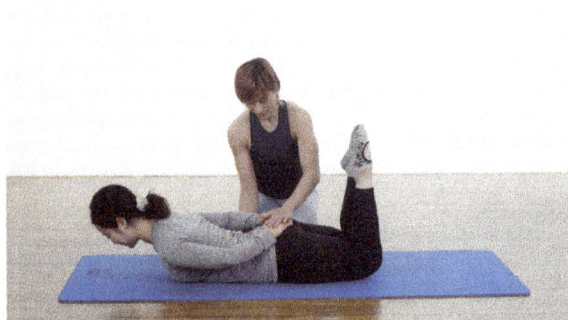

Guided cue for Double Leg Kick exercise

M16 - Swan

The Swan movement is sometimes broken down into 3 levels of difficulty. IN this version we will look at the intermediate level version.

The Swan has the potential to place considerable stress through the postural back muscles so it is imperative to maintain good alignment between the ribcage and pelvis to protect the lower back.

Contraindications & Precautions

Extension exercises may be contraindicated for persons with stenosis.
Persons with low back pain should avoid this exercise.

Set Up

Prone position as if attempting the prone extension exercise. The arms are extended in a wide position overhead and the normal checklist is followed :

- *Ankles plantar flexed with feet on the floor*
- *Knees lifted from the floor*
- *Pubic bone pushes into the mat*
- *Left and right ASIS 1 finger width from the floor*
- *Abdominals pulled in (ice cube under the belly)*
- *Face down with nose 5 - 10 cm from the floor*

Movement

Begin with a thoracic extension using the extended arms to help lift you until the last couple of ribs.
Now bring the hands next to your chest without dropping the upper body. Press into the floor to go further into the spinal extension until you are on your pubic bone or thighs.
Inhale to quickly release the hands from the floor bringing them towards your sides of your chest. As you do so roll though the abdominals towards the chest and 'throw your legs to the ceiling' as though trying to move against gravity and keep the upper body from the mat.
When you reach the sternum with the legs pointed to the ceiling return to the high chest spinal extension position and pause for a moment before repeated the same rolling movement.
After completing the required number of repetitions bring the spine to a 'Childs pose' position for 5 breaths breathing into the back of the ribcage.

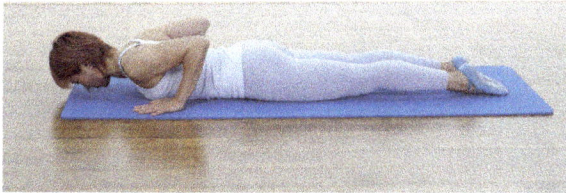

1

Start position

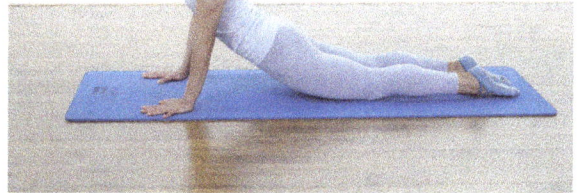

2

Extend into high position

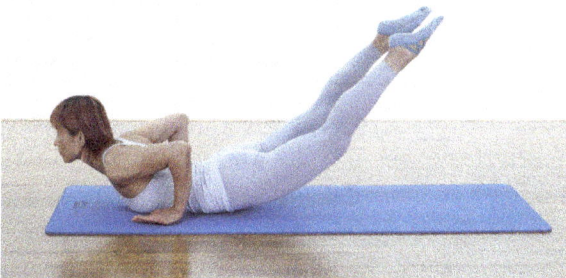

3

'Throw' the legs into the air and roll along the abdomen

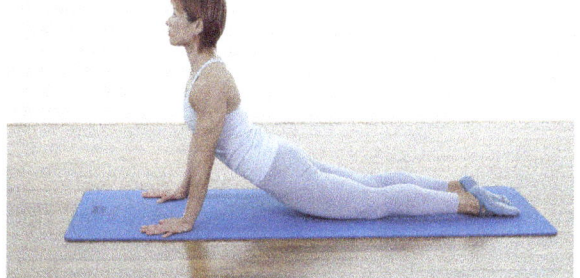

4

Use hands to decelerate and then push to high position

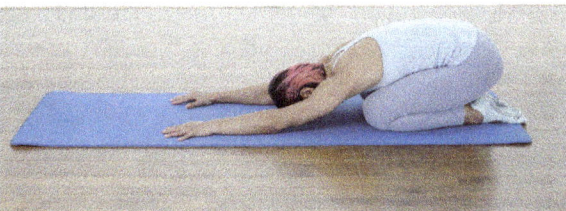

5

Take minimum 5 breaths in Childs Pose

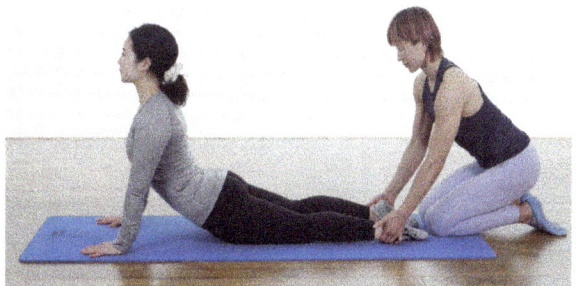

Teacher gives assisted cue by scooping and helping to 'throw' legs into the air on forwards dive.

Scan the QR code to view the exercise Swan II

The more you lift your legs in the dive the more of a roll you achieve.

M17 - Mermaid

Benefits

Strengthens the back muscles
Helps release tension at front of hips

Contraindications & Precautions

Persons with shoulder pathologies may find Version 1 difficult to perform and should only practice Version 2.

Principles

Core Control
Organization of shoulder girdle
LPHC stability
Spinal articulation in extension

Cues

Verbal : Throw your legs to the ceiling as the chest goes down
Pull your shoulder blades into your back pockets
Squeeze the abdominals to make as much length as possible between your chin and pubic bone.
Imagine your whole body to like the rocker on a rocking chair as you roll up and down

Tactile : Teacher can help 'lift / throw' the legs up to keep momentum for the 'dive'.

The Mermaid is a very interesting mat exercise in that it is probably one of the most recognisable Pilates exercises however it does not have it's own position in the classical mat sequence !

The Mermaid can be practiced or taught on all of the Pilates studio equipment. It is very often taught on the mat as a single variation with the spine starting in an upright position however here we will look at 2 versions.

Version 1 has a narrow base of support and places greater emphasis on shoulder stability and would be a great preparation for getting the client ready for more advanced exercises such as the Side Lift. It also allows for some pelvic integration into the lumbar spine.

Version 2 has a wider base of support and differs in that an emphasis is placed on the side bending articulation of the spine and also has an emphasis on the stability of the pelvis as well as needing hip mobility.

Benefits

Helps to mobilize the thoracic spine and therefore help to improve : breathing, spinal articulation movements in all planes.
Stretches the latissimus dorsi muscle and thoracolumbar fascia thereby helping with low back pain and improving shoulder mobility
Extremely good exercise for good posture due to the movements of the spine and stability and mobility of the shoulder girdle

Version 1

Set Up

Sit with the hips and knees flexed to the same side and the right hand placed in the same line as your right hip. You should have approximately 70-80% of body weight over your right arm supporting you from the side. The pelvis is at an angle to the floor with the spine 'stacked' vertically over the the pelvis when looking from the front or back.

Movement

Maintain the 'right angle' of the spine to the pelvis whilst slowly lowering the right elbow to the floor. The spine should remain stable with no side bending, rotation or translation of the rib cage to the side.
Press the hand into the floor to extend the elbow and lift back up to the start position maintaining the stable pelvis and spine.
Repeat 8-10 times.
Return to the down position and with an inhalation, reach the left arm overhead.
With an exhalation rotate the upper body and inhale once more to feel stretch from the tip of your left fingers across the upper back and to the right lower back.
Move the right arm slightly more lateral (out to the side) and then bring the left arm and elbow to the floor parallel to the right arm.
In this position perform 5 'Cat / Camel' (extension / flexion) movements of the spine.
Straighten the arms in this position and perform 5 more 'Cat / Camel' movements with the exhalation and inhalation.
Rotate the upper body to return to the extended arm side pose position.
Bring the left hand to clasp the left lower leg just above the ankle and with an inhalation perform a 'counter stretch' of the right side.

Scan the QR code to view the exercise - Mermaid version 1

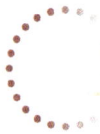
❶
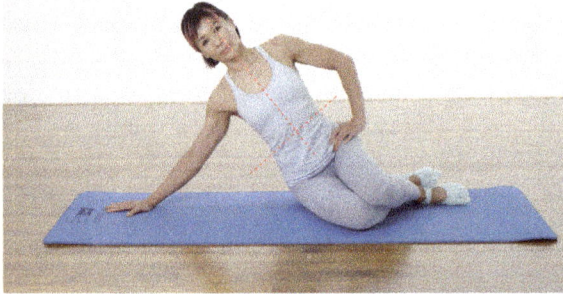

Start position

❷
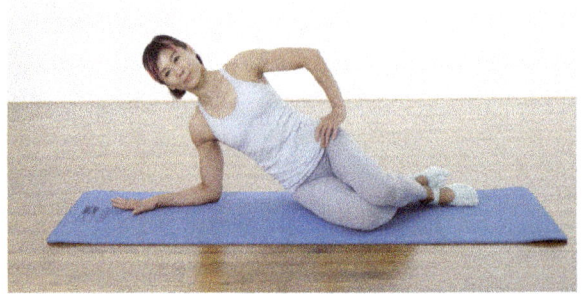

Elbow down

❸
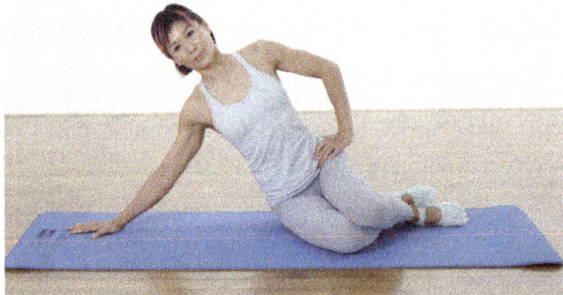

Elbow up

❹
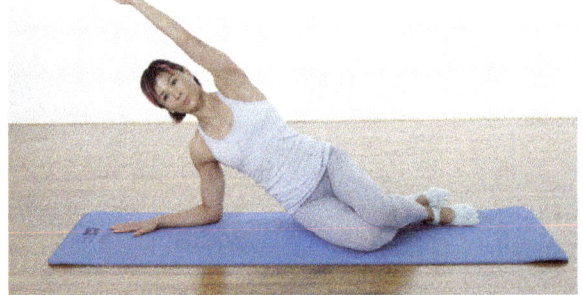

Elbow down - reach arm up

❺
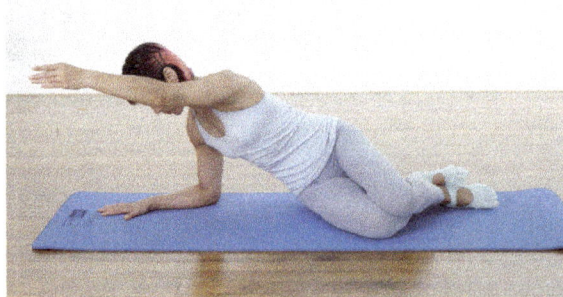

Elbow down - reach arm away

❻
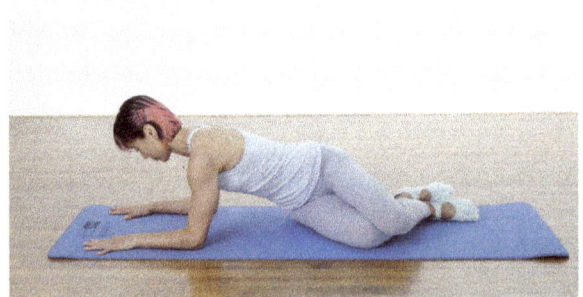

Both elbows down

7

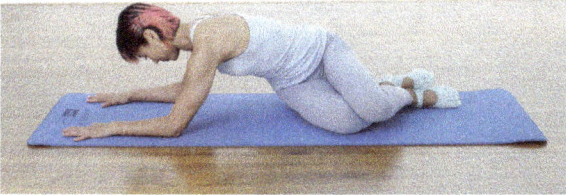

Camel - spine rounds

8

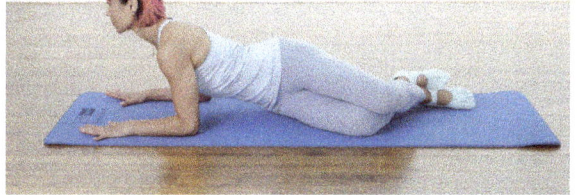

Cat - spine arches

9

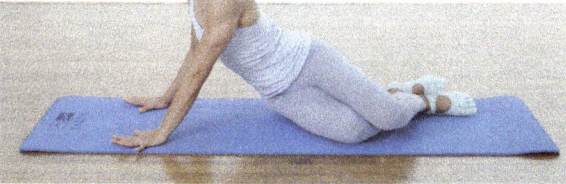

Elbows up - cat - spine arches

10

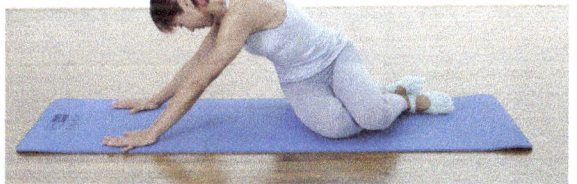

Elbows up - Camel - spine rounds

11

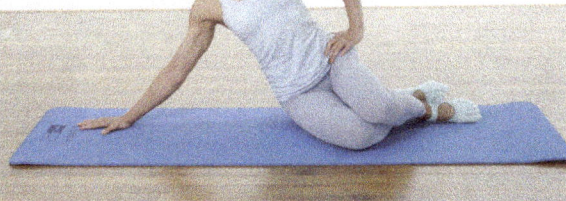

Return to start position

12

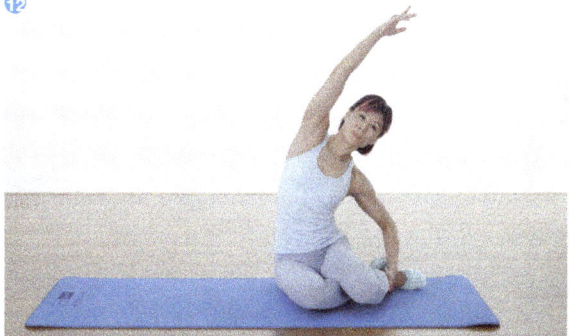

Counter stretch

Principles

Breathing
Core control
Shoulder Girdle Mobility
Shoulder Girdle Stability
Spinal Articulation in sidebending, rotation, flexion & extension

Tactile : Run the fingers down the upper spine for extension cue
Gently lift/stroke the top of the manubrium with 1 finger for extension cue
Gently depress the manubrium with 2 fingers for flexion cue
Gently hold and lift lower ribs with both hands for flexion cue

Experiment with exhalation & inhalation for both the flexion & extension part of the movement. How do they compare ?
What is the difference between the 2 ?

Can you feel how the pelvis moves when the arms are extended compared to when the elbows are down ?

Version II - wide support

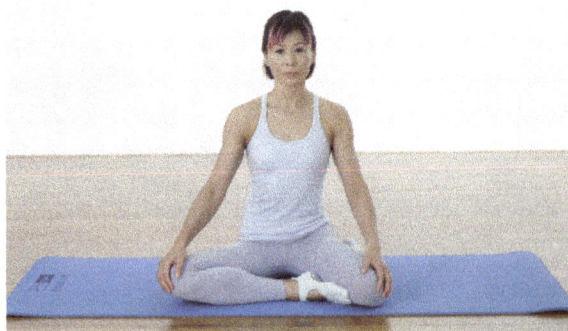

Cues

Verbal : Draw the shoulder blades towards the back pockets
Pull your elbow towards the ribcage to lower the body
Reach the tail and top of the head in opposite directions
Imagine holding a noodle in the heel of the hand to cup the hand onto the floor
Press evenly through all 5 fingers
Imagine your armpit as a vacuum cleaner sucking up the floor
Hold an imaginary tennis ball in your armpit

Sit with the right knee flexed and hip externally rotated and the left knee flexed and hip internally rotated. Sometimes referred to as the 'Z' sitting position.
Extend the arms out to the sides almost to shoulder height.
Inhale to reach the right arm to the floor and lift the left arm overhead.
Press into the floor with the right hand to maintain a connection to the ribcage with the right shoulder blade.
Rotate the upper body to reach the left hand through

the space created by the right arm and ribcage.

Return to the sidebend position and repeat the rotation movement 5 - 8 times.

Move the right arm slightly more lateral (out to the side) and bring the left hand parallel to the right arm. Perform 5 - 8 Cat / Camel (extension / flexion) movements in this position.

Return to the side bend position with left arm overhead.

Hold the left lower leg above the ankle with the left hand and perform a side bend to the left side to stretch the right side of the torso.

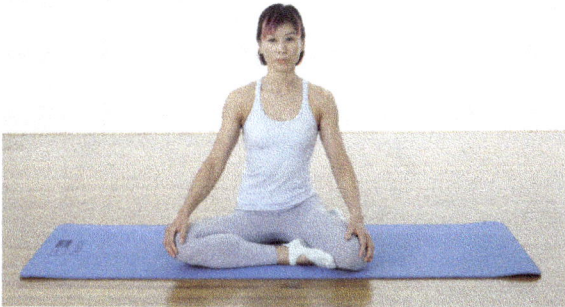

Start position

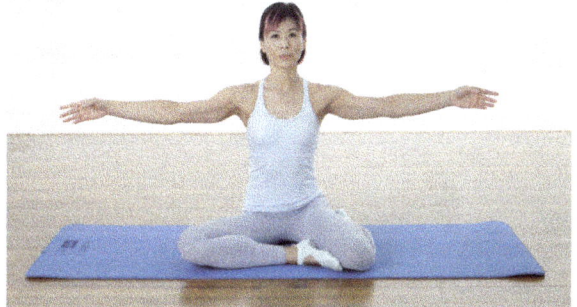

Arms lift to the side

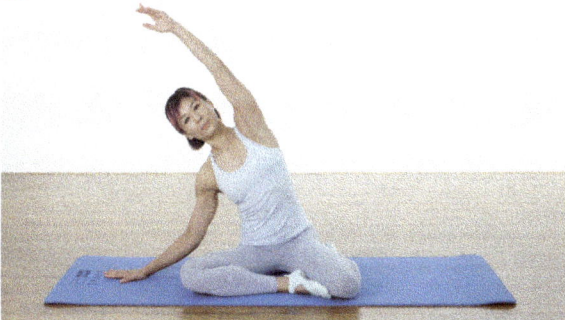

Side bend right with left arm up
Breathe into left ribs

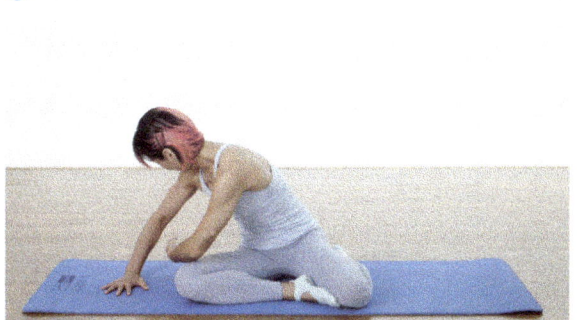

Rotate right

⑤

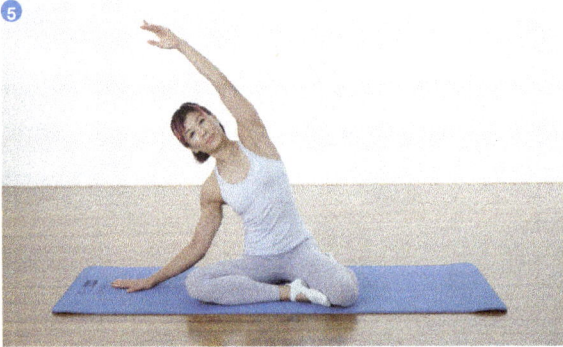

Return to side bend position

⑥

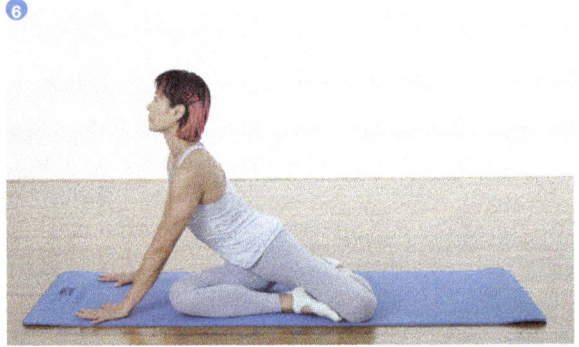

Cat / Camel in rotation position

⑦

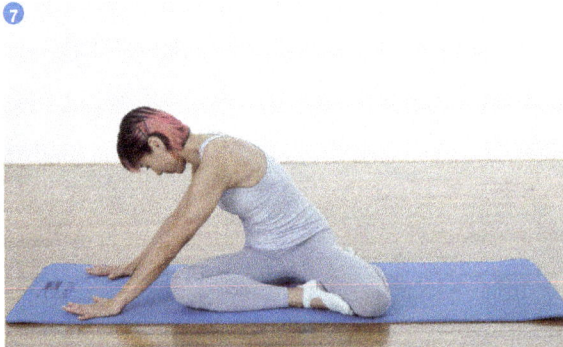

Cat / Camel in rotation position

⑧

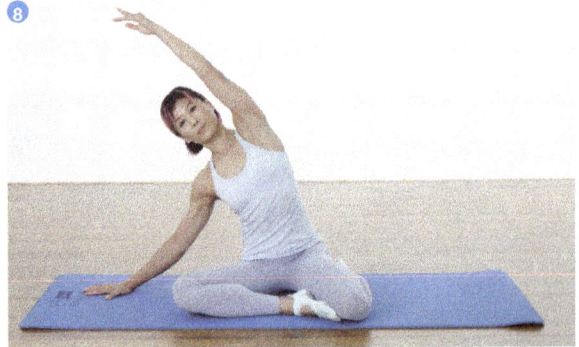

Return to side bend position

⑨

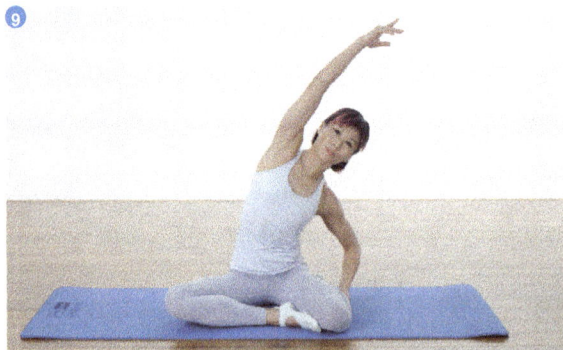

Hold shin and side bend left

Perform the rotation movement starting at the head and also starting from the lower ribs.

How do the movements compare ?

Cues

Can you think of any other verbal cues or imagery to help these movements ?

Scan the QR code to view the exercise - Mermaid version 2

Tactile Cues for the Mermaid Exercise

①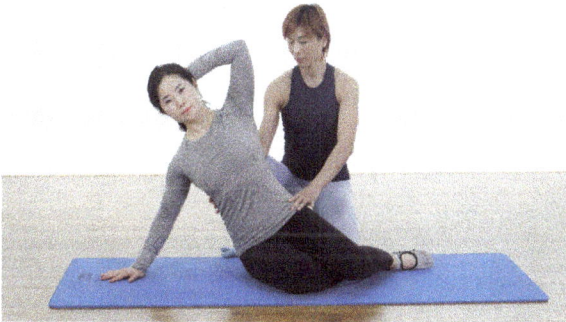

Guided for spine stability

②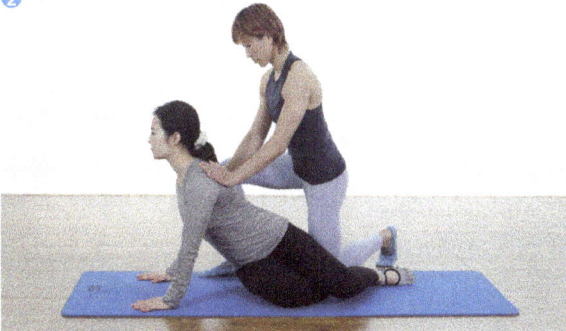

Guided for scapula movement

③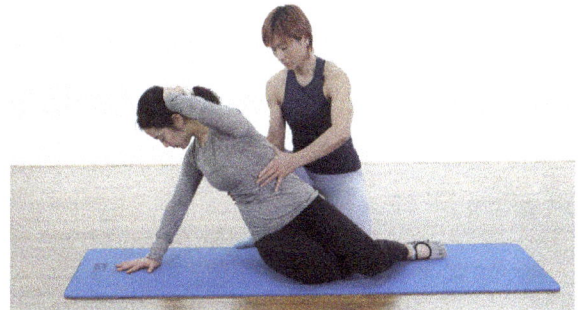

Assisted for rotation

④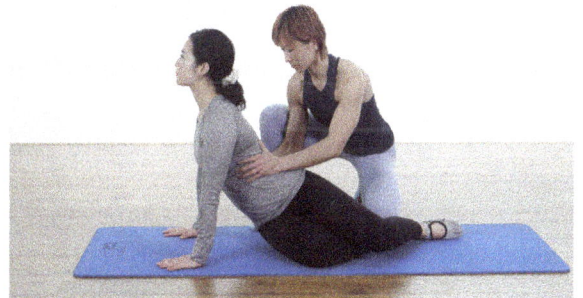

Assisted for extension

⑤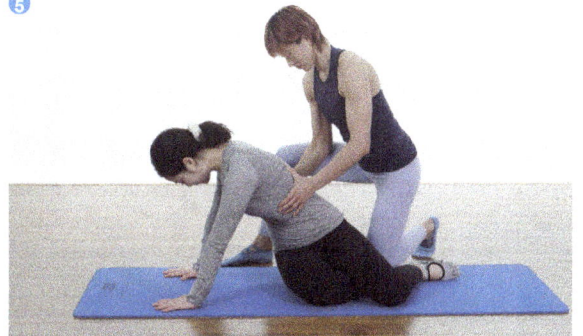

Assisted for flexion

M18 - Side Kick Series

> ### Contraindications & Precautions
>
> Persons with shoulder pathologies may find Version 1 difficult to perform and should only practice Version 2.

The Side Kick series is another classic instantly recognisable exercise in the Pilates Mat repertoire with many variations and subtle differences depending on whom you ask.

This is however a very important set of exercises to strengthen the gluteus medius and minimus muscles of the hip that are required for hip stability and consequently so that the gluteus maximus muscle can fire up efficiently. Basically a lack of gluteus medius and minimus strength may contribute significantly to a lack of gluteus maximus activity and / or back pain.

Because of the importance of these muscles we will look at not only the traditional method of this exercise but also some of the variations that are easily incorporated into the matwork as well as a 'functional' movement for the same muscles.

Basic Kick

Set Up

Side lying on the mat with the spine parallel and close to the back of the mat. The hips are slightly flexed so that the legs can extend in front of the body with the feet stacked at the corner of the mat.

The top arm is bent with the palm on the mat for added support and the bottom arm is extended high to allow the head to rest on it. The waist should be clear of the floor the whole time during the exercise.

Movement

Lift the top leg until it is parallel to the floor. Dorsi flex the ankle and kick / sweep the extended leg to the front so that the thigh is 90 degrees to the hip or slightly higher.

Plantar flex the ankle and sweep the leg back behind you. You are looking for an angle of approximately 10 - 15 degrees of hip extension in this movement however the amount you bring the leg back behind you should be limited by the passive extensibility of the hip joint plus the ability to stabilize the pelvis when the leg is moving.

For instance a person with short tight hip flexors should not even go to 'neutral' position of the leg in line with the spine as the short hip flexors will in fact not allow this range of motion and he or she will compensate by unwanted movement in the spine leading to issues with instability.

The foot should be dorsi flex first before repeating the kick movement to the front.

The name of the exercise is called 'Side Kicks' - meaning there should be an element of 'kicking the leg out in front of you' thereby the challenge becomes stabilizing the pelvis and spine against the momentum of the kick.

Things to watch out for :

• *The leg should move parallel to the floor*
• *The pelvis should remain stable*
• *Dorsi flex forwards - plantar flex backwards*
• *Keep the neck and shoulders relatively relaxed - it is very easy to compensate through the neck muscles.*
• *The under side of the waist should be lifted away from the floor at all times.*

①

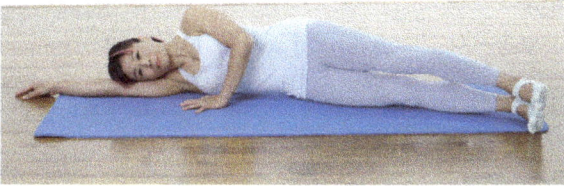

Start position

②

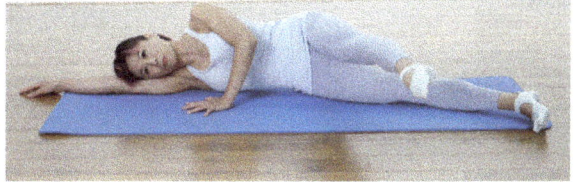

Plantar flex

③

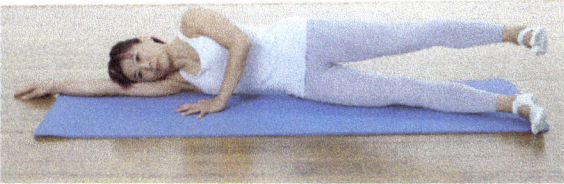

Lift top leg

④

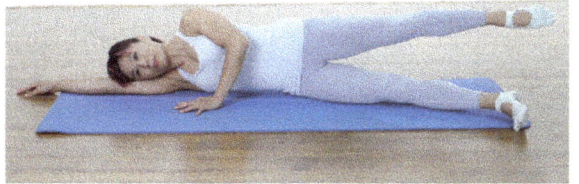

Sweep back into extension

⑤

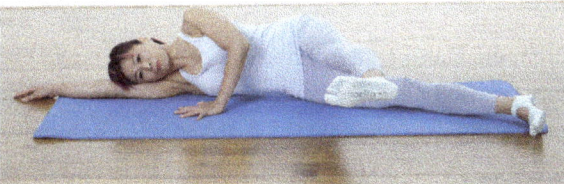

Dorsi flex and kick

Benefits

Strengthens the Gluteus minimus and medius muscles
Improves stability of the hip and pelvis
Allows greater recruitment of the gluteus maximus muscle
Helps stabilize the Sacral iliac joint

Scan the QR code to view the exercise
Side Kick Series - Kick

Principles

Breathing
Core control
LPHC mobility
LPHC stability

Cues

Verbal : Lift your waist away from the floor - imagine space for a mouse to run under the waist
Imagine putting on a really tight pair of jeans as you stabilize the pelvis
Draw a line across the opposite wall with your foot
Quickly forwards and slowly back
Maintain the leg parallel to the floor.

Tactile : Teacher places hand under the waist to remind client of the waist lifted
Teacher can place a hand in front of the pelvis to cue the pelvis NOT to rotate backwards.
Teacher can place a hand or fingers under the leg to cue the height from the floor
Teacher can place a hand at the place for maximum extension for the client and ask him/her to press into the hand at the end of the extension movement.

Experiment with the bottom leg in different positions.

Swing / kick the top leg at various intensities and speeds.

Experiment with the top hand in different positions

Up & Down (Abduction)

Set Up

Side lying on the mat with the spine parallel and close to the back of the mat. The hips are slightly flexed so that the legs can extend in front of the body with the feet stacked at the corner of the mat.
The top arm is bent with the palm on the mat for added support and the bottom arm is extended high to allow the head to rest on it. The waist should be clear of the floor the whole time during the exercise.

Movement

From the start position externally rotate the hip of the top leg and lift the leg towards the ceiling whilst plantar flexing the ankle. If the hip is externally rotating then the knee will rotate upwards and point towards the ceiling.
Decelerate the leg downwards to the start position whilst dorsi flexing the ankle.
Repeat the up and down movements again whilst dorsi flexing the ankle when the leg goes up and plantar flexing the ankle when the leg comes down.

• *Ensure the pelvis remains stable and does not rotate with the leg*
• *Maintain the space under the waist*

• *The position of the top leg relative to the pelvis in extension will depend on the individuals own hip flexor length. The shorter and tighter the hip flexors* *the more flexion is needed in both the top and bottom leg to ensure pelvic stability.*

①

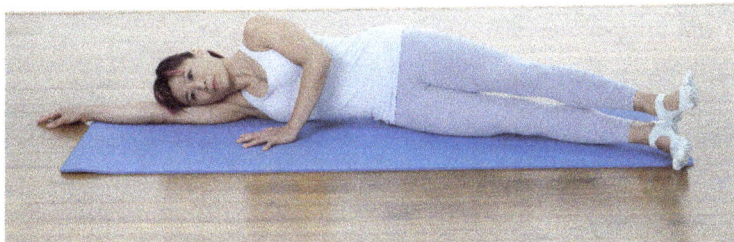

Start position

②

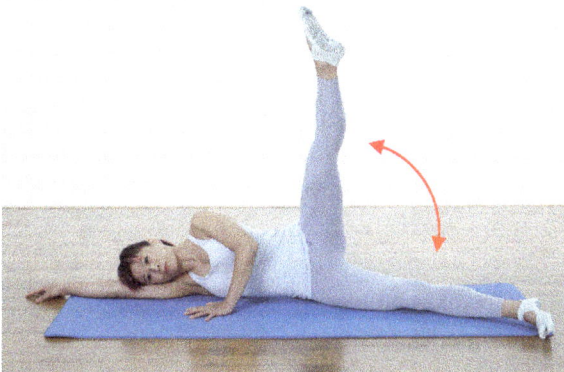

Plantar flexed ankle

③

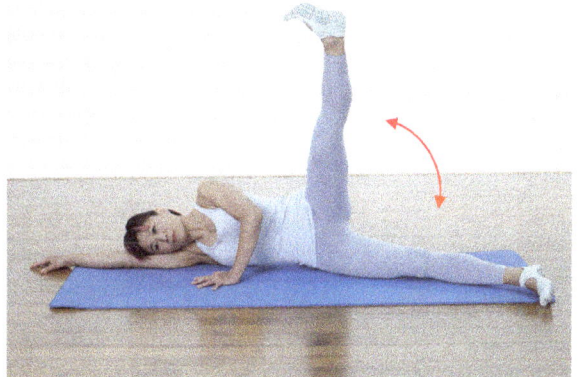

Dorsi flexed ankle

Benefits

Strengthens the Gluteus minimus and medius muscles
Improves stability of the hip and pelvis
Allows greater recruitment of the gluteus maximus muscle
Helps stabilize the Sacral iliac joint

Scan the QR code to view the exercise Side Kick Series - Abduction

Leg Circles

Set Up

Side lying on the mat with the spine parallel and close to the back of the mat. The hips are slightly flexed so that the legs can extend in front of the body with the feet stacked at the corner of the mat.
The top arm is bent with the palm on the mat for added support and the bottom arm is extended high to allow the head to rest on it. The waist should be clear of the floor the whole time during the exercise.

Movement

From the start position imagine your foot is a paintbrush and you can draw a circle on the wall closest to your feet.
Begin with small circles in a clockwise manner and slowly increase the diameter of the circle and the tempo of the movement depending on the ability of your lumbar spine and pelvis to remain stable.

Benefits

Strengthens the Gluteus minimus and medius muscles
Increases hip mobility
Improves stability of the hip and pelvis
Allows greater recruitment of the gluteus maximus muscle
Helps stabilize the Sacral iliac joint

Scan the QR code to view the exercise Side Kick Series - Leg Circles

As the leg abducts add external rotation and as the leg adducts add internal rotation.
Repeat the movements in an anti clockwise direction.

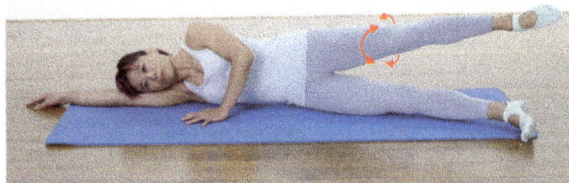

Développé

The développé is a wonderful classical exercise from ballet that requires a large of amount of both stability and mobility of the pelvis - especially in external rotation.

Set Up

Side lying on the mat with the spine parallel and close to the back of the mat. The hips are slightly flexed so that the legs can extend in front of the body with the feet stacked at the corner of the mat.
The top arm is bent with the palm on the mat for added support and the bottom arm is extended high to allow the head to rest on it. The waist should be clear of the floor the whole time during the exercise.

Movement

Begin in the side lying position. Externally rotate and flex the knee of the upper leg to slide the foot along the inside of the lower leg. Stop when the foot reaches the knee. The hip of the upper leg is now in a considerable externally and abducted position.
Maintain the hip in this position and quickly straighten the leg towards the ceiling with the ankle in a plantar flexed position.

Slowly lower the leg on top of the bottom leg whilst dorsi flexing the ankle.

Now quickly abduct the top leg again, flex the knee to bring the foot back on top of the bottom knee and then with control slide the foot back to the start position.

All of the above movements are performed with the hip of the top leg in maximal external rotation.

1

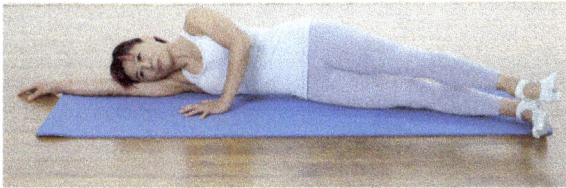

Start position

2 *slow*

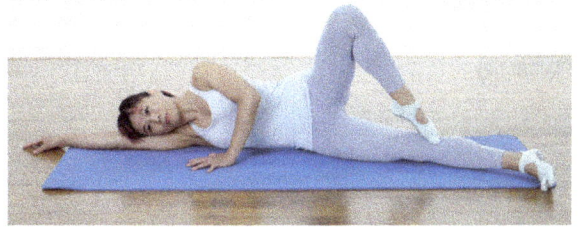

Bend leg - slide foot

3 *quick*

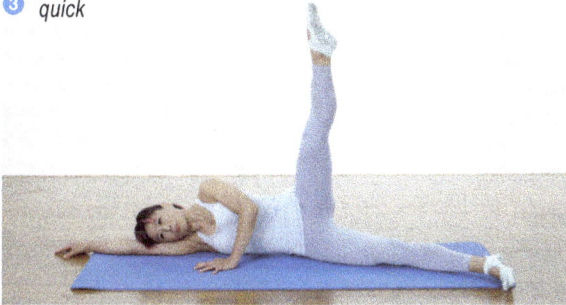

Abduct leg in externally rotated position

4 *quick*

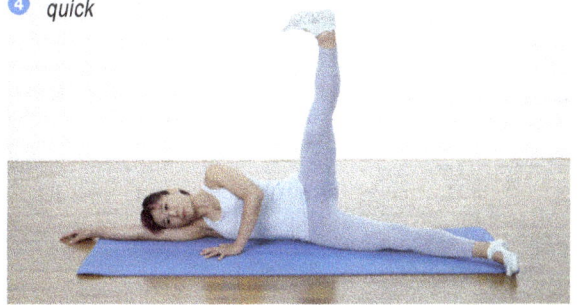

Abduct in externally rotated position

5 *slow*

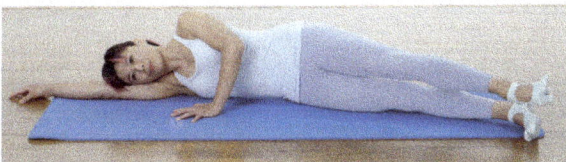

Squeeze legs together

6 *quick*

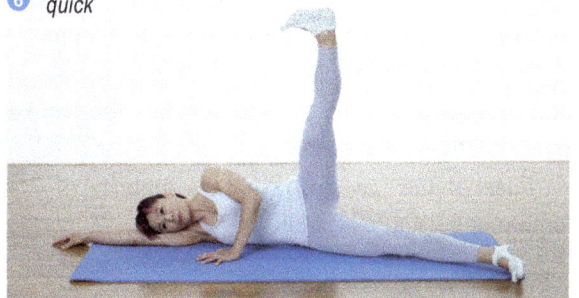

Dorsi flex and abduct

7 *quick*

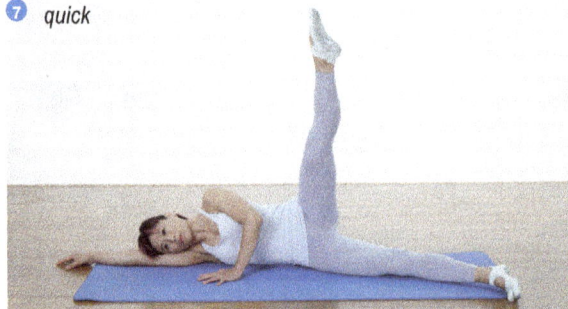

Plantar flex

9 *slow*

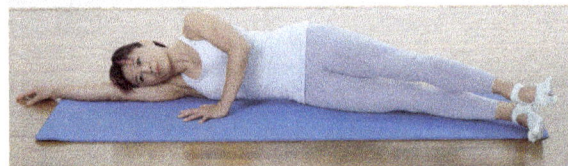

Return to start position

Scan the QR code to view the exercise Side Kick Series - Développé

Scissor Kicks

For the Scissor Kicks we need to add an extra element that we didn't use yet and that is the lower leg will adduct or lift from the floor and remain in approximately 10 cm in the air for the whole movement which will challenge both the inner thigh muscles of the lower leg and the stability of the lumbar spine and pelvis.

Set Up

Side lying on the mat with the spine parallel and

8 *quick*

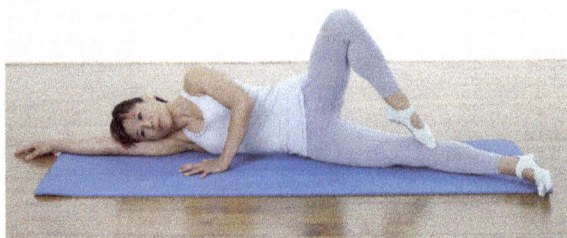

Flex knee - foot goes to lower knee

Benefits

Strengthens the Gluteus minimus and medius muscles

Improves stability of the hip and pelvis

Allows greater recruitment of the gluteus maximus muscle

Helps stabilize the Sacral iliac joint

Improves external rotation

close to the back of the mat. The hips are slightly flexed so that the legs can extend in front of the body with the feet stacked at the corner of the mat.

The bottom leg is adducted / lifted from the mat with the 2 legs squeezed together using the inner thigh muscles

The top arm is bent with the palm on the mat for added support and the bottom arm is extended high to allow the head to rest on it. The waist should be clear of the floor the whole time during the exercise.

Movement

Flex the hip of the top leg whilst extending the bottom leg. Now 'switch' so that the bottom leg comes forwards and the top leg goes backwards. Dorsi flex the ankle for the leg coming forwards and

plantar flex for the leg going backwards.
Begin with a slow movement and increase the tempo

to challenge the stability of the spine and pelvis.

①

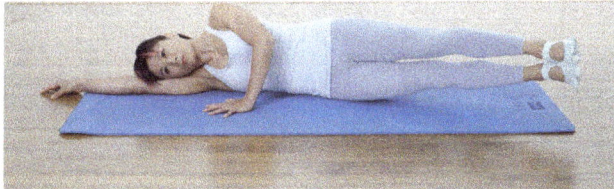

Start position

②

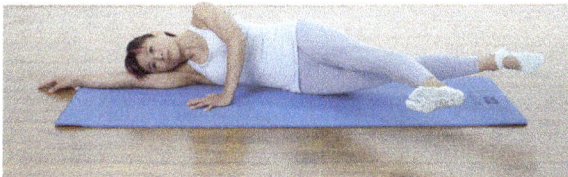

Kick left leg forwards - right leg backwards

③

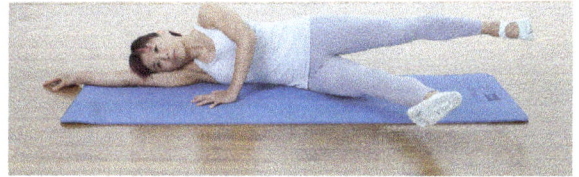

Kick left leg backwards - right leg forwards

Benefits

Strengthens the Gluteus minimus and medius muscles
Improves stability of the hip and pelvis
Allows greater recruitment of the gluteus maximus muscle
Helps stabilize the Sacral iliac joint
Strengthens inner thigh muscles

Bicycle

The Bicycle challenges the stability of the lumbar spine and pelvis whilst challenging the coordination with the 2 legs performing different movements as one leg extends with a straight leg whilst the other leg flexes with a bent leg.

Set Up

Side lying on the mat with the spine parallel and

Scan the QR code to view the exercise Side Kick Series - Scissor Kicks

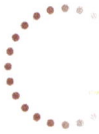

close to the back of the mat. The hips are slightly flexed so that the legs can extend in front of the body with the feet stacked at the corner of the mat.

The top arm is bent with the palm on the mat for added support and the bottom arm is extended high to allow the head to rest on it. The waist should be

1

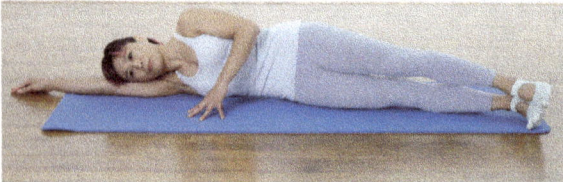

Start position

2

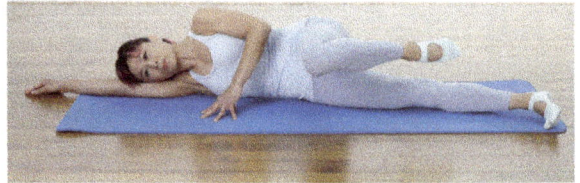

Hip and knee flexes

3

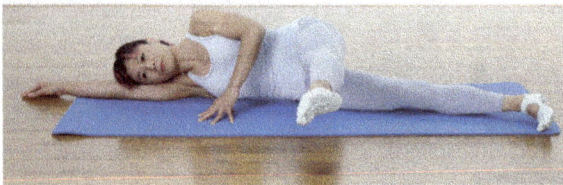

Knee extends in hip flexion

4

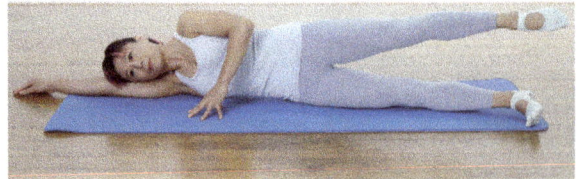

Hip extends

5

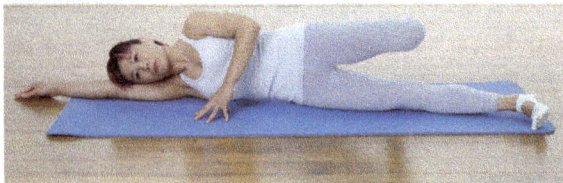

Knee flexes in hip extension

6

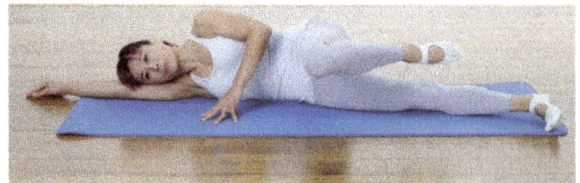

Continue.......

Scan the QR code to view the exercise Side Kick Series - Bicycle

clear of the floor the whole time during the exercise.

Movement

The top leg performs ad smooth continuous cycling movement by flexing at the hip and knee, extending at the knee and then extending a straight leg backwards. Continue is a smooth controlled manner and increase the tempo as appropriate.

Lower Leg Lifts

This is a great exercise to activate the adductor muscle group whilst challenging the stabilization of the spine and pelvis.

Set Up

Side lying on the mat with the spine parallel and close to the back of the mat. The bottom leg is in line with the spine and the top leg is placed with the sole of the foot on the mat with the knee flexed and the hip abducted, flexed and externally rotated.
The top arm is bent with the palm on the mat for added support and the bottom arm is extended high to allow the head to rest on it. The waist should be clear of the floor the whole time during the exercise.

Movement

Engage the inner thigh muscles of the bottom leg to

lift the leg (adduct) as much as possible whilst maintaining the stability of the pelvis.
Watch out for :

• Rotating the pelvis backwards as this is a common compensation due to lack of external rotation of the top hip and / or internal rotation of the bottom hip.

❶

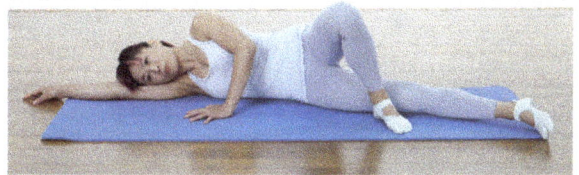

Start position

❷

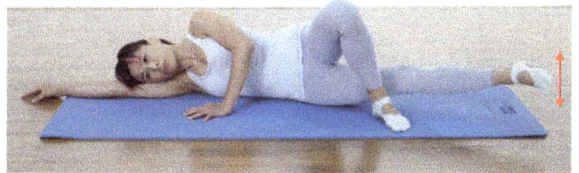

Lower leg moves up and down

Scan the QR code to view the exercise Side Kick Series - Lower Leg Adduction

• *Waist dropping to the floor.*
• *Lower back arching due to lack of hip flexor mobility*

Clam

This is a very popular and recognizable exercise practiced to strengthen the butt muscles.
However care must be taken not to 'overdo' this

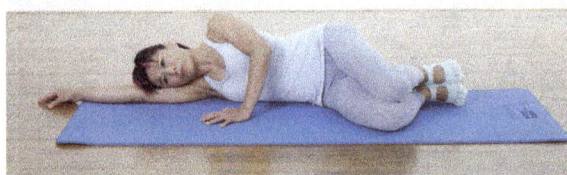

Start position

Benefits

Strengthens the Gluteus minimus and medius muscles
Improves stability of the hip and pelvis
Allows greater recruitment of the gluteus maximus muscle
Helps stabilize the Sacral iliac joint
Improves external rotation

Scan the QR code to view the exercise Side Kick Series - Clam

exercise because the rotation is performed with the hip in flexion which can cause overuse of some muscles that we wish to actually 'turn off' !

Set Up

Side lying position with the head rested on an out stretched arm and waist lifted from the mat. Both hips are flexed approximately 30 degrees and both knees flexed 90 degrees with the top leg stacked directly over the bottom leg.

Movement

Using both the hip and the heels as a fulcrum or pivot point lift (abduct) the top leg away from the bottom leg.
Externally rotate the hip joint and squeeze the butt muscles at the end of the range of motion for 3 seconds before lowering the leg to the start position. As with all the other movements in this series ensure :

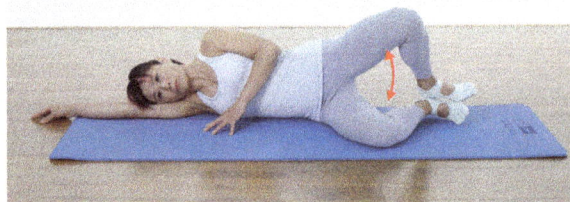

Pivot on hip and heel

• *The pelvis does not rotate but stays fixed in position*
• *The lower back does not arch*
• *The waist remains lifted away from the mat.*

Gluteus Medius Muscle

Due to prolonged sitting in modern life many of us

suffer from dysfunctions that have common root causes causing many ailments and musculo skeletal problems. Probably the 3 most targeted culprits for dysfunctional behaviour are the Gluteus Medius (and minimus), Gluteus Maximus and Psoas muscles.

The poor old gluteus medius muscle in particular quite often doesn't know if its coming or going as it needs to constantly act as either a prime mover or a stabilizer and as a result over time it basically gives up and lets other 'people' do the work.

The Side Kick series does a lot of Gluteus Medius activation but it is still good to know that there are a couple of moves left that can target the different fibers of the muscle depending on ones needs.

The anterior and posterior fibers are 2 such areas that will usually benefit from some more specific movements as follows.

Gluteus Medius Anterior & Posterior

Set Up

Side lying position with the head rested on an out stretched arm and waist lifted from the mat. Both hips are flexed approximately 30 degrees and both knees flexed 90 degrees with the top leg stacked directly over the bottom leg.

Movement

Using both the hip and the heels as a fulcrum or pivot point lift (abduct) the top leg away from the bottom leg as in the clam exercise but stop halfway when the

Scan the QR code to view the exercise Side Kick Series - Hip Rotations

1

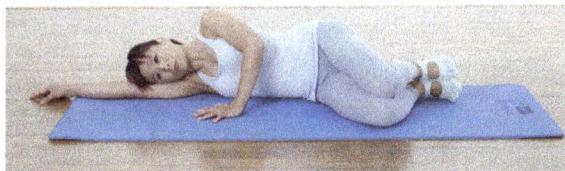

Start position

2

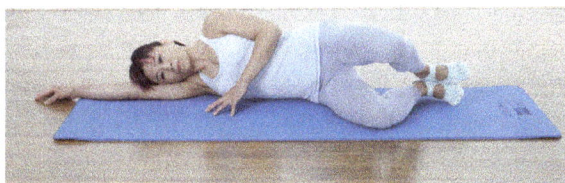

Top leg externally rotates

3

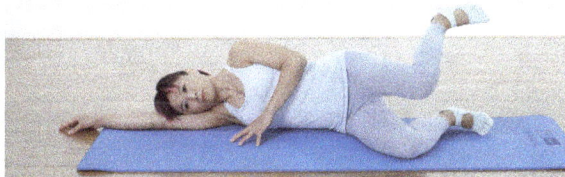

Top leg internally rotates around knee axis

4

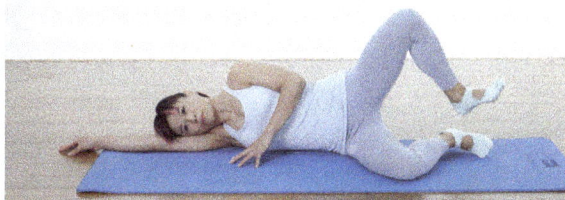

Top leg externally rotates around knee axis

Benefits

Strengthens the Gluteus medius muscle in rotation

Improves stability of the hip and pelvis

Allows greater recruitment of the gluteus maximus muscle

Helps stabilize the Sacral iliac joint

knee is level with the height of the hip.

At this point now use the 'knee' as a pivot point to lift the top foot away from the bottom foot until it is higher than the top knee.

The hip joint will now be in full internal rotation.

Slowly allow the foot to pivot through the top knee towards the foot (external rotation) and then repeat the action of lifting and lower the foot using the knee as a pivot point even though it is not supported on any base from below but rather the knee is 'hanging in the air'.

Functional Movement of Gluteus Medius

All of the previous exercises are great for single joint muscle recruitment however

The gluteus medius muscles just don't work like that in real life so it's probably worth while just to stick a more functionally orientated exercise at the end to enable the client to integrate what has just been learned with the other exercises.

Set Up

Standing on the right leg which is on a small block or thick book - the left foot is the same height as the right foot when viewed from the side.

Movement

Move the left leg up and down by pivoting on the raised right hip.

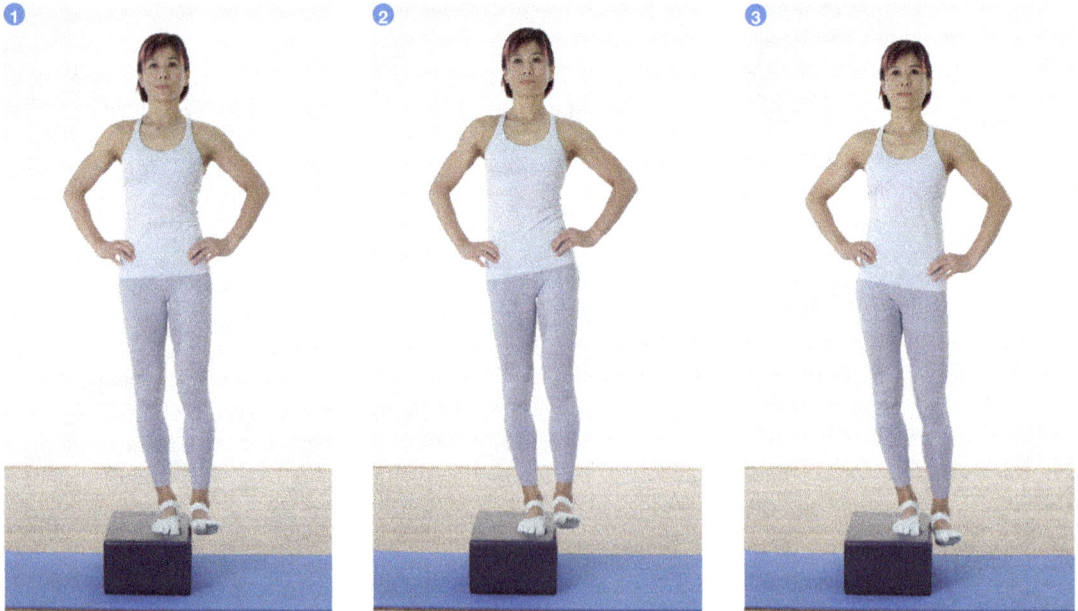

| Start position - Hips level | Left hip up | Left hip down |

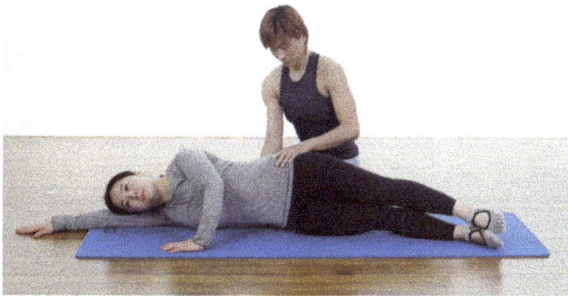

Guided cue for the Sidelying Leg Kicks series

M19 - Teaser

Affectionately known as the 'Mother of all Sit Ups' the Teaser is a demanding exercise that will challenge many of the principles you have learned up till now in one movement.

Set Up

Sitting position with the hands placed on the mat behind you and hips and knees flexed with feet on the floor.

Movement

Extend the legs up and out in front of you. Find the point of balance behind your sit bones and reach the arms out straight parallel to the legs so that when viewed from the side your legs and body form a 'V' position.

Curl your tail towards your pubic bone and initiate a backwards movement of the pelvis to slowly roll and articulate the spine onto the mat. As you roll the spine down to the mat also bring the legs down with you similar to the 'Double Straight Leg Stretch' and stop the legs at the appropriate distance (depending on your core stability and / hip flexor flexibility) from the floor.

Your upper body is now on the mat with the legs held out straight away from the floor.

Reach the arms up over the top of the head and make a circular motion of the arms to bring them down towards your sides however as the arms pass the 90 degrees mark with the shoulders begin to lift the head, chest and legs at the same time to curl the spine back off the mat and into the 'V' sitting position.

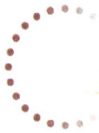

1

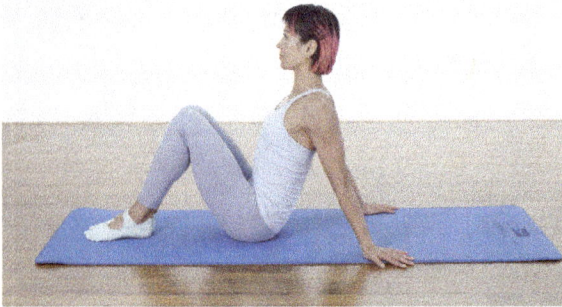

Start position

2

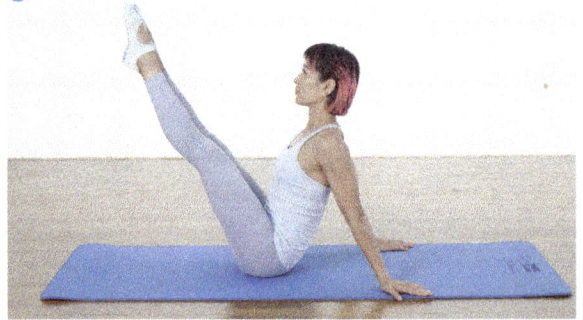

Lift and extend legs

3

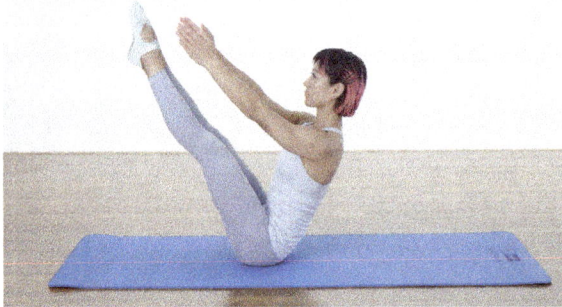

Reach the arms out in front

4

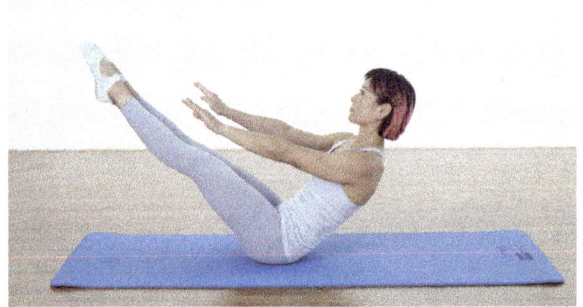

Articulate spine to mat

5

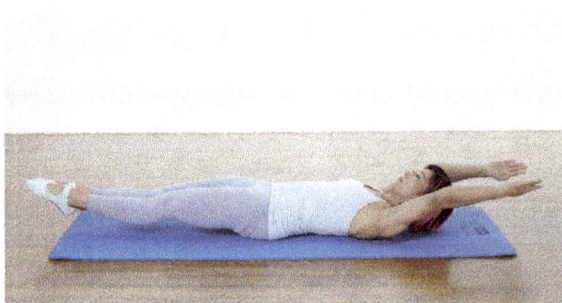

'Big stretch' with legs lifted

6

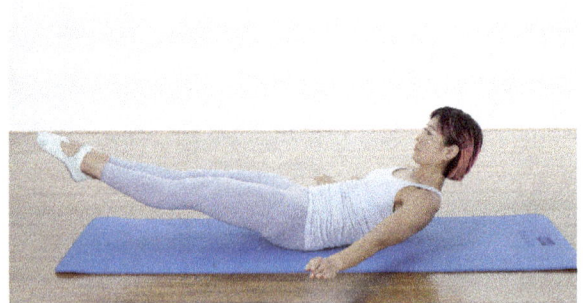

Sweep arms around and lift head and chest

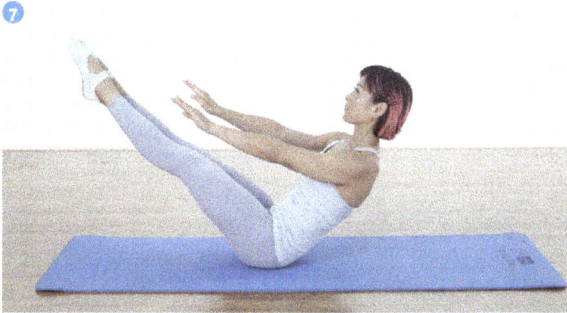

Articulate spine from the mat

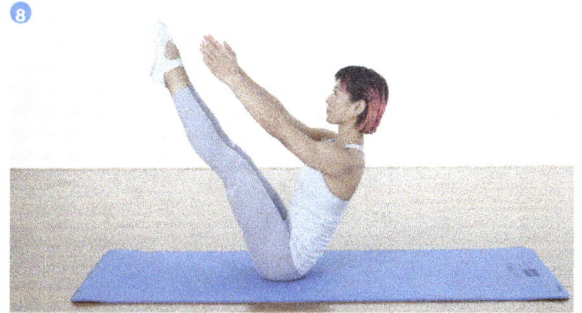

Return to 'Teaser position'

Benefits

Strengthens the abdominal muscles
Improves abdominal core muscle recruitment
Strengthens hip flexors
Improves quadriceps activation (knee extension)

Principles

Breathing
Core control
LPHC mobility & stability
Helps differentiate hips from pelvis
Shoulder girdle organization

Practice the different elements of the exercise separately :
Roll Up
Roll up with legs bent and lifted
Double Straight Leg Stretch
Sitting with arms behind you in the start position with leg extensions.

Cues

Verbal : imagine your spine is a strip of sticky tape being stuck down and then lifted from the mat
Imagine your spine is a bicycle chain being laid down on the mat and lifted up again one link at a time.
See if you can count the number of bones in your spine being placed down on the mat one by one
Imagine each bone in the spine being lifted away and up from the one below it as you sit up

Tactile : Assisted, Resisted and Guided cues are all very useful for helping to lift the legs with a beneficial strategy.
Guided cue with the fingers can be used for spinal articulation

Scan the QR code to view the exercise - Teaser

Tactile Cue Options for Teaser exercise

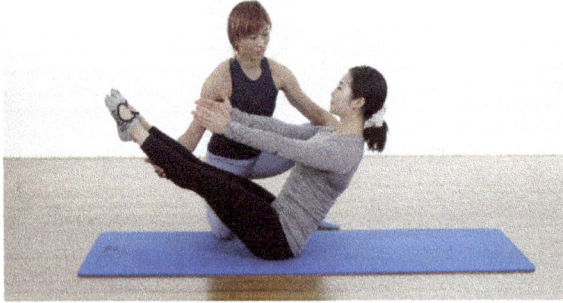

Assisted for articulation

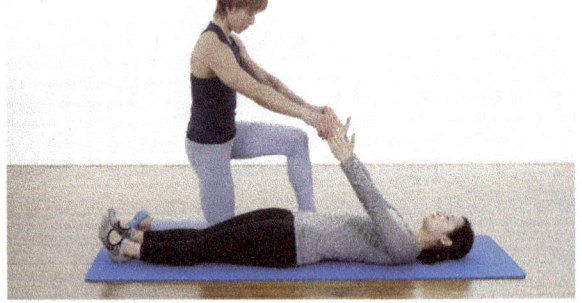

Assisted for articulation

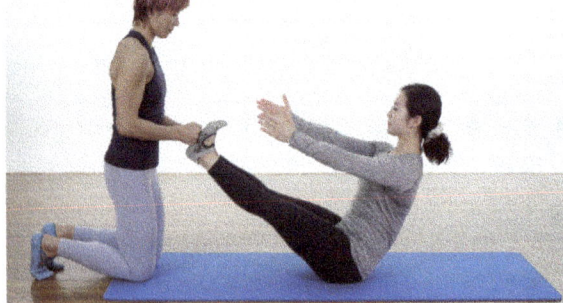

Resisted for articulation

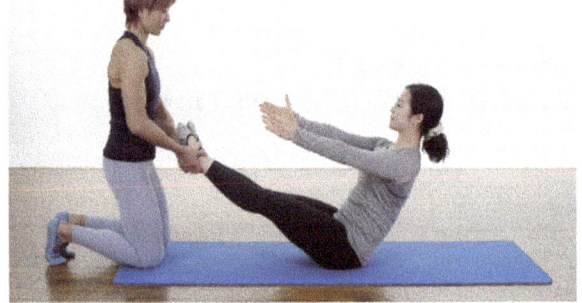

Assisted for articulation

M20 - Can Can

Can Can builds on the skills learned in the Teaser exercise for the lower extremities and now adds a rotational component as an advanced version of the Side to Side exercise.

Particular care must be taken in this exercise to ensure the rotation is made with appropriate organization of the abdominal and musculature and pelvis in order to protect the lower back. If any discomfort in the lower back is felt during this exercise you should stop immediately as it probably means there is too much stress with rotation in the

Contraindications & Precautions

This exercise may be contraindicated for persons with disc pathologies due to the rotational component under load.

Persons with chronic back should approach this exercise with caution

extend.

Summary :

1. *Bent legs left - body right*
2. *Bent legs right - body left*
3. *Straight legs left - body right*

4. *Bent legs right - body left*
5. *Bent legs left - body right*
6. *Straight legs right - body left*

lumbar spine and/or lumbar spine - sacral junction.

Set Up

Sitting position with the hands placed on the mat behind you and hips and knees flexed with feet on the floor with inner thighs activated pressed together.

Movement

Draw in deeply through the abdominals and lift the heels from the floor so that the big toes of each foot are barely touching the paint on the mat.

Slowly lower the legs to the left side as in the Side to Side exercise ensuring that the left leg is 'glued' to the right leg and makes a small 'slide' up the leg as they are lowered to one side.

At the same time turn the upper torso to the left side to create a counter rotation.

Now take the legs to left side and the upper body to the right side.

Now take the legs to the right side again with the torso turning left however this time extend the knees without dropping the thighs so that the legs point to the ceiling.

Pause in this position for 1 second and then continue with bent legs to the left and body turning to the right.

Legs move right and body rotates left

Legs move left and body rotates right - however legs

Practice the different elements of the exercise separately :

Double Straight Leg Stretch
Sitting with arms behind you in the start position with leg extensions.
Practice with different drivers - what difference does it make ?
Bottom up (pelvic floor / pelvic half)
Top down (eyes & head)

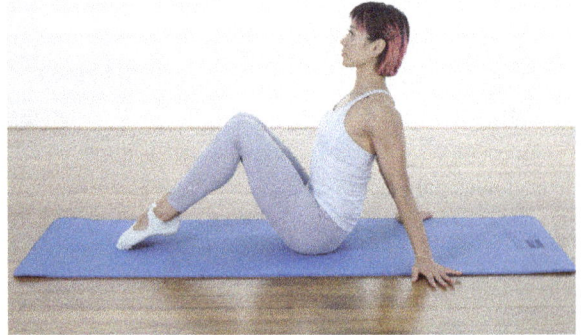

❶

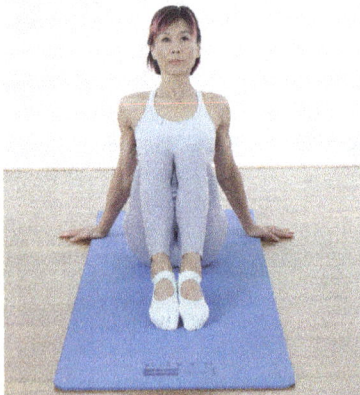

Start position

❷

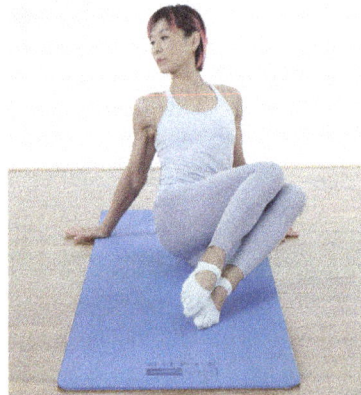

Bent legs left
Body turns right

❸

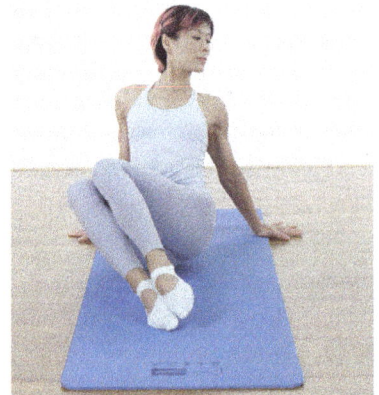

Bent legs right
Body turns left

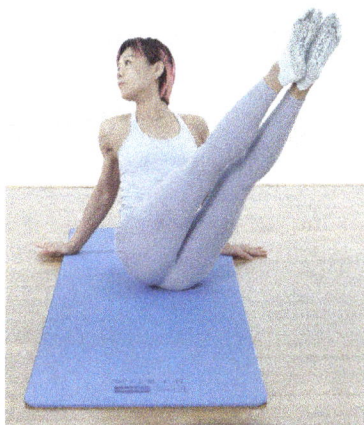

④

Straight legs left
Body turns right

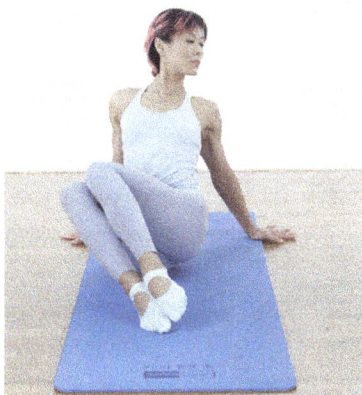

⑤

Bent legs right
Body turns left

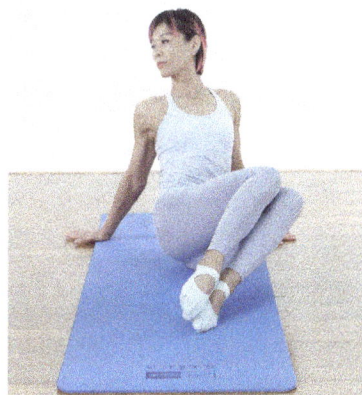

⑥

Bent legs left
Body turns right

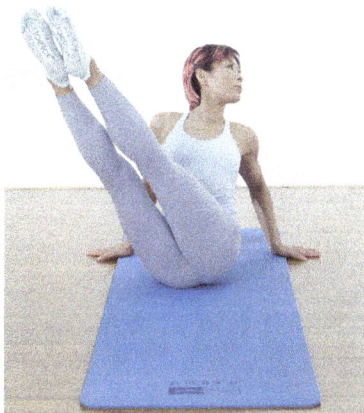

⑦

Straight legs right
Body turns left

Scan the QR code to view the exercise - Can Can

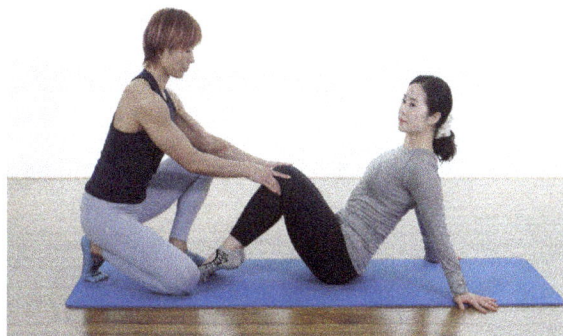

Guided cue for the Can Can exercise

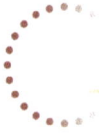

M21 - Hip Circles

The Hip Circles exercise is a nice progression from the Can Can as the skills learned in the Can Can are now put to the test with a continuous long lever load from the lower extremities into the pelvis and core.

Contraindications & Precautions

Do not attempt this exercise until you are proficient in the Can Can first.

Set Up

Sitting position with the hands placed on the mat behind you and hips and knees flexed with feet on the floor with inner thighs activated pressed together.

Movement

Bring the legs and upper body immediately to the end position of the Can Can exercise with legs extended to the right side and head and torso rotated to the left side.

Sweep the legs across to the left side with a slight lowering of the legs to create a rotational counter clockwise movement. At the same time rotate the head and torso to the right.

Continue sweeping the legs in a counter clockwise circle to lift and bring them back to the right side as the head and torso rotates back to the left.

Pause for 1 second

Repeat this circular rotational movement 2 more times for a total of 3 circles and then repeat in the other direction 3 times.

❶

❷

❸

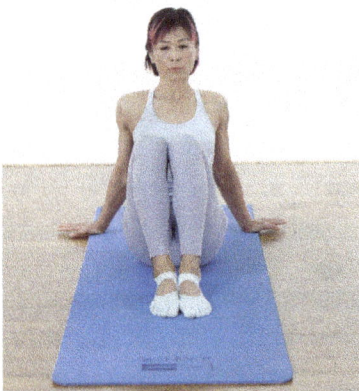

Start position

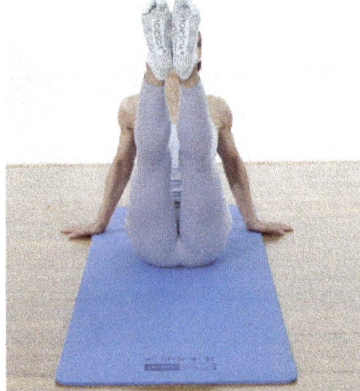

Extend legs up

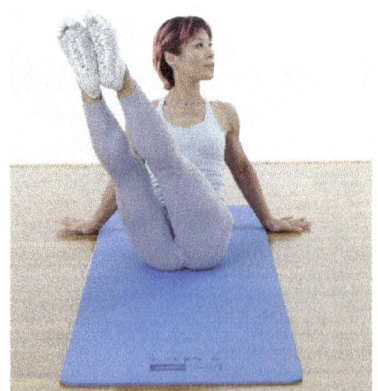

Look left - legs right

④

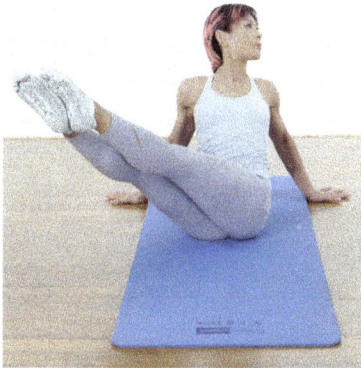

Look left - legs lower to the right

⑤

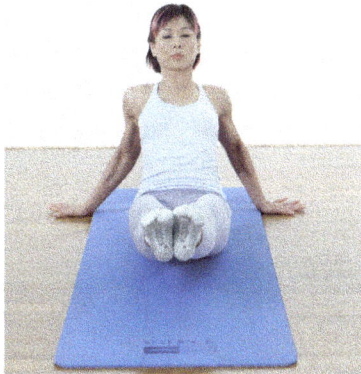

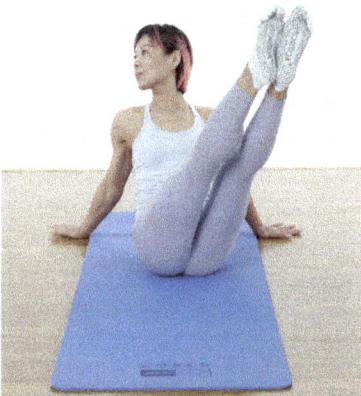

Look straight - legs straight

⑥

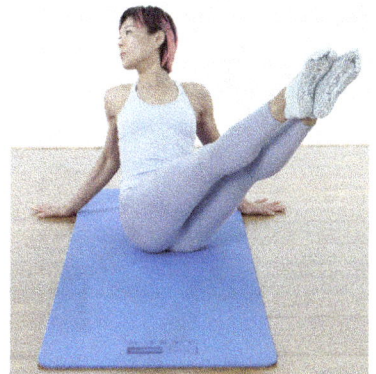

Look right - legs lift left

⑦

Look right - legs straight

⑧

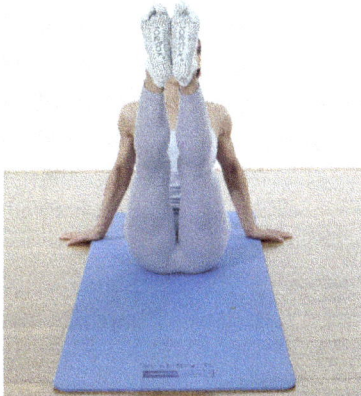

Look straight - legs up and straight
Repeat in other direction

Scan the QR code to view the exercise - Hip Circles

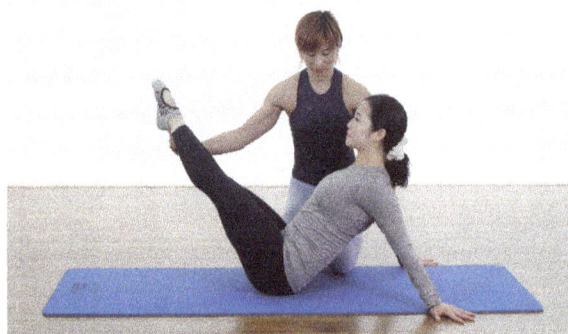

Guided / assisted cue for the Hip Circles exercise

Cues

Verbal : Maintain your ribcage over pelvis alignment
Keep inner thighs activated throughout the movement
Feel the lower abdominal connection from belly button to ASIS
Keep the legs light and let them float

Tactile : Assisted, Resisted and Guided cues are all very useful for helping to lift the legs with a beneficial strategy.
Guided cue with the fingers can be used for spinal articulation in rotation

Benefits

Strengthens the abdominal muscles
Improves abdominal core muscle recruitment
Strengthens hip flexors
Improves quadriceps activation (knee extension)
Improves integration of torso into pelvis

Practice the different elements of the exercise separately :

Double Straight Leg Stretch
Sitting with arms behind you in the start position with leg extensions.
Practice with different drivers - what difference does it make ?
Bottom up (pelvic floor / pelvic half)
Top down (eyes & head)
Practice with hands in various positions - what difference does it make ?

Principles

Core control
LPHC mobility & stability
Helps differentiate hips from pelvis
Torso - pelvis integration

M22 - Side Lift

The Side Lift is an interesting exercise that really calls for your 'Pilates Face'. When seeing somebody perform this well it is hard to appreciate the core and shoulder girdle stability needed to perform the exercise.

The classic mistake here is to constantly lift the pelvis too high so bear in mind that the correct position is to have the spine and pelvis in line to place greater demand into the butt and waist muscles. We will look at 4 versions including one with a twist.

> **Contraindications & Precautions**
>
> Persons with shoulder pathologies should approach this exercise with caution

Version 1

Set Up

Lying on your side propped up on the right elbow with the elbow in line with the hip. The hips, knees and ankles are stacked and on the mat. The ideal position for the knees is also to be in line with the hips however the majority of persons are unable to find this 'neutral position' due to too much tension in the hip flexors generated by the need to stretch the quadriceps with the flexed knee position. For these persons the knees will need to be placed slightly in front of the pelvis.

Movement

Lift the pelvis from the mat to support yourself on the right elbow and right knee so that the head, spine and legs form a single straight line when viewed from the front or back. The right elbow should now be immediately under the right shoulder when viewed from the front.

Hold for 5 breaths and return to start position.

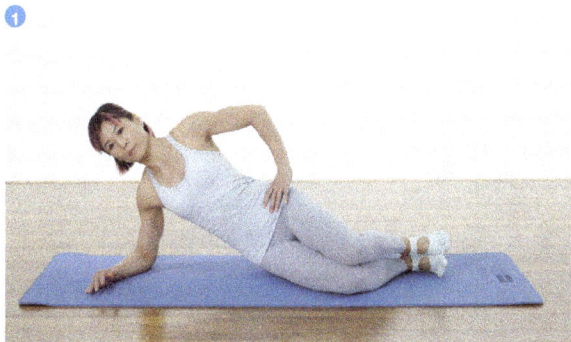

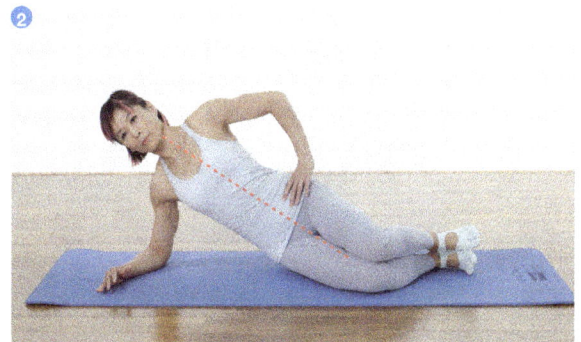

Knees in front of hips / pelvis

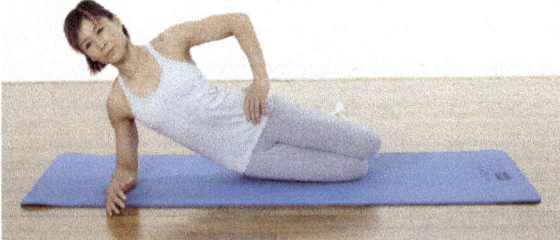

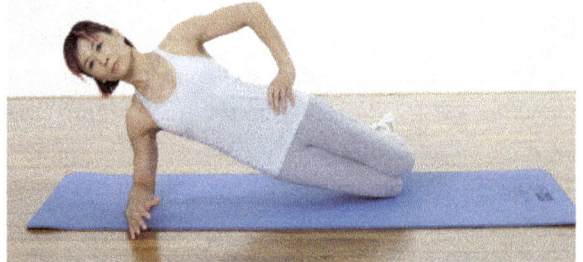

Knees in line with hips / pelvis

Version 2

Set Up

Lying on your side propped up on the right elbow with the elbow in line with the hip. The hips, knees and ankles are stacked and on the mat. The feet are placed in alignment with the elbow and hips so that the knee are in front of the body. The elbow should be slightly abducted so that it is under the right ear as opposed to the right shoulder when viewed from the front.

Movement

Lift the pelvis and knees to come to a 'plank' position supported by the right elbow and outside of the right foot.

As you lift into position the body should travel in a direction that takes the head towards the top of the mat so that the knees can extend and move backwards to form a perfect straight line with the spine. The shoulders should also move in the direction of the head so that the right shoulder is now directly over the right elbow.

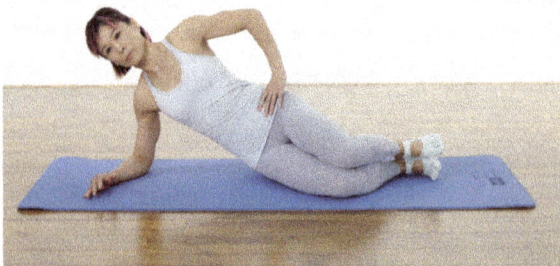

Start position

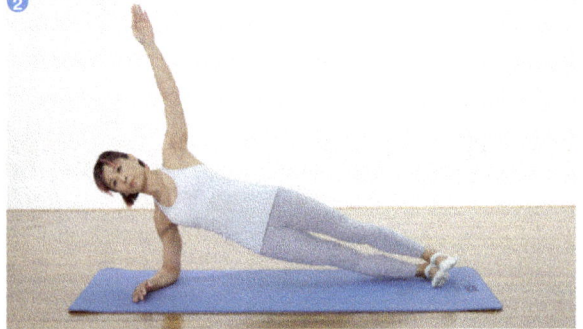

Right shoulder over right elbow
Knees move back into line with the spine, pelvis and feet

Hold for 5 breaths and lower back down again.

Version 3

Set Up

Sitting on your right side with the hand in line with the hip. The hips, knees and ankles are stacked and on the mat. The feet are placed in alignment with the elbow and hips so that the knees are in front of the body.

Now shift the top (left) foot forwards so that it is placed on the mat in front of the right foot.

The shoulder should be in a position under the right ear with the hand placed further towards the top of the mat.

Movement

Lift the pelvis whilst moving in a direction to take the head towards the top of the mat, the right shoulder over the right hand and the knees backwards in line with the hand, hips and feet.

You should now be in a side plank position with the weight over the right arm, outside of the right foot and inside of the left foot.

The left arm is in a line with the right arm pointing

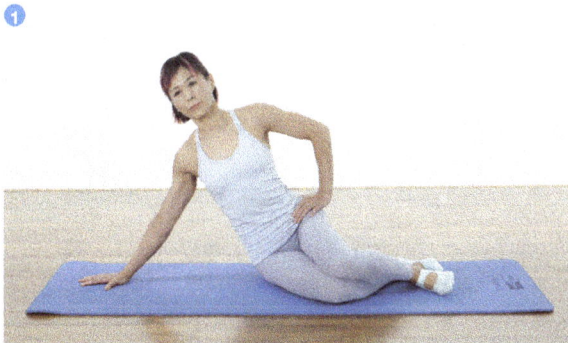

Start position

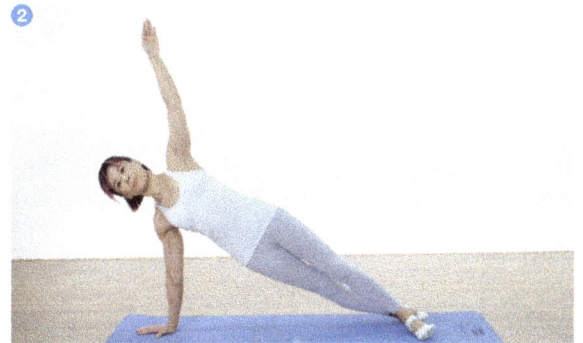

Pelvis lifts

towards the ceiling.
Return to the start position.

An alternative position is to have the top leg slightly behind the bottom leg whcih will challenge the stability through the pelvis due to the added stretch through the hip flexors pulling the pelvis into a transverse plane rotation.

Version 4 - Side Lift with Twist

Set Up

Sitting on your right side with the hand in line with the hip. The hips, knees and ankles are stacked and on the mat. The feet are placed in alignment with the elbow and hips so that the knees are in front of the body.

Now shift the top (left) foot forwards so that it is placed on the mat in front of the right foot.

The shoulder should be in a position under the right

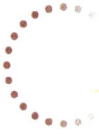
ear with the hand placed further towards the top of the mat.

Movement

Lift the pelvis whilst moving in a direction to take the head towards the top of the mat, the right shoulder over the right hand and the knees backwards in line with the hand, hips and feet.

You should now be in a side plank position with the

weight over the right arm, outside of the right foot and inside of the left foot.

The left arm is in a line with the right arm pointing towards the ceiling.

Rotate the upper body to bring the left arm under the chest in a 'big hug'.

Now imagine a rope attached to a hook on your pelvis lifting your tail bone towards the ceiling. As the pelvis floats to the ceiling continue to reach the left

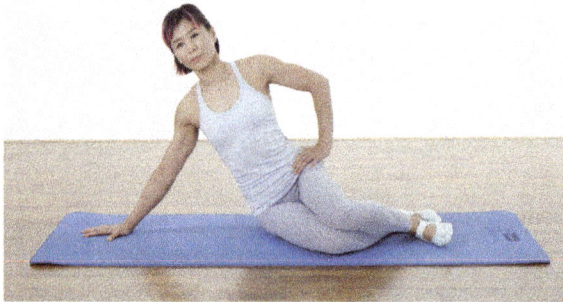

Start position

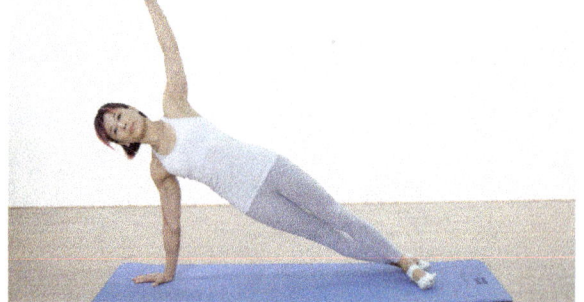

Pelvis lifts

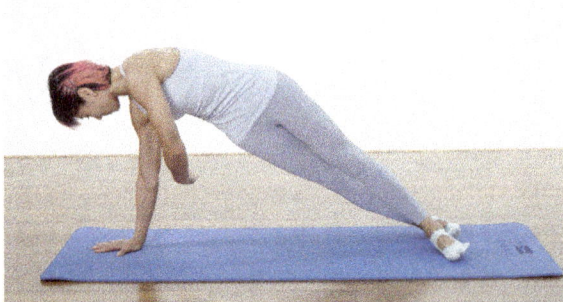

Rotate upper body

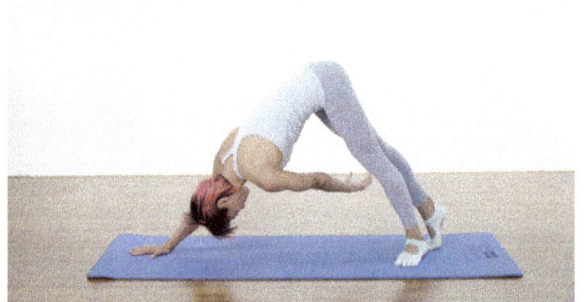

Reach towards right foot

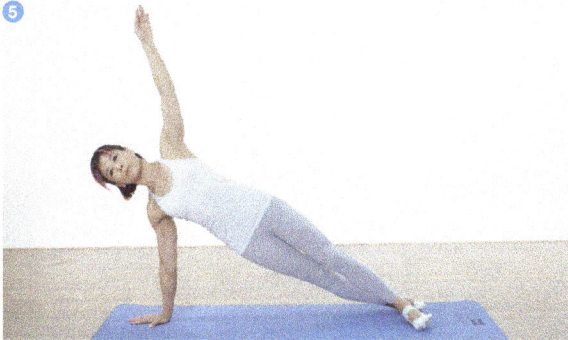

❺

Return to plank

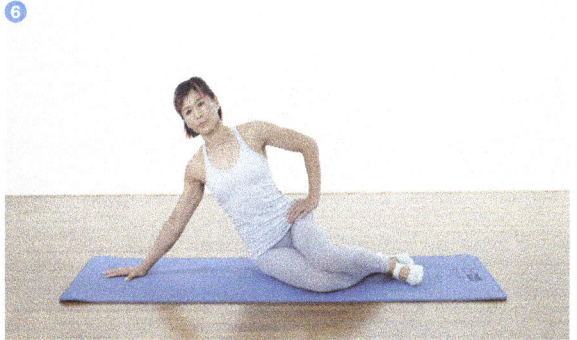

❻

Return to start position

In all of the versions of the Side Lift ensure you do not initially lift too far by bringing the pelvis higher than it should go.

Practice using an inhalation to lift.

Practice using an exhalation to lift.

What is the difference between using inhalation and exhalation for the lift ?

Principles

Core control
LPHC & stability
Shoulder girdle stability & mobility
Integration of upper extremities into the core
Integration of lower extremities into the core

Benefits

Strengthens the abdominal muscles
Improves abdominal core muscle recruitment
Strengthens shoulder girdle
Improves shoulder stability
Improves integration of upper extremity into the 'core'.

Cues

Verbal : Float the pelvis
Imagine balloon lifting the pelvis
Imagine balloons attached to the tailbone to lift the pelvis
Squeeze from the sides as you lift
Imagine pulling yourself out of a tube as you lift

Tactile : Teacher can guide the ribcage in wanted direction on the lift
Teacher place to assist or guide the pelvis

Scan the QR code to view the exercise - Side Lift

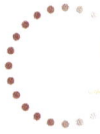

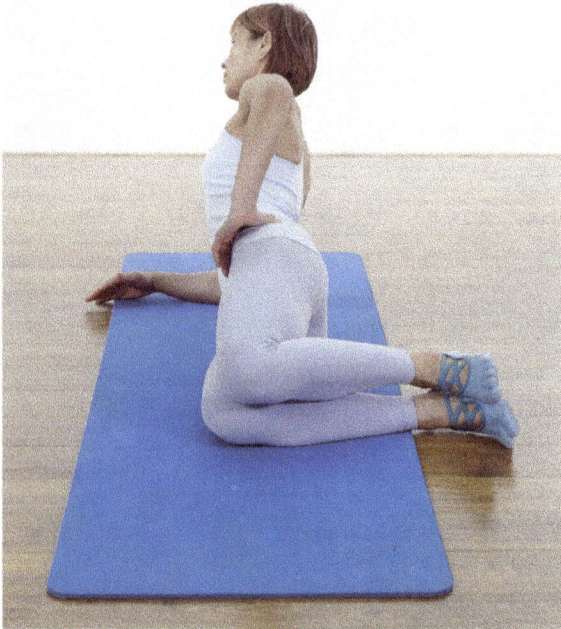

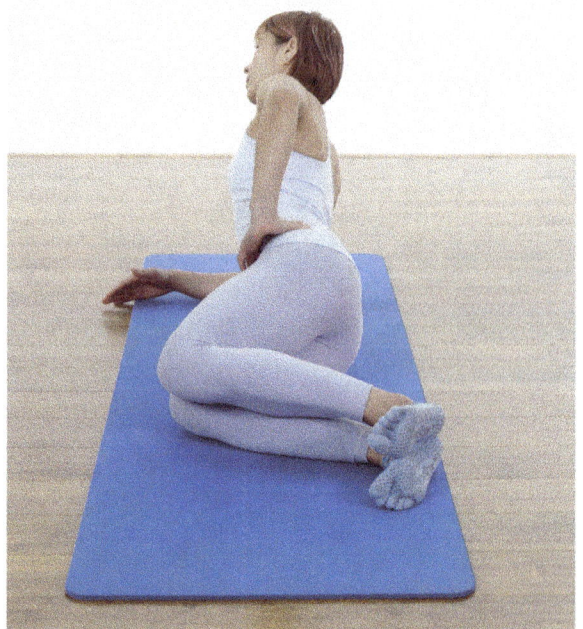

Optional leg positions for the Side Lift on Elbows exercise according to hip flexor flexibility

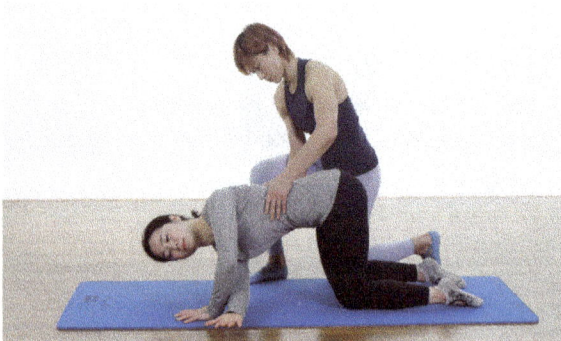

Rotation may be easily regressed by performing the exercise in the quadruped position

M23 - Kneeling Side Kicks

The Kneeling Side Kicks exercise progresses the Side Kick series through a number of differences :

- *The balance of the body is challenged*
- *There is a need for flexibility through the trunk muscles on the side making the kicks.*
- *The pelvis is challenged for stability on top of the femur heads in all 3 planes of movement.*
- *The hips need to have mobility for both adduction and abduction.*
- *The position of the body increases the leverage into the hip joint*
- *There is considerable challenge for core stability.*

Set Up

Begin in a high kneeling position facing the side of the mat with thighs hip width apart.

Slide your left leg out to the side so that the knee is fully extended and the sole of the foot is on the mat.

Abduct and lift both arms out to the side just below shoulder height.

Pivot the body sideways over the right hip lifting the extended left leg and lowering the right hand towards the floor.

Make contact with the palm of the right hand on the mat. The right hip should be directly over the right knee without 'sticking your butt out' and the left leg is extended and held parallel to the floor.

Bring the left hand so that the fingers are held behind the head.

Movement

From this position you may perform the 'Side Kick' variations as follows :

- *Kick to front and back*
- *Leg circles*
- *Bicycle*

When the movements are completed return the body to an upright position with the left leg extended out to the side and arms outstretched to the sides.

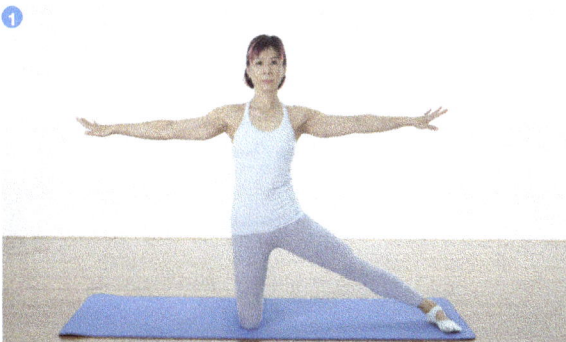

Lift arms and slide left leg to side

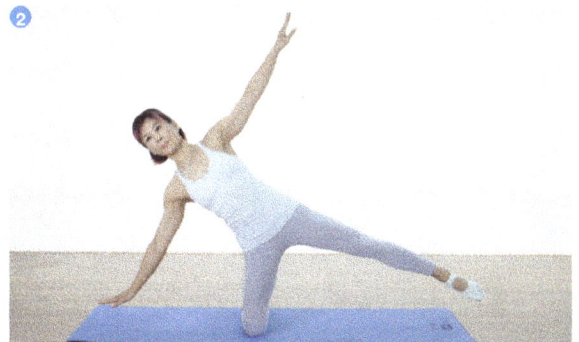

Pivot over right hip

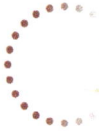
③

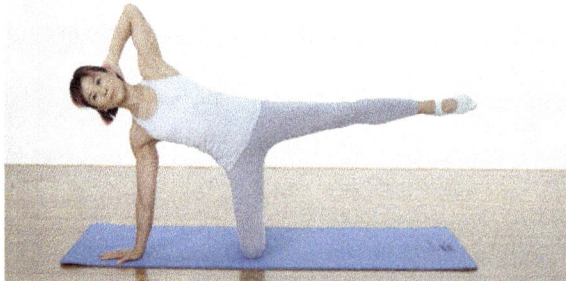

Lift arms and slide left leg to side

④

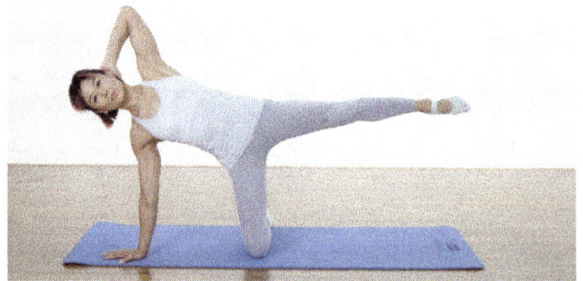

Kick to back

Kick to Front & Back

⑤

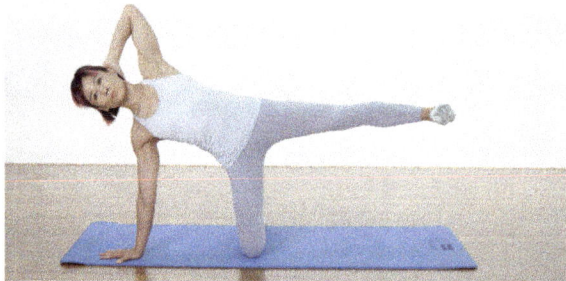

Dorsi flex ankle

Leg Circles

⑥

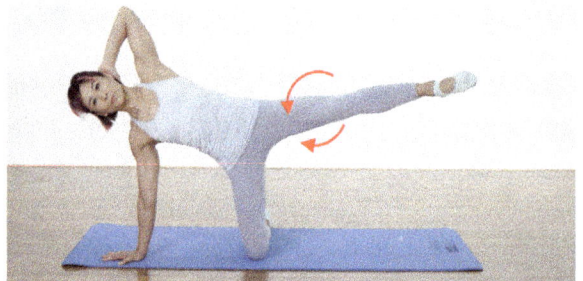

Clockwise & Anti clockwise direction

⑦

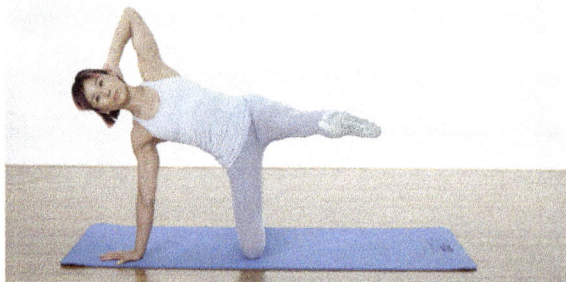

Kick to front

Bicycle

⑧

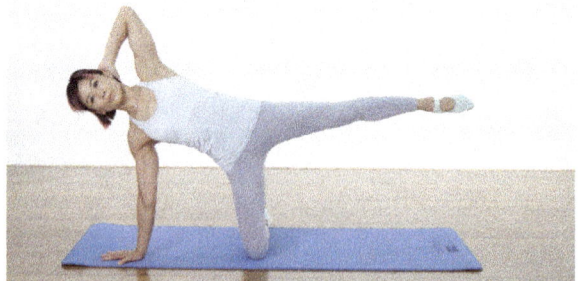

9

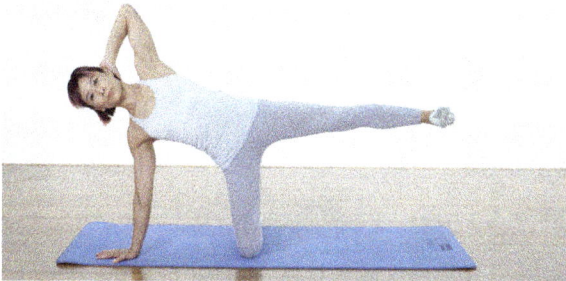

Dorsi flex ankle

10

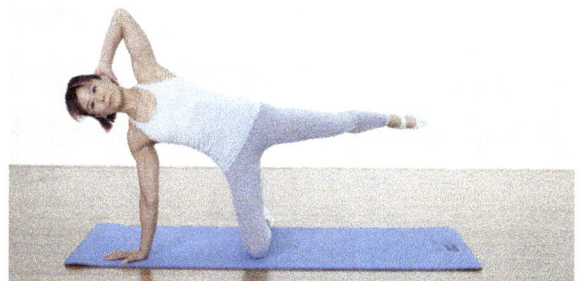

Kick to back

11

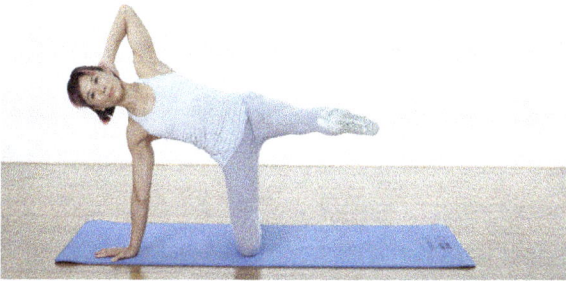

Kick to front

12

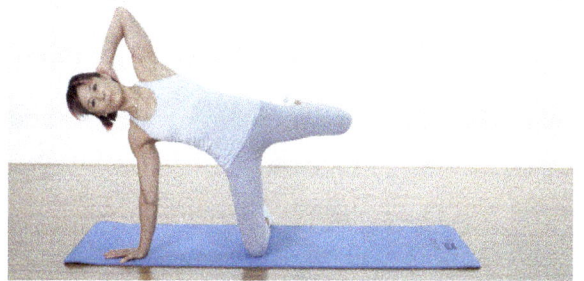

Flex knee behind

13

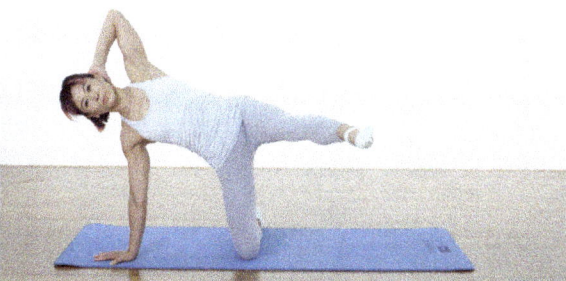

Plantar flex ankle

14

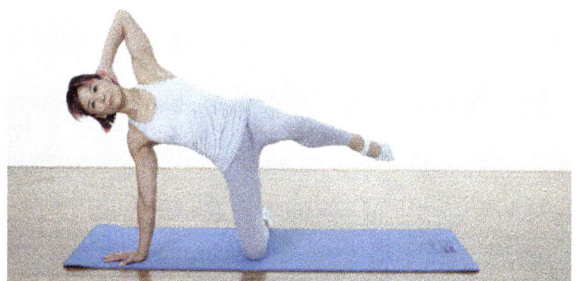

Flex hip with flexed knee

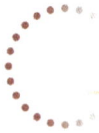

⑮

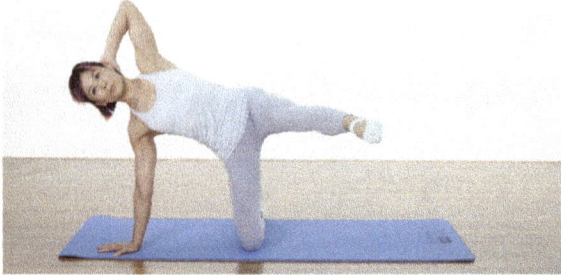

Extend knee

Cues

Verbal : Imagine your pelvis an spine is flat against the wall

Visualise a ball in the socket of your hip with oil being added to lubricate

Imagine a piece of elastic from your left ear to the left hip - keep it stretched out

Imagine your pelvis being suspended by a rope attached to the left hip bone

When you pivot on the knee to place the hand on the mat see if you can hold and balance in mid position

Tactile : Teacher places hands against abdominals and pelvis for feedback

Teacher give guided, assisted or resisted cue for leg

Benefits

Strengthens the abdominal muscles
Improves hip stability
Improves hip mobility
Integrates the lower extremity to the core
Strengthens hip muscles

Principles

Core control
LPHC & stability
Shoulder girdle stability
Integration of lower extremities into the core

Practice with various tempos for the kicks and circles.

Scan the QR code to view the exercise - Kneeling Side Kicks

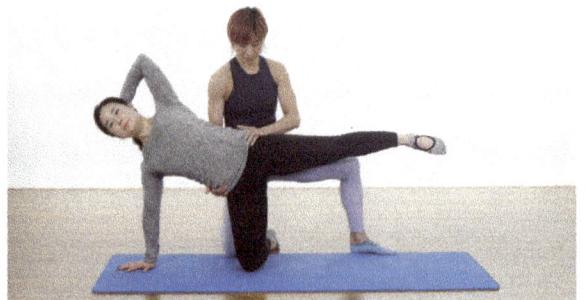

Guided cue for the Kneeling Side Kicks exercise

M24 - Side Bend

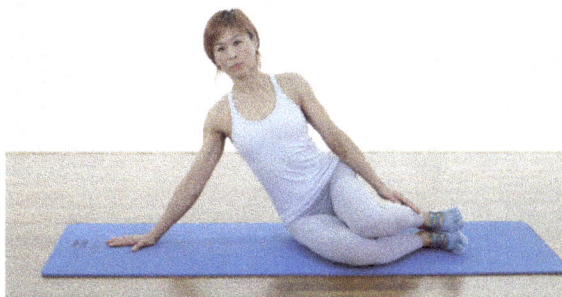

Start position

The Side Bend follows on from the Side Lift and challenges the stability of the shoulder girdle whilst the body is taken in a frontal plane movement.

Set Up

Sitting on your side propped up on the right arm with the hand in line with the right hip. The hips, knees and ankles are stacked and on the mat with the knees placed in front of the body.
The left hand rests on the left hip.

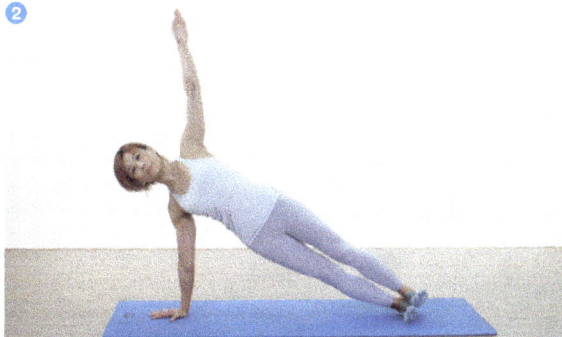

Lift to side plank

Movement

Raise the left arm overhead.
Lift the pelvis from the mat to to a side plank position with the weight supported by the right arm and outside of the right foot. As you lift the pelvis adduct the left arm to bring the extended straight arm down to the left side of the body.
Turn your head and look towards the left.
Side your left hand down the outside of the left leg towards the left foot creating a left side bend of the spine.
Return to the straight plank position and lift the left arm up and over the head to create a side bend to the right side of the body. Pause for a moment before returning to the side plank position and then lower the body to the start position.

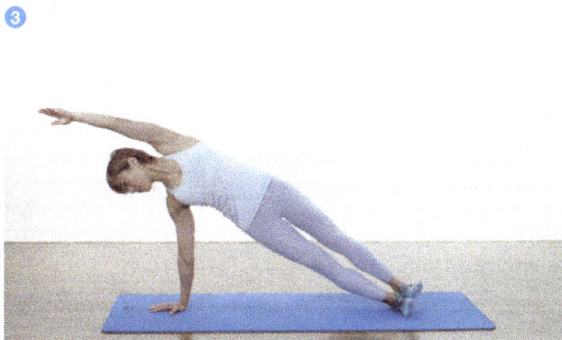

Reach arm overhead and side bend torso

④

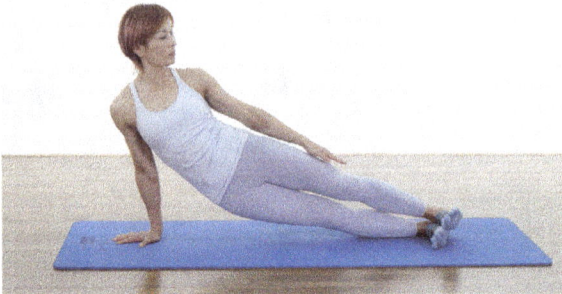

Place hand on outer side of knee and slide
hand towards ankle to side bend other side.

⑤

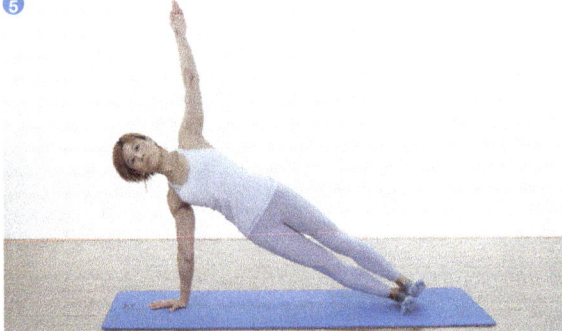

Return to side plank position

Benefits

Strengthens the abdominal muscles
Improves abdominal core muscle recruitment
Strengthens shoulder girdle
Improves shoulder stability
Improves integration of upper extremity into the
'core'.

Principles

Core control
LPHC & stability
Shoulder girdle stability & mobility
Integration of upper extremities into the core
Integration of lower extremities into the core

Cues

Verbal : Float the pelvis
Imagine balloon lifting the pelvis
Imagine balloons attached to the tailbone to lift
the pelvis
Squeeze from the sides as you lift
Imagine pulling yourself out of a tube as you lift

Tactile : Teacher can guide the ribcage in wanted
direction on the lift
Teacher place to assist or guide the pelvis

In all of the versions of the Side Lift ensure you do
not initially lift too far by bringing the pelvis higher
than it should go.
Practice using an inhalation to lift.
Practice using an exhalation to lift.
What is the difference between using inhalation
and exhalation for the lift ?

Scan the QR code to view the
exercise - Side Bend

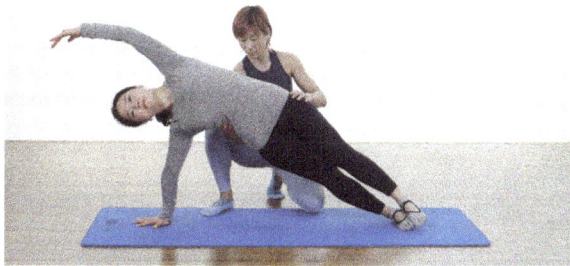

Guided / assisted cue for the Side Bend exercise

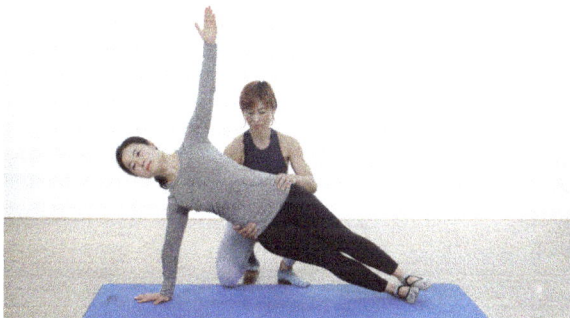

Contraindications & Precautions

Persons with hip, shoulder or spinal pathologies should approach this exercise with caution

M25 - Swimming

The Swimming exercise is a great exercise to work all the muscles in the back kinetic chain needed for both posture and locomotion.
However care should be taken to focus on quality of movement rather than range of motion by keeping unwanted tension away from the lower spine.

Set Up

Prone position with the arms overhead.
The feet make contact with the mat - the knees are lifted from the mat.
The pubic bone presses gently into the mat
The abdominals are drawn in
The head is lifted away from the mat

Movement

Raise the head so that you are looking approximately 1 - 2 meters in front of you. Draw your left shoulder blade down into the back pocket to lift the left arm feeling a retraction of the shoulder blade and the myofascial connection into the pelvis.
At the same time extend the right leg with reciprocal activation of the abdominals to float the leg from the mat.
See if you can feel the connection between the left arm and right leg.
Move the left arm up and down in unison with the right leg.
Perform 8 repetitions and then repeat with the right arm and left leg.
Now put the two movements together keeping both arms and legs raised from the mat the whole time and maintaining a thoracic extension the whole time. Right arm and left leg followed by the left arm and left leg.
Start slowly and gradually build up to a fast tempo for up to 30 seconds.

Cues

Verbal : Draw the shoulder blades into the back pockets as you feel retraction of the scapula

Imagine you are on a surf board - keep your head up and don't get your hear wet

Imagine you are on a surf board - keep looking over the top of the waves

Maintain contact with your lower ribs and pubic bone on the mat

Tactile : Teacher can guide the movement of the shoulder blades to help arm movement

Use guided cues to help pelvic position

Benefits

Strengthens the back muscles

Helps improve posture

Integrates the upper and lower extremities into the core

Helps improve hip extension

Strengthens the gluteus muscles

Principles

Core control

LPHC & stability

Shoulder girdle stability & mobility

Integration of upper extremities into the core

Integration of lower extremities into the core

How does your breathing pattern affect the movement ?

Practice with slight rotation of the thoracic ribcage and with no rotation. How do they compare ?

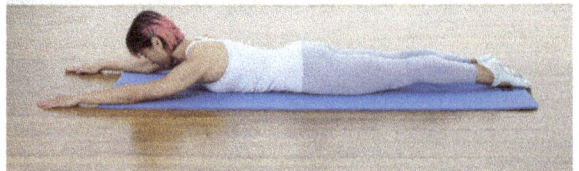

Arms overhead with legs extended

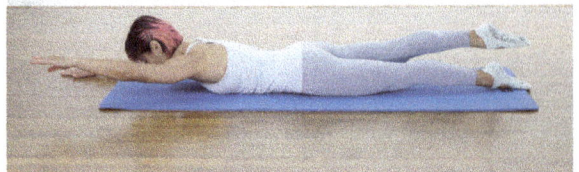

Left arm - Right leg

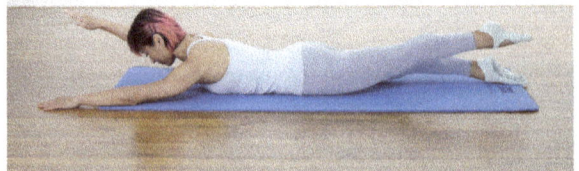

Right arm - Left leg

4

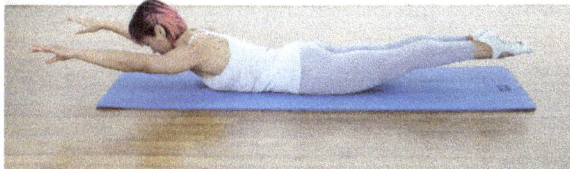

Both arms & legs up

5

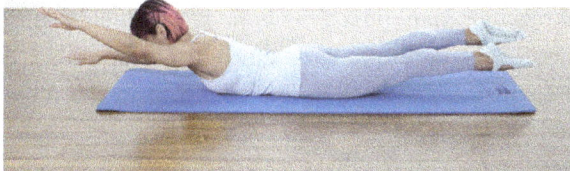

6

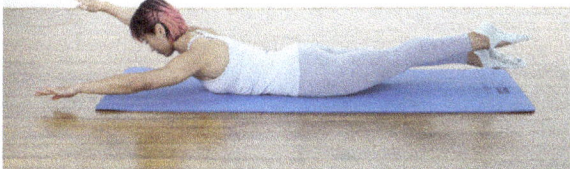

Alternating arms and legs - begin slowly and then progress to quick tempo

Scan the QR code to view the exercise - Swimming

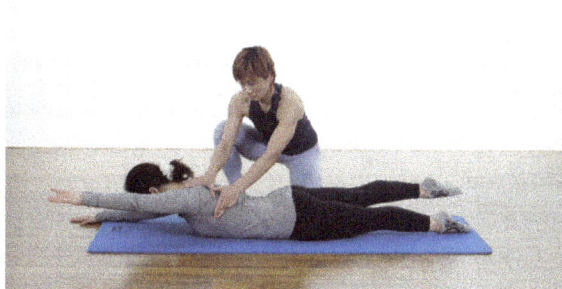

Guided cue for the Swimming exercise

M26 - Shoulder Bridge

The Shoulder Bridge exercise is a great exercise to progress a Pelvic Lift or Pelvic Curl and challenge the connection of the inner thighs through the legs and into the pelvis so that the glutes can work to stabilize your body and not have to use unnecessary tension from the lower back.

So that being said one of the most important things in this exercise is to ensure that the glutes (butt) is doing the work along with the hamstrings without that unwanted lower back tension.

Contraindications & Precautions

Persons with high or low blood pressure, hip, shoulder or spinal pathologies should approach this exercise with caution

Set Up

Supine with both legs in triple flexed position and arms by your sides.

Walk your heels close to your sit bones and lift the pelvis.

Lift on to the balls of the feet so that the pelvis moves higher.

Slide the heels of your hands under the back of the pelvis lateral (slightly away) from the PSIS's with your elbows directly underneath.

Allow your heels to return to the floor. Your pelvis is now nicely supported through the butt muscles and the lower arms connection into the floor through the elbows.

Take a moment to adjust the pelvis so that there is no excessive tension in the lower back and that the chest is 'open' with a big wide 'grin' across your collar bones.

Ensure the weight is evenly distributed between the outside/ inside and front/back of the feet to balance out the inner and outer thigh support.

Movement

Press through the sole of the right foot and float the left leg into the air with the knee flexed positioned vertical over the left hip.

Extend the left leg straight to the ceiling and take a moment to bring your attention to the position of the pelvis.

Plantar flex the left ankle and smoothly extend the hip so that the left leg dips just below horizontal to the left hip. Dorsi flex the left hip and return the leg to the vertical position.

Repeat 5 times and then continue the same movement with the leg but dorsi flexing the ankle to go down and plantar flexing the ankle to come up.

Repeat 5 more times before changing to the other leg.

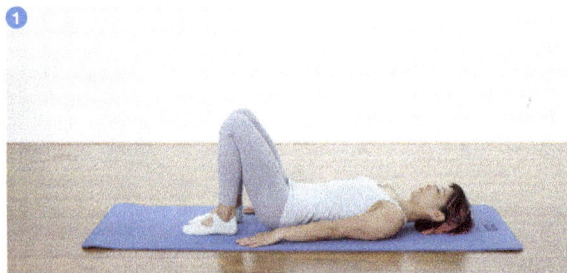

Supine position

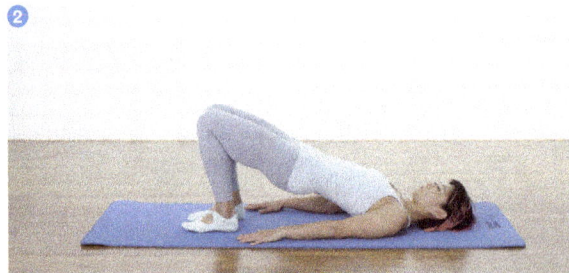

Lift the pelvis

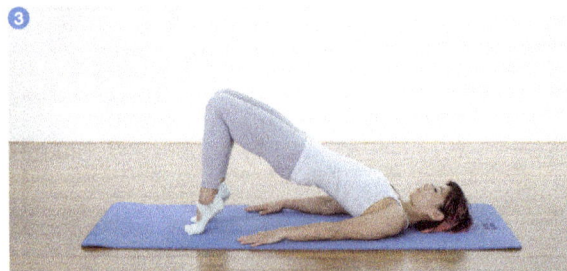

Balls of feet

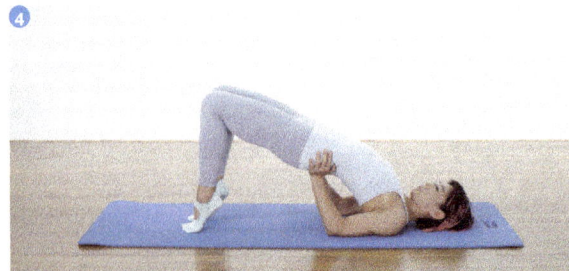

Hands under pelvis

318

⑤

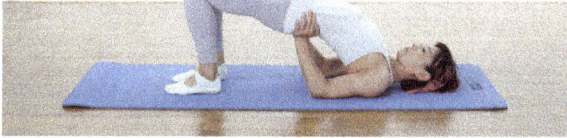

Heels back down

⑥

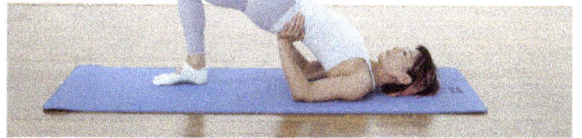

Left leg up

⑦

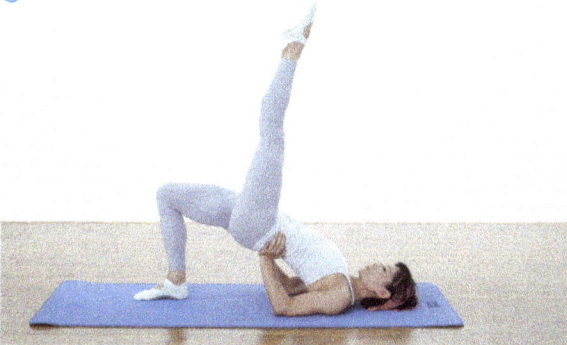

Extend left leg

⑧

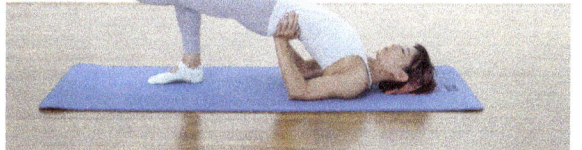

Extend left hip

⑨

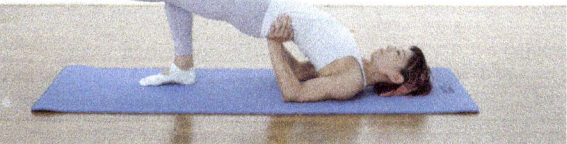

Dorsi flex left ankle

⑩

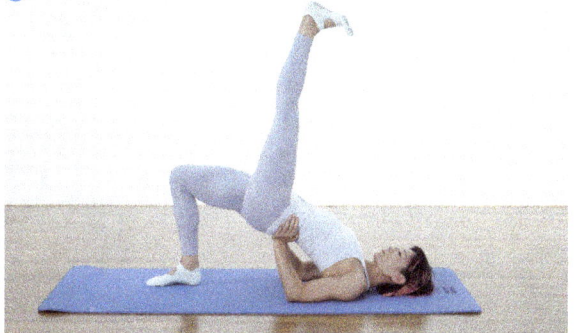

Flex left ankle

Benefits

Strengthens the gluteus muscles
Stabilizes the hips
Helps release the front of the hip
Strengthens hamstrings
Helps in stabilization of the pelvis

Principles

Core control
LPHC & stability
Integration of lower extremities into the core

Cues

Verbal : Lift the heels to place the hands under the pelvis
Hollow the abdominals and lengthen the sides
Squeeze our waist from the sides
Press the soles of the feet firmly into the mat
Push the mat away with your feet downwards.
Take your pubic bone as far away from your collar bone as you can

Tactile : Teacher tries to lift the feet vertically from the floor - gluteus Maximus test

How does your breathing pattern affect the movement ?
Practice lifting the pelvis on an inhalation and an exhalation
How does the ankle position change the movement ?
Can you feel the difference between over using the lower back and using the gluteus muscles ?

Scan the QR code to view the exercise - Shoulder Bridge

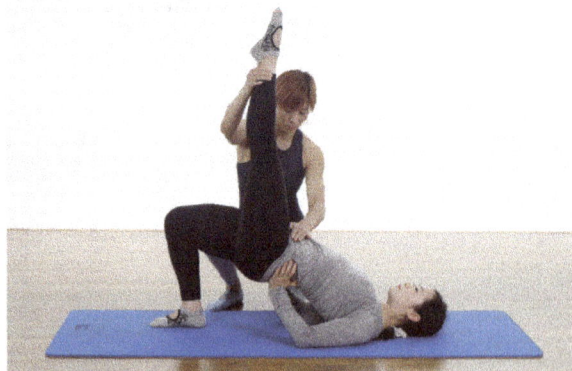

Guided / assisted cue for the Shoulder Bridge exercise

M27 - Scissors

The Scissors exercise is a great way to challenge the core stability whilst having the opportunity to lengthen the front of the body especially through the hip flexors and front of the hip.

Note: Because of the inverted position and pressure placed on the upper spine persons with blood pressure or neck and shoulder problems should consult an exercise specialist before attempting this exercise.

Set Up

Supine with the legs in the triple flexed position.

Flex both hips to bring the thighs vertical to the mat and then extend both legs so the feet are pointing to the ceiling.

Press into the floor with both arms to initiate a roll backwards through the spine bringing the legs towards the floor over the top of your head.

In this 'roll over' position place the palms of each hand over the lower back area so that the heels of each hand can feel the rib cage and the finger tips of each hand can feel the top of the pelvis. Further support to this body position is given by the elbows in contact with the floor directly underneath each hand.

Extend the left hip so that the left leg points away from the body approximately 15 degrees below the line of the spine and pelvis depending on hip flexor flexibility.

When viewed from the side the left and right leg make a 90 degree angle.

Movement

In one smooth fluid movement switch the positions of the left and right leg :

Focus on the stability of the pelvis whilst the hips make dynamic movements for 10 - 20 repetitions.

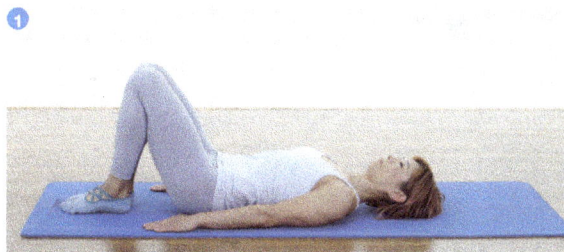

Starting position

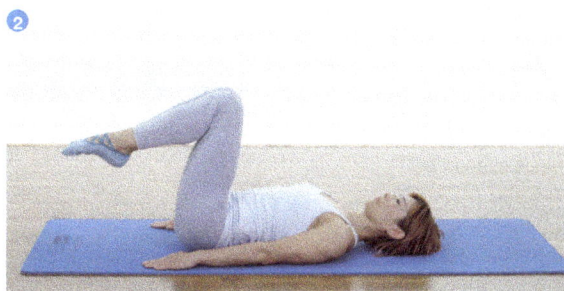

Flex hips

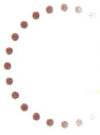

3

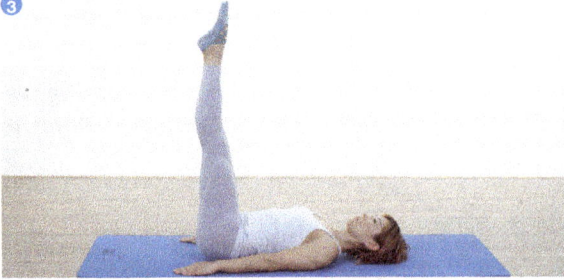

Straighten legs

4

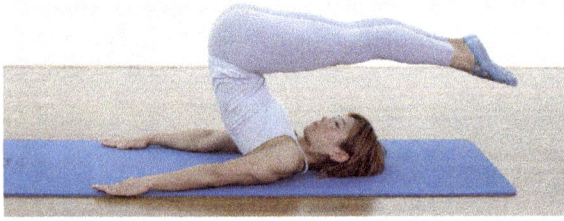

Roll over position

5

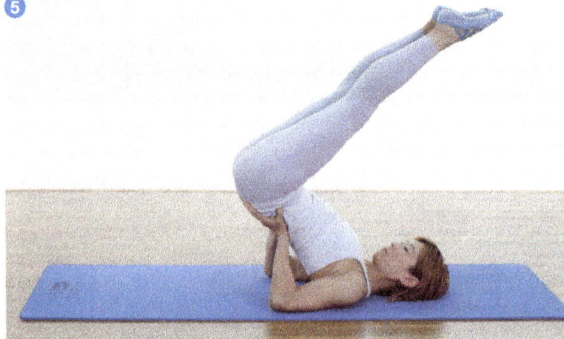

Hands support pelvis

6

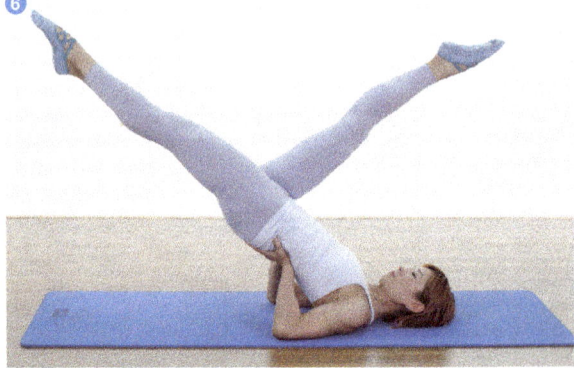

Extend left hip

7

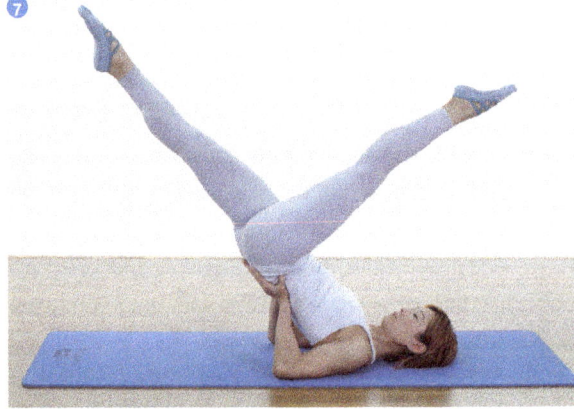

'Scissor' - flex left hip / extend right hip

Benefits

Strengthens the core
Improves hip mobility
Improves lumbo pelvic hip stability
Can help release tension in the lower back for
chronic conditions

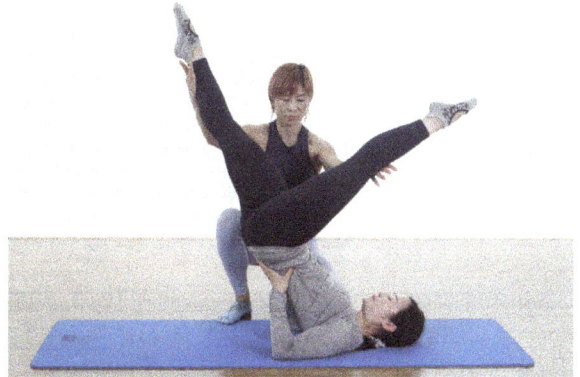

Guided / assisted cue for the Scissor exercise

Play with the different leg positions - how does this affect the pelvis and spine ?
What happens if you focus on trying to hold the extended leg up in the air ?
What happens if you focus on flexing the hip and no extension through the other hip ?

Scan the QR code to view the exercise - Scissors

M28 - Bicycle

The Bicycle exercise is a natural follow-on from the Scissors allowing for a more circular motion through the hips and the opportunity to release tension and shortness created by some of the accessory hip flexors such as the rectus femoris, tensor fascia latae and sartorius muscles - all of which may have a significant contribution towards low back pain.

Set Up

The set up is the same as for the Scissors exercise.
Supine with the legs in the triple flexed position.
Flex both hips to bring the thighs vertical to the mat
and then extend both legs so the feet are pointing to
the ceiling.
Press into the floor with both arms to initiate a roll
backwards through the spine bringing the legs
towards the floor over the top of your head.
In this 'roll over' position place the palms of each hand
over the lower back area so that the heels of each hand
can feel the rib cage and the finger tips of each hand
can feel the top of the pelvis. Further support to this
body position is given by the elbows in contact with the
floor directly underneath each hand.

Extend the left hip so that the left leg points away
from the body approximately 15 degrees below the
line of the spine and pelvis depending on hip flexor
flexibility.
When viewed from the side the left and right leg
make a 90 degree angle.

Movement

Flex the left knee without flexing the hip ! This will
stretch the front of the thigh without shortening the
muscles at the front of the hip.
Flex the left hip whilst extending the the left knee.
At the same time extend the right hip whilst flexing
the right knee.
Continue this 'bicycle' movement for as many
repetitions as needed focusing on the stability of the
pelvis with a fluidity of movement in the hips and

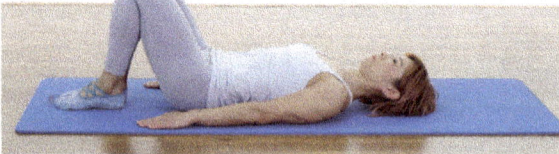

Starting position

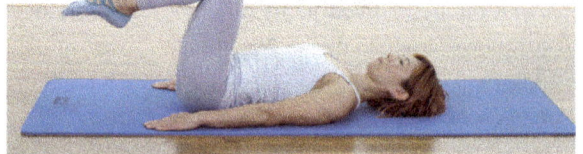

Flex hips

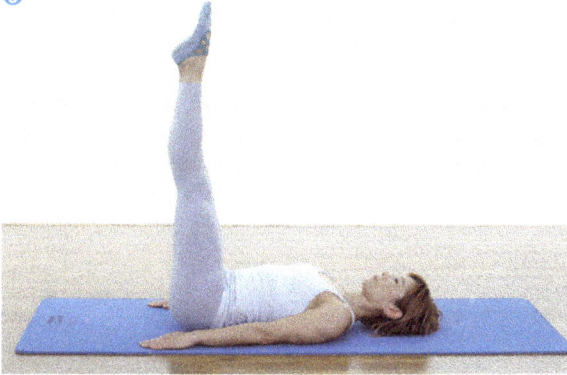

3 Straighten legs

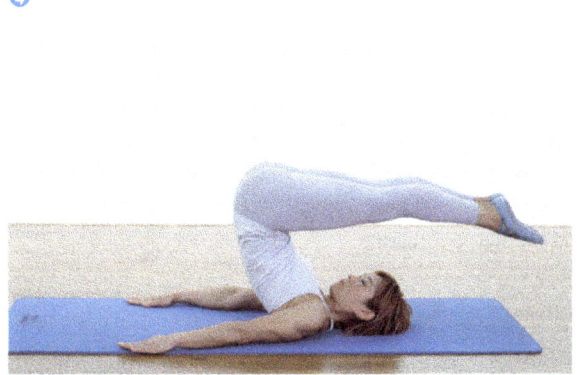

4 Roll over position

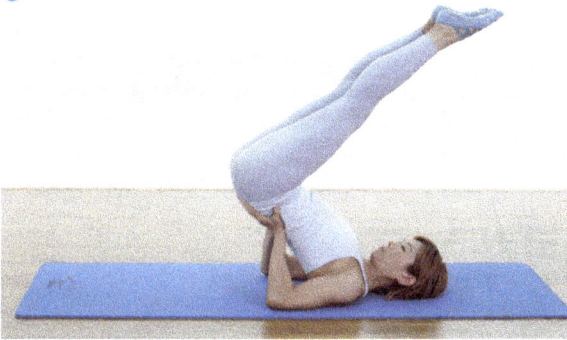

5 Hands support pelvis

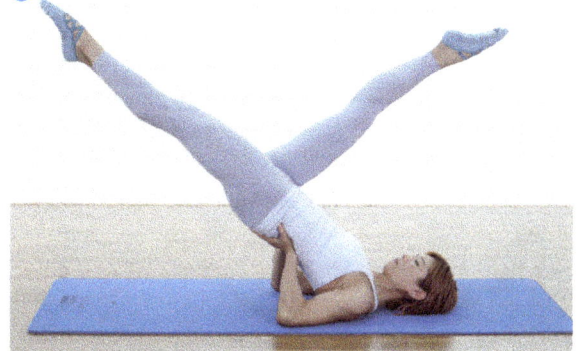

6 Extend left hip

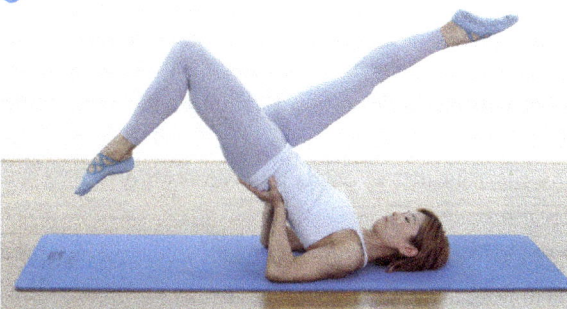

7 Flex left knee

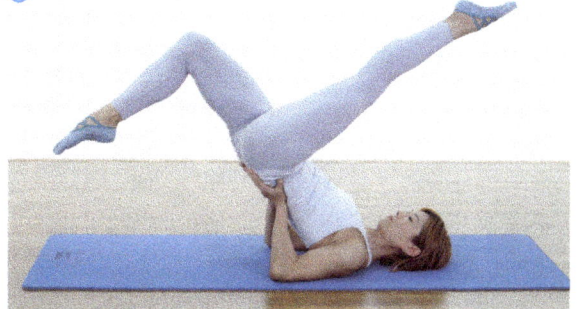

8
1) Flex left hip   2) extend left knee
3) Extend right hip   4) Flex right knee

Benefits

Strengthens the core
Improves hip mobility
Improves lumbo pelvic hip stability
Can help release tension in the lower back for chronic conditions

Play with different leg positions - how does this affect the pelvis and spine ?
Use slightly different hand positions and see how it affects your support

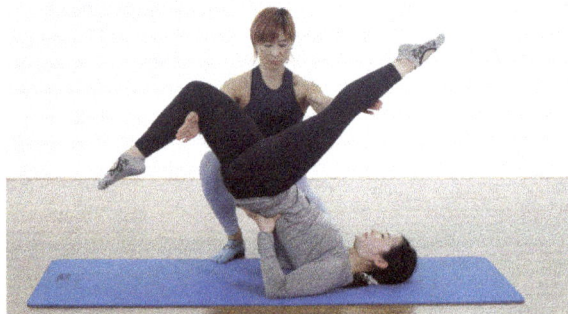

Cues

Verbal : Feel the dynamic balance created through the position of both legs
Use the leg of the flexed hip to help balance out the extended leg
Reach the extended leg to the ceiling - don't try and 'hold it up'
When flexing the extended leg don't just let the lower leg drop - use the muscles in the back of the leg to pull the lower leg into position
When extending the knee on the flexed leg maintain the hip position

Tactile : Teacher can give guided cue with both hands for the lumbo pelvic position
Teacher can give assisted or resisted cue to the extended leg.

Guided / assisted cue for the Bicycle exercise

Scan the QR code to view the exercise - Bicycle

Principles

Core control
LPHC & stability
Integration of lower extremities into the core

M29 - Leg Pull - 'Back'

Whilst it may not look so difficult to the viewer the Leg Pull Back is an extremely challenging exercise to the stability of the pelvis and strength and stability for the hamstring muscles.
Persons with short tight hip flexors will most certainly 'not enjoy' this exercise !

Set Up

Sitting position with the legs extended and pressed

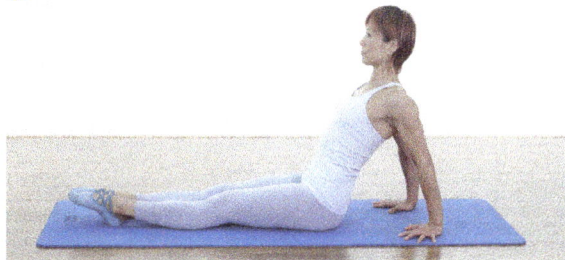

Start position

together in front of you. The arms are placed behind you to help open the chest and collar bones. The hands are on the mat with fingers pointing away from you.

Movement

Lift the pelvis so that it comes in line with the legs and spine. Press the feet firmly into the floor.
Hold this position and flex the left hip to lift an extended left leg towards your chest. Ideally you want this leg to move past the 90 degree position. Perform 3 kicks as follows :

one kick with plantar flexion - one kick dorsi flexion - one kick plantar flexion

Repeat on the other leg.
Things to watch :

• *The pelvis should stay 'lifted' at all times - do not allow the pelvis to drop*
• *Avoid transverse plane rotation of the pelvis*

A Very Special Note :

The supporting leg should have the foot fully plantar flexed with the sole of the foot in contact with the floor. In fact this position is not possible for a vast

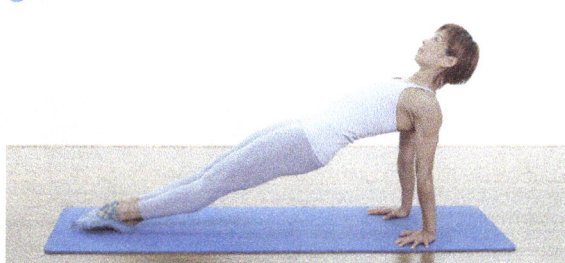

Lift pelvis - press feet into floor

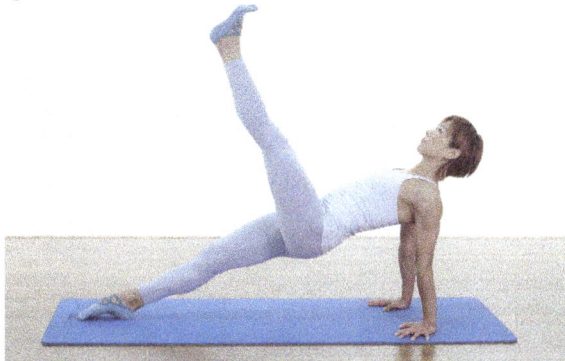

Flex left hip with dorsi flexed ankle

④

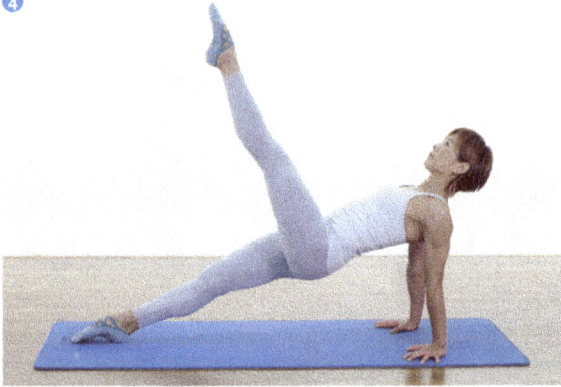

Plantar flex left ankle

⑤

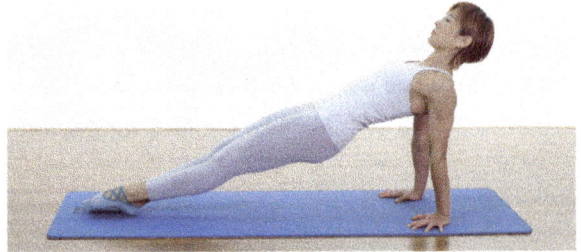

Lower left leg

⑥

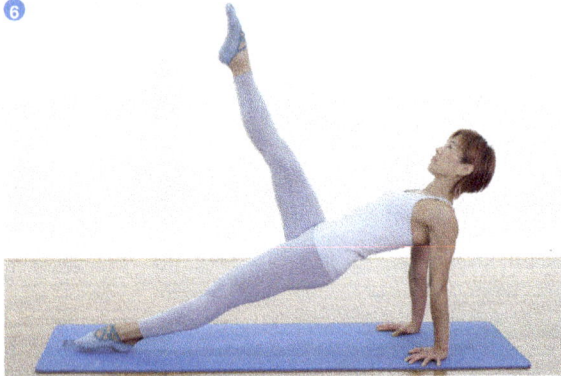

Plantar flex right ankle

⑦

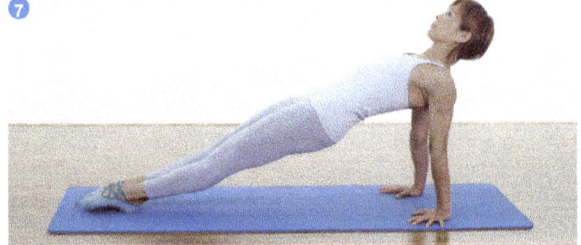

Lower right leg

⑧

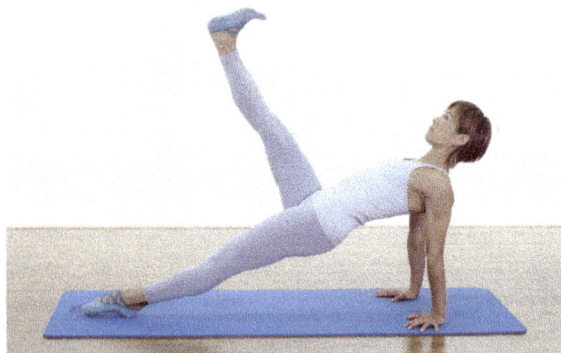

Flex right hip with dorsi flexed ankle

majority of the population but is extremely important for the exercise. If the sole of the foot is not in contact with the floor then this will compromise the myofascial chain into the pelvis and usually results in an outwards rotation of the tibia as the persons tries to stabilize through the outside of the heel.

This compensation should be avoided at all costs if possible and one of the best methods I have found is to use either a rolled up towel or wedge under the foot. In this way you are helping to set up your client to succeed in he exercise and find an extremely important kinetic chain link through the posterior aspect of the body.

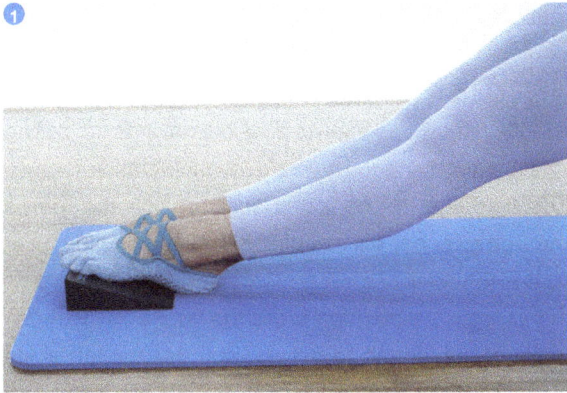

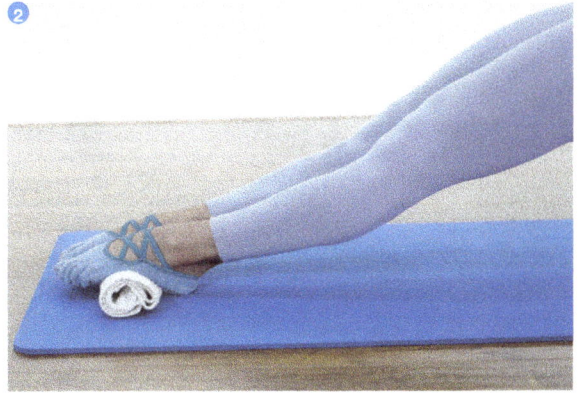

A wedge or rolled towel may be used to support the foot and ankle

Benefits

Strengthens the core
Improves hip mobility
Helps release tension on front of the thighs
Improves hamstring strength
Improves hamstring flexibility

Principles

Core control
LPHC & stability
Integration of lower extremities into the core

Practice using different hand positions and see how it affects your support and ability to open the chest.

Cues

Verbal : Press the sole of the foot into the floor
Push the floor away with the foot
Hollow your abdominals to draw the leg up
Open the collar bones to lift the chest

Tactile : Teacher can give guided cue with both hands for the lumbo pelvic position
Teacher can give resisted cue to the extended leg on the mat.
Teacher can give guided cue for collar bones and chest

Scan the QR code to view the exercise - Leg Pull Back

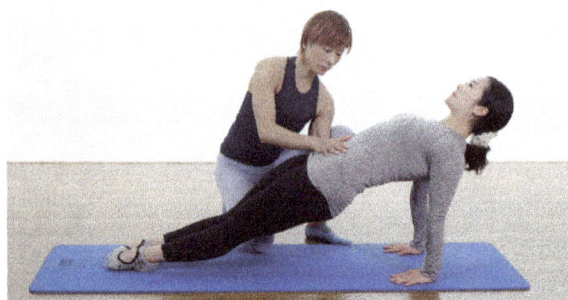

Guided / assisted cue for the Leg Pull Back exercise

M30 - Leg Pull - Front

The Leg Pull Front challenges the stability of your shoulder girdle, core muscles, and pelvis in a 'plank position'.

Benefits

Strengthens the core
Improves hamstring strength
Improves strength of the gluteus muscles
Helps balance the hamstring, gluteus, paraspinal muscle relationship
Improves shoulder girdle stability
Helps upper body strength

Set Up

Begin in quadruped position with the knees under the hips and hands under the shoulders.
Slide the left leg back so that it is fully extended on the ball of the foot.
Slide the right leg back to fully extended on the ball of the foot.
You are now in a full plank position with strong activation of the shoulder girdle, hamstring and glute muscles.

Movement

Pull the right leg as high as possible towards the ceiling whilst maintaining the whole body stabilization.
Ensure there is no compensation of the pelvis through rotation, side shifting or hoiking on hip closer to the shoulder.
In this leg lifted position press the floor away with the ankle of the left leg to fully plantar flex the left ankle and drive the head and body forwards along the mat a few centimeters.
Pause in this position and then strongly dorsi flex the left ankle to bring the head and body backwards along the mat.
Bring the right leg back down to the mat and repeat the whole movement 3 - 5 times.

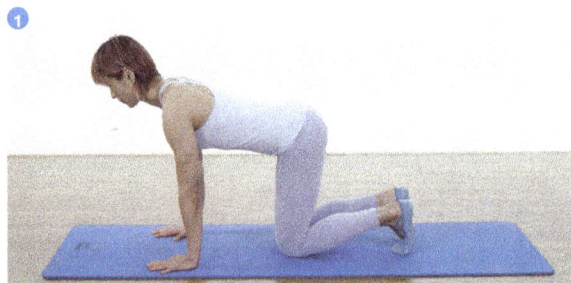

Starting position

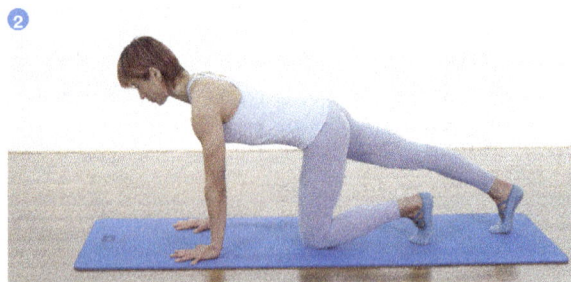

Extend right leg

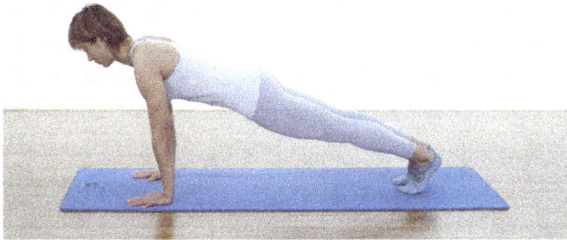

Plank position

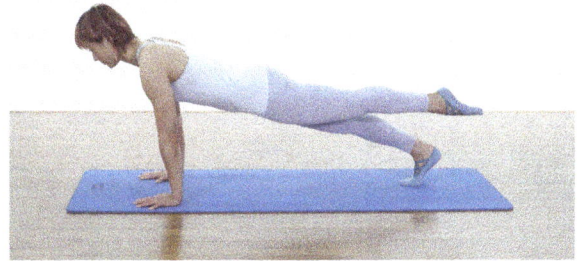

Lift left leg

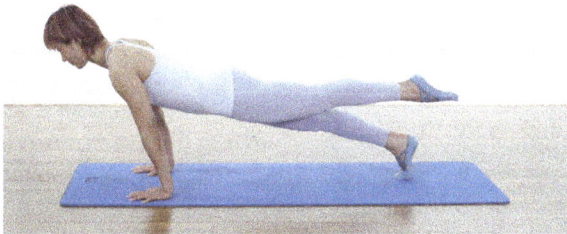

Plantar flex - pull upper body - push feet into the floor

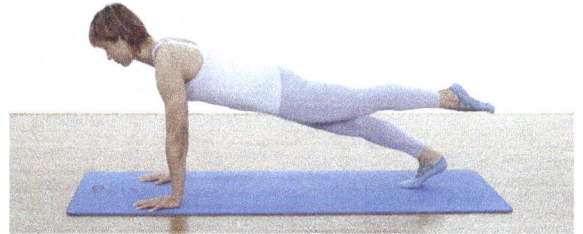

Dorsi flex - push with upper body - push feet into the floor and hollow abdominals

Principles

Core control
LPHC & stability
Integration of lower extremities into the core
Shoulder girdle stability

Practice using both an exhalation and an inhalation to lift the leg. What difference do you feel ?

Cues

Verbal : Press the ball of the foot into the floor
Push the floor away with the foot
Hollow your abdominals to draw the leg up
Open the collar bones to lift the chest
Reach the top of your head and tail bone away from each other

Tactile : Teacher can give guided cue with both hands for the lumbo pelvic position
Teacher can give guided cue for collar bones/ chest and thoracic spine

Scan the QR code to view the exercise - Leg Pull Front

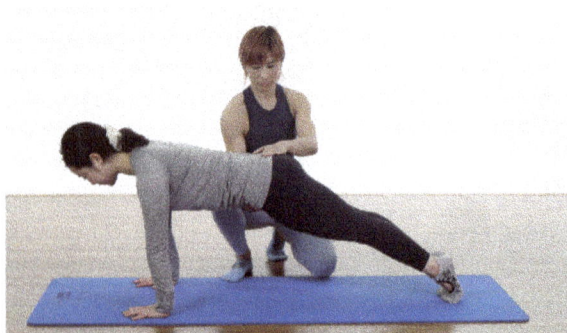

Guided cue for the Leg Pull Front exercise

Benefits

Strengthens the core

Improves hamstring strength

Improves strength of the gluteus muscles

Helps balance the hamstring, gluteus, paraspinal muscle relationship

Improves shoulder girdle stability with mobility

Helps upper body strength

Improves arm strength

M31 - Push up - 5 positions

The Push Up or Press Up is an integral part of all physical fitness programs and it's no surprise to see it in the Pilates Mat repertoire.

Here we will practice a variation on the traditional version and you will find many variations elsewhere in studios around the world.

The hand position for a Push Up greatly influences how the muscles of the lower, upper arm and shoulder girdle are use and so it makes sense to practice in a manner that will recruit and use as many combinations as efficiently as possible.

Set Up

Begin in quadruped position with the knees under the hips and hands under the shoulders.

Slide the left leg back so that it is fully extended on the ball off the foot.

Slide the right leg back to fully extended on the ball off the foot.

You are now in a full plank position with strong activation of the shoulder girdle, hamstring and glute muscles.

Movement

Move into a 'down dog' position by pressing the floor away with the arms whilst lifting the tail bone towards the ceiling.

Pause for a moment and then return to the plank position.

Lower the whole body towards the mat maintaining a straight line from head through the spine through the pelvis and through the legs.

Stop just before the chest is about to touch the mat and then press back up to the plank position.

Move back into the down dog position and then repeat the push up 3 - 5 times to complete 1 set.

In this manner the hands stay close to the chest with the fingers pointed to the top of the mat producing a lot of work through the tricep muscles and more stabilization work through the spinal muscles due to the narrow base of support.

Continue the exercise for 5 sets of 3 - 5 repetitions with the hands in different positions :

Fingers face top of mat - narrow position
Fingers face bottom of mat - narrow position
Fingers face each other - medium position

Fingers point outwards to the sides - wide position
Fingers form a triangle with each thumb - very narrow position

The exercise can be easily regressed by simply performing on the knees for the press up and down phase.

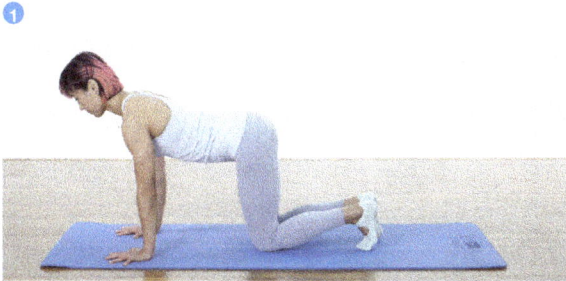

Start position

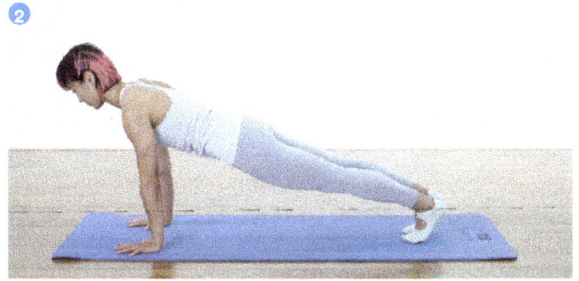

Plank position

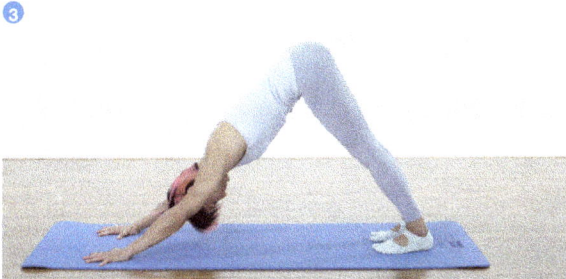

'Down Dog'

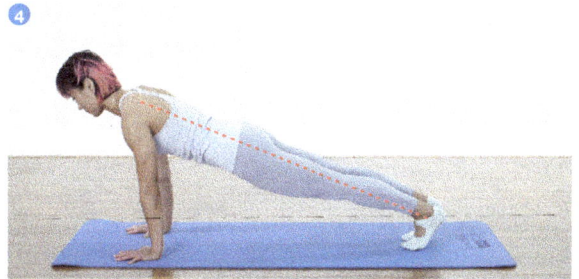

Plank position

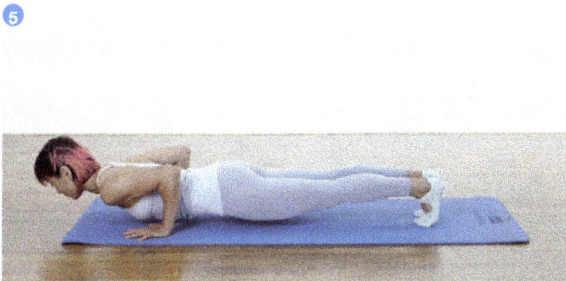

Body Down

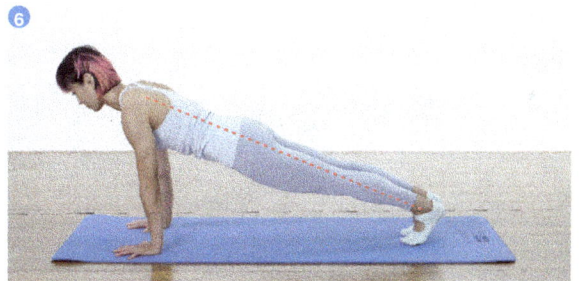

Press Up

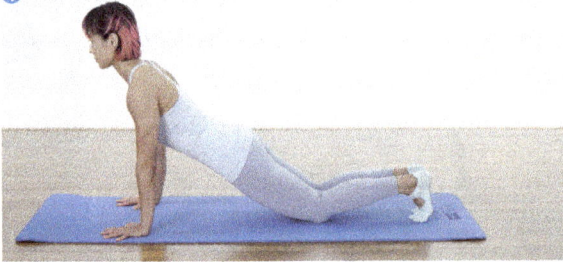

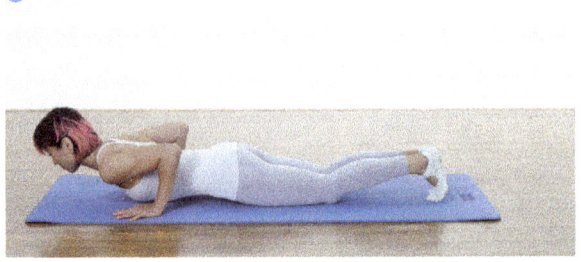

Regression practiced on knees

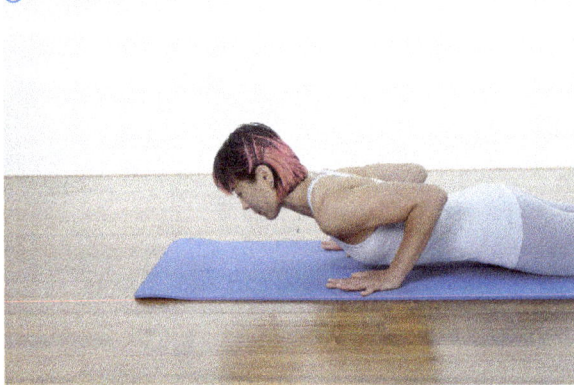

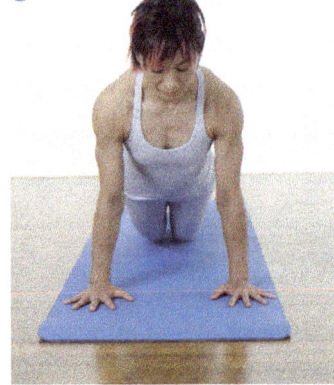

Fingers point upwards

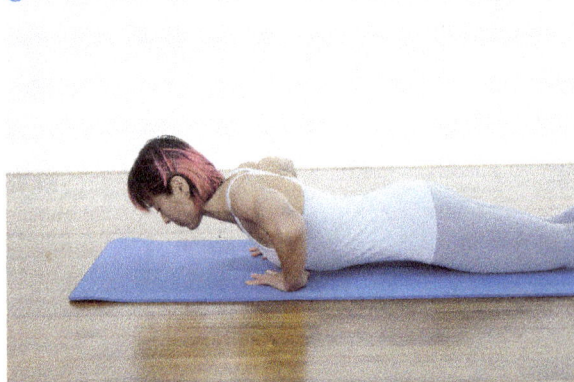

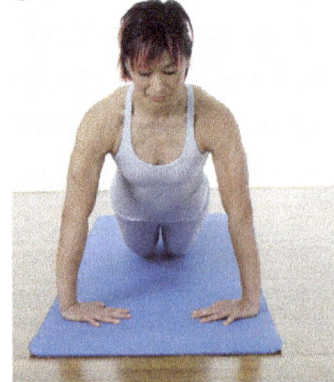

Fingers point inwards

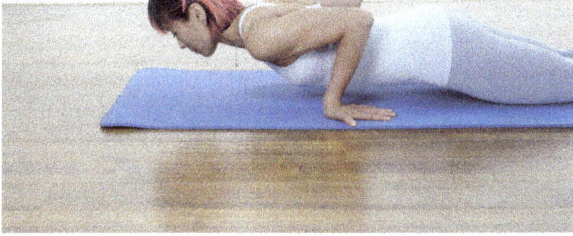

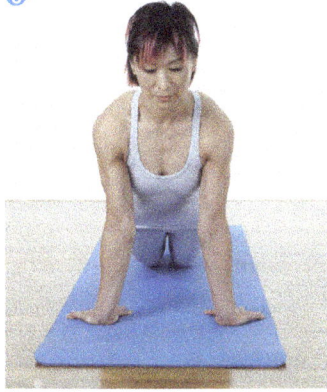

Fingers point downwards

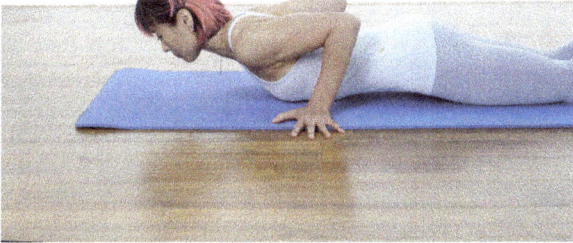

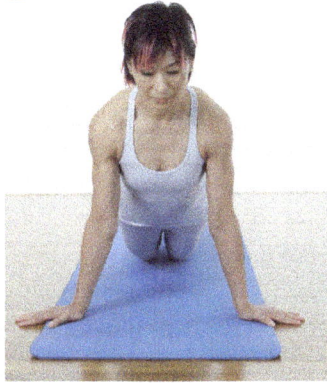

Fingers point outwards

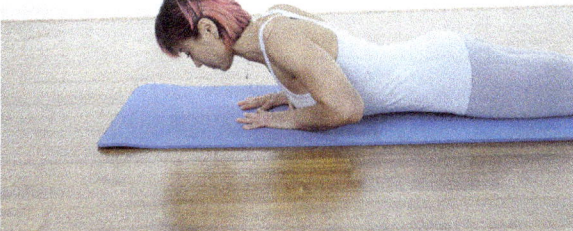

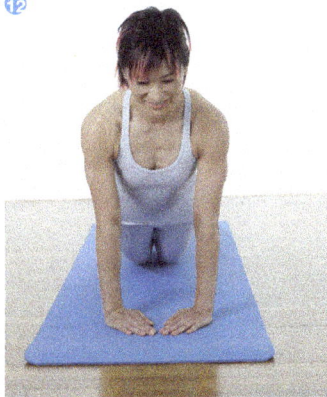

Fingers make triangle

Principles

Core control
LPHC & stability
Integration of lower extremities into the core
Shoulder girdle stability
Shoulder girdle mobility

Practice using both an exhalation and an inhalation when lowering the body down and pressing back up. What difference do you feel ?

Cues

Verbal : Press the ball of the foot into the floor
Lift your tail to the ceiling
Hollow your abdominals to lift the pelvis
Imagine your spine and pelvis like an iron bar - straight that can't bend
Reach the top of your head and tail bone away from each other

Tactile : Teacher can give guided cue with both hands for the lumbo pelvic position

Scan the QR code to view the exercise - Push Up

Scan the QR codes below to view the related exercise video

Hundred exercise

Roll Over exercise

Corkscrew exercise

Neck Pull exercise

Jack Knife exercise

Boomerang exercise

Seal exercise

Crab exercise

Rocking on Stomach exercise

Control Balance exercise

The Traditional Pilates Mat Sequence

1	Hundred
2	Roll Up
3	Roll Over
4	Single Leg Circles
5	Rolling Like a Ball
6	Single Leg Stretch
7	Double Leg Stretch
8	Single Straight Leg Stretch / Scissors
9	Double Straight Leg Stretch
10	Criss Cross
11	Spine Stretch
12	Open Leg Rocker
13	Corkscrew
14	Saw
15	Swan Dive
16	Single Leg Kick
17	Double Leg Kick
18	Neck Pull
19	Scissors
20	Bicycle
21	Shoulder Bridge
22	Spine Twist

23	Jack Knife
24	Side Kick
25	Teaser
26	Hip Circle
27	Swimming
28	Leg Pull Front
29	Leg Pull
30	Kneeling Side Kick
31	Side Bend
32	Boomerang
33	Seal
34	Crab
35	Rocking on Stomach
36	Control Balance
37	Push Up
38	Neck Pull
39	Scissors
40	Bicycle

Appendix II

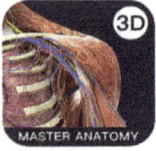

Muscle Images courtesy of Vesal

Appendix III

Recommended reading

Anatomy Colouring Book	Joe Muscolino
Anatomy Trains	Thomas Myers
Born to Walk	James Earls
Centered	Madeline Black
CORE	Owen Lewis
Functional Anatomy of Movement	James Earls
Return to Life Through Contrology	Joseph Pilates
The Complete Pilates Tutor	Alan Herdman
The Pilates Effect	Stacy Redfield & Sarah Holmes
Trail Guide to the Body	Andrew Biel
Understanding the Human Foot	James Earls

www.ingramcontent.com/pod-product-compliance
Lightning Source LLC
Chambersburg PA
CBHW080244030426
42334CB00023BA/2697